Gayle ❤

The Family Practice
Desk Reference

Second Edition

The Family Practice Desk Reference
Second Edition

Charles E. Driscoll, M.D.
Professor and Head
Department of Family Practice
College of Medicine
University of Iowa
Iowa City, Iowa

Edward T. Bope, M.D.
Director, Family Practice Residency Program
Riverside Methodist Hospital
Columbus, Ohio

Charles W. Smith, Jr., M.D.
Executive Associate Dean for Clinical Affairs
Professor of Family and Community Medicine
Medical Director
The University Hospital of Arkansas
University of Arkansas for Medical Sciences
Little Rock, Arkansas

Barry L. Carter, Pharm. D.
Associate Professor
College of Pharmacy
University of Houston
Adjunct Associate Professor
Department of Family Medicine
Baylor College of Medicine
Houston, Texas

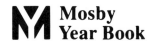

Mosby Year Book

St. Louis   Baltimore   Boston   Chicago   London   Philadelphia   Sydney   Toronto

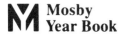 **Mosby
Year Book**

Dedicated to Publishing Excellence

Sponsoring Editor: Kevin M. Kelly
Assistant Director, Manuscript Services: Frances Perveiler
Production Project Coordinator: Yvette Sellers
Proofroom Supervisor: Barbara M. Kelly

Mosby–Year Book, Inc.
11830 Westline Industrial Drive
St. Louis, MO 63146

4 5 6 7 8 9 0 Y R 95 94 93

Library of Congress Cataloging-in-Publication Data

The Family practice desk reference / [edited by] Charles E. Driscoll
. . . [et al.].—2nd ed.
    p. cm.
  Rev. ed. of: Handbook of family practice, c1986.
  Includes bibliographical references and index.
  1. Family medicine—Handbooks, manuals, etc. I. Driscoll,
Charles E. II. Title: Handbook of family practice.
RC55.H26 1991
610—dc20   91–6604
                                                CIP

To the memory of Nicholas J. Pisacano, M.D.,
our mentor and friend

PREFACE TO THE SECOND EDITION

When first conceived, this quick-reference text was envisioned as a pocket-sized handbook for family physicians that would serve to hold all those facts one needs for daily practice. As the first edition proved, pocket size is unattainable if the reference is to be comprehensive and readable. With its new title, *The Family Practice Desk Reference* remains a complete reference that will quickly assist the student, resident, or practicing family physician to make diagnostic and treatment decisions—a desk reference for everyday practice in the office, nursing home, or hospital. For practicing physicians, it will help to increase efficiency in ambulatory care and provide a single source for reference values needed from day to day. For residents, it will help to guide their emerging skills in the practice of ambulatory medicine.

Readers will discover tables on topics such as pulmonary function testing and the characteristics of cerebrospinal fluid, and refer to them time and again to refresh their memories of normal values. Others, such as the treatment for chemical burns of the eye, will be helpful for medical decision making, while still others will help with quick patient education—the illustration of dermatomes, for example, to explain the referred pain of a herniated lumbar disc. Whenever information could be condensed into tabular format or an algorithm, we have done so to spare the reader a lot of time in sorting through texts to find quick answers.

We have also attempted to pass along "pearls" of wisdom given to us by our teachers and colleagues to be recalled and reviewed when needed. Such bits of information often mean the difference between an average practitioner of medicine and one who appears more polished. We hope the material in this book will on one occasion jog the memory, while on another provide some new insight.

The second edition brings together the best work from the first edition and new material reflecting the latest developments in medical science.

Topics not formerly covered include AIDS and HIV infection, new essentials for advanced cardiac life support, changes in treatment for STDs, and many more. Most drug information has now been moved to a single chapter on drug therapy, and we have attempted to eliminate outdated material and items of limited usefulness. Finally, many good suggestions have come to us from our readers, and we have tried to include some of these as well. We greatly appreciate your ideas and hope you will keep them coming for the next revision.

Charles E. Driscoll, M.D.
Edward T. Bope, M.D.
Charles W. Smith, Jr., M.D.
Barry L. Carter, Pharm. D.

CONTENTS

1 *Family Practice*

Charles E. Driscoll, M.D.

CONTENT OF FAMILY PRACTICE

Family physicians provide care for patients of all ages, both sexes, and in a variety of settings for up to one third of the ambulatory medical visits in the United States.

TABLE 1–1.—Most Common Reasons for Ambulatory Visits to a Physician*

RANK	PRINCIPAL REASON FOR VISIT	PERCENT
1	General medical exam	4.8
2	Prenatal exam	4.0
3	Well baby exam	2.6
4	Throat symptoms	2.6
5	Postoperative visit	2.6
6	Cough	2.5
7	Progress visit/follow-up	2.1
8	Ear symptoms	1.8
9	Back symptoms	1.8
10	Skin rash	1.6
11	Blood pressure test	1.5
12	Visual disturbance	1.5
13	Fever	1.4
14	Upper respiratory tract infection	1.4
15	Abdominal cramps	1.4
16	Hypertension	1.4
17	Headache	1.4
18	Chest pain	1.3
19	Knee symptoms	1.2
20	Eye exam	1.1

*Adapted from McLemore T, Delozier J: *NCHS Advance Data* 128: Jan 23, 1987.

TABLE 1–2.—Age-Sex Distribution of Patients Making Office Visits*

Female (3.2 visits/yr)	
< 15 yr	9.2%
15–24 yr	7.7%
25–44 yr	18.6%
45–64 yr	12.9%
> 65 yr	12.5%
	60.9% of total
Male (2.2 visits/yr)	
< 15 yr	9.5%
15–24 yr	3.9%
25–44 yr	9.0%
45–64 yr	8.7%
> 65 yr	8.0%
	39.1% of total

*Adapted from McLemore T, Delozier J: *NCHS Advance Data* 128: Jan 23, 1987.

SCREENING AND HEALTH MAINTENANCE

TABLE 1–3.—Recommended Schedule for Active Immunization of Infants, Children, and Adults

AGE	IMMUNIZATION
2 mo.	Diphtheria-tetanus-pertussis (DTP) #1
	Trivalent oral polio (TOPV) #1
4 mo.	DTP and TOPV #2
6 mo.	DTP #3
12 mo.	Hematocrit and tuberculin PPD tine
15 mo.	Measles-mumps-rubella (MMR), DTP #4, OPV #3
18 mo.	Hemophilus B conjugate vaccine
5 yr	Diphtheria-tetanus pediatric type (DT), TOPV #4, MMR #2
>5 yr, every 10 yr	Diphtheria-tetanus adult type (Td)
>65 yr and high-risk adults	Inactivated influenza virus vaccine annually
High-risk adults	23-Valent polysaccharide pneumococcal vaccine
IV drug users, homosexual adults, and high-risk health care workers	Inactivated hepatitis B surface antigen vaccine

FIG 1-1.
Screening flow sheet for children.

Test/Intervention	Weeks		Months							Years										Comments
	2	4	2	4	6	9	12	15	18	2	3	4	5	6	8	10	12	15	20	Age
Complete History & Physical	•	•	•	•	•	•	•	•	•	•	•	•	•	•	•	•	•	•	•	assess each time a major change is to occur (ie enter junior high)
Height & Weight	•	•	•	•	•	•	•	•	•	•	•	•	•	•	•	•	•	•	•	
Head Circumference	•	•	•	•	•	•	•	•	•											
Blood Pressure										•	•	•	•	•	•	•	•	•	•	
Developmental Assessment	•	•	•	•	•	•	•	•	•	•	•	•	•	•	•	•	•	•	•	developmental milestones, school progress, anticipatory guidance
Automobile Safety Education	•		•	•	•	•	•	•	•	•	•	•	•	•	•	•	•	•	•	for parents initially, later child
Alcohol/Smoking Education																	•	•	•	
Teach Self Exam Breasts/Testes																	•	•	•	
Immunization Review/Update	•		•	•	•	•	•		•	•		•	•					•		(see immunization schedule)
PKU, Thyroxine	•																			if not done at birthing facility
Hematocrit					•		•				•									less than 33 is anemic; age 16 important if menstruating
Sickle Cell Test					•		•													if black race, affects 1 in 300
Uricult									•				•							females only
Tuberculosis Test													•		•		•			at any change of schools or locale to aid in epidemiology
Hearing/Vision					•	•		•			•	•	•						•	screening audiometry, tympanometry, vision screening

FIG 1-2.
Screening flow sheet for adults.

Test/Intervention	Age in Years	Comments
	21 22 23 24 25 26 27 28 29 30 31 32 33 34 35 36 37 38 39 40 41 42 43 44 45 46 47 48 49 50 51 52 53 54 55 56 57 58 59 60 61 62 63 64 65 70 75+	
Complete History & Physical	• •	**if not previously examined ***q 2 yr. until 75, then annually
MD Breast Exam	• •	annually after age 40
Pelvic Exam	• •	annually after age 40; palpation of adnexa
Rectal Exam	• •	(*earlier and annually if sexually active or high risk)
Ht, Wt, & Blood Pressure	• •	
Influenza Vacination		annually after age 60
Immunization Review & Update	• •	annually after age 65
PAP Smear	• •	every 2 years
Serum Lipid Screening	• •	
VDRL	• •	
PPD	• •	
Stool for Occult Blood		annually after age 50
Tonometry & Fundoscopy		
Sigmoidoscopy with Anoscopy		more often if positive family history
Mammography		annually after age 50
Teach Self Exam Breast/Testes	•	

TABLE 1–4.—Health Education Topics for All Patients

1. Eat each of the basic four food groups, decrease red meat intake, decrease animal fat intake, and choose low-fat dairy products. Choose polyunsaturated and monosaturated fats.
2. Eat more fish and poultry; remove skins. Bake or broil; do not fry.
3. Increase soluble fiber content in diet, such as oat bran, dry beans, and peas, and eat high-fiber vegetables such as peas and corn.
4. Seek calcium and potassium; avoid sodium and phosphate.
5. Drink 3 or more glasses of water daily.
6. Eat one main meal daily (prior to activity, not sedentary period) and two smaller ones; maintain ideal weight, plus or minus 10 lb.
7. Be physically active: 30 min, 3–5 times/wk at 75% max pulse.*
8. Avoid excess alcohol (3 drinks or less/wk).
9. Do not smoke or use smokeless tobacco.
10. Know your blood pressure (keep it <100 + age/90) and cholesterol (keep <200 mg/dl).
11. Maintain immunity with up-to-date boosters.
12. *Always* wear seatbelts.
13. Do not act irresponsibly in sexual activity; use safe-sex practices.

*Max. pulse = 220 − Patient's age (yr).

OCCUPATIONAL HEALTH

The occupational history is an integral part of delivering total care to the family. Emotional and physical concerns may arise secondary to the occupation, or preexisting problems may adversely affect the work role. Use all occupational health encounters to screen for risk factors (e.g., tobacco, seatbelts) and health advice (see Table 1–4).

TABLE 1–5.—OCCUPATIONAL AND ENVIRONMENTAL ASSESSMENT

1. Describe any health problems or injuries arising from past or present jobs.
2. Has any substance you work with caused a rash on your skin?
3. Has an illness related to work caused you to lose more than 1 day of work?
4. Have you ever worked in a job that caused you to have difficulty breathing?
5. Have you ever had a TB skin test or chest x-ray film as screening for your work?
6. Have you ever had to change jobs because of illness or injury?
7. Do you have frequent low back pain, or have you ever had to see a doctor for back care?
8. Do you come into direct contact with liquid, gaseous, powdered, or other toxic substances?
9. Are you aware of sensory (hearing, visual, smell, taste, touch) disturbances connected to your work?
10. Have you ever had to change homes because of a health problem?
11. Have you in the past or present lived very near an industrial plant?
12. Which hobbies or crafts do you do at home?
13. Do you use home and garden chemicals?
14. Do you have (air conditioning, humidifier, fireplace) at home?

THE FAMILY LIFE CYCLE AND FAMILY FUNCTION

The patterns of development in most families are relatively consistent and predictable. The family physician can use this knowledge to solve puzzling diagnoses, provide anticipatory guidance, and detect deviations from the norm. The family life cycle is a composite of the individual developmental changes of its members and the marital relationship itself.

A family crisis may occur abruptly or gradually and can have profound effects on the emotional and physical well-being of individuals in the family. Assessment of family function and coping abilities aids in efficient management of these problems. Family function should also be studied whenever (1) a new family enters your practice, (2) family members must render care for chronic illness, (3) psychosomatic illness is suspected, and (4) patient-physician relationships are strained.

TABLE 1–6.—Types of Family Crises*

Dismemberment
  Hospitalization
  Loss of child
  Loss of spouse
  Prolonged separation (military service, work, etc.)
Demoralization
  Disgrace (alcoholism, crime, delinquency, drug addiction, etc.)
  Infidelity
  Prolonged unemployment
  Sudden impoverishment
  Progressive dissention
Accession
  Adoption
  Relative moves in
  Stepmother/stepfather marries in
Demoralization plus dismemberment or accession
  Desertion
  Divorce
  Illegitimacy
  Imprisonment
  Institutionalization
  Runaway
  Suicide or homicide

*From Rakel RE: *Principles of Family Medicine.* Philadelphia, WB Saunders Co, 1977, p 351. Reproduced by permission.

TABLE 1-7.—DEVELOPMENTAL STAGES OF THE FAMILY*

MAJOR STAGES OF THE FAMILY	AVERAGE LENGTH	DEFINITION	TASKS
Newly married	2 yr	Union of man and woman; no children	Disengage from family of origin; adjust to each other's personality; meet social, economic, and sexual needs; establish effective methods of communication.
Birth of first child	2.5 yr	Oldest child age 0–30 mo.	Assume parental role while maintaining marital role; institute new schedule; deal with fatigue, financial stress, home confinement, and decreased leisure activity.
With preschool children	3.5 yr	Oldest child age 30 mo. to 6 yr	Socialization of the children; child learns to relate emotionally to others, undergoes early individuation and sexual identity.
With children in school	7 yr	Oldest child age 6–13 yr	First official separation from home; parents' social activities widen to include school activities; child develops physically, socially, emotionally, and intellectually.
Families with teenagers	7 yr	Oldest child age 13–20 yr	Stressful stage; family must maintain closeness and cohesiveness while simultaneously encouraging child's development of independence; child begins disengagement process; adolescent sexual feelings conflict with social restriction.
Launching years	8 yr	First child leaves home to last child gone	Parent-child relationship changes to adult-adult type; parents face prospect of time alone and need to reinvest in each other instead of children.
Parents alone in middle years	15 yr	Last child leaves; empty nest	Reappraisal of lifetime goals, realignment of priorities; couples who have remained together for sake of children divorce; most difficult time for women, causing emotional crises; adaptation to grandparent role.
Retirement and later years	10–15 yr	Retirement—death of both spouses	Coping with aging process; loss of occupation; societal disengagement; depression may arise.

*Adapted from Duvall EM: *Family Development*, ed 4. Philadelphia, JB Lippincott Co, 1971.

TABLE 1–8.—Five Components of Family Function
(Family Apgar)*

The family Apgar is a five-item family function screening questionnaire where the patient is asked to describe how family members communicate, eat, sleep and carry out home, school, and job responsibilities.

Adaptation: The utilization of intra- and extrafamilial resources for problem-solving in times of crisis.

Partnership: The sharing of decision-making and nurturing responsibilities by family members.

Growth: The physical and emotional maturation and self-fulfillment that are achieved by family members through mutual support and guidance.

Affection: The caring or loving relationship that exists among family members.

Resolve: The commitment to devote time to other members of the family for physical and emotional nurturing, involving a decision to share wealth and space.

*From Rosen GM, Geyman JP, Layton RH: *Behavioral Science in Family Practice.* New York, Appleton-Century-Crofts, 1980, p 145; Smilkstein G: The family APGAR: A proposal for a family function test and its use by physicians. *J Fam Pract* 1978; 6:1231–1239. Reproduced by permission.

TABLE 1–9.—Family Apgar Questionnaire*

	ALMOST ALWAYS	SOME OF THE TIME	HARDLY EVER
I am satisfied that I can turn to my family when something is troubling me.	————	————	————
I am satisfied with the way my family talks over things with me and shares problems with me.	————	————	————
I am satisfied that my family accepts and supports my wishes to take on new activities or directions.	————	————	————
I am satisfied with the way my family expresses affection and responds to my emotions, such as anger, sorrow, and love.	————	————	————
I am satisfied with the way my family and I share time together.	————	————	————

Scoring: The patient checks one of three choices, which are scored as follows: "Almost always" (2 points), "Some of the time" (1 point), or "Hardly ever" (0). The scores for each of the five questions are then totaled. A score of 7–10 suggests a highly functional family. A score of 4–6 suggests a moderately dysfunctional family. A score of 0–3 suggests a severely dysfunctional family.

*From Rosen GM, Geyman JP, Layton RH: *Behavioral Science in Family Practice.* New York, Appleton-Century-Crofts, 1980, p 147; and Smilkstein G: The family APGAR: A proposal for a family function test and its use by physicians. *J Fam Prac* 1978; 6:1231–1239. Reproduced by permission.

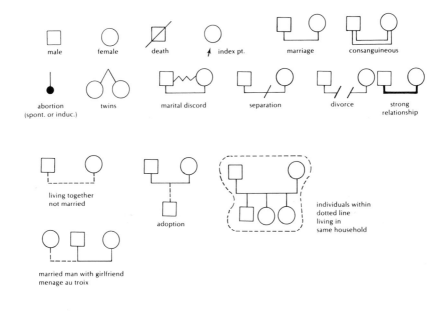

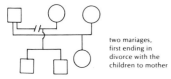

FIG 1–3.
Using a family genogram to understand family structure. Standard symbols are illustrated. Genograms help to (1) record data on repetitive conditions (e.g., bipolar illness, Down's syndrome), (2) understand family interactions and relationships (e.g., conflict, enmeshment, roles), and (3) establish a plan for follow-up and screening (e.g., familial poliposis, cancer family syndrome). Completion of the genogram often supplies the "missing link" to diagnosing illness or family dysfunction. (See McGoldrick M, Gerson R: *Genograms in Family Assessment.* New York, WW Norton & Co, 1985.)

FAMILY-CENTERED CARE

TABLE 1–10.—GUIDELINES FOR INVOLVING THE FAMILY IN A PATIENT'S CARE

See patient only	Minor acute problems (URI, laceration)
	Routine self-limiting problems (back strain, influenza, fracture)
Family conference desirable	Treatment failure or regular recurrence of symptoms
	Routine preventive/educational visits (premarital exam, prenatal care, well child care)
Family involvement essential	Chronic illness (diabetes, obesity, cancer, hypertension)
	Serious acute illness (major trauma, acute myocardial infarction)
	Psychosocial problems (anxiety and depression, trouble with the law, substance abuse)
	Diagnostic or treatment errors, undiagnosed cases
	Death

TABLE 1–11.—BASIC STRATEGIES FOR FAMILIES COPING WITH CHRONIC ILLNESS

1. Provide regular physician contact for empathetic guidance; explain the diagnosis and management (carefully, clearly, slowly and repeatedly).
2. Have a family meeting—involve all members in decisions and care.
3. Involve competent assistants in the family's care (social worker, visiting nurse, minister).
4. Assist family in recognizing financial and legal issues.
5. Suggest resources that can provide respite for the care-givers (hospice, church groups) and places available for placement if it should eventually be needed.
6. Focus on the needs of the entire family, not just the patient. Have family develop a "coping notebook" with names and phone numbers (doctor, friends), agencies, self-help support groups or societies, and emergency care services.
7. Strive to maintain patient's general health, mental status, and skills for independent activities.
8. Insure patient safety. Reduce objects that may cause falls, install tub/toilet rail, reduce bathwater temperature, wear ID bracelet, install intercom or call bell system, use lifeline system (automatic dialing of emergency number by single button push).
9. Provide names of other families who have successfully dealt with a similar medical problem.
10. Provide periodic written summary of patient's course and your assessment and plans to family care-givers and any other physicians or professionals involved in patient's care.

COMMUNITY RESOURCES

To provide comprehensive health care, the family physician must utilize community resources to serve physical, emotional, sociological, and rehabilitative needs. Use appropriate referral and consultation request letters to provide information, ask questions, and give notice that the family physician will remain involved in the patient's care. Written documentation of services or care provided should be requested.

TABLE 1–12.—COMMUNITY RESOURCES UTILIZED BY FAMILY PHYSICIAN'S PATIENTS

Physical health care
   Planned Parenthood and family planning clinics—contraception and venereal disease treatment.
   County Health Department—TB and STD case follow-up.
   WIC (women-infants-children) programs providing food supplements.
   Community dental services
   Veterinarian—zoonoses control.
   Public Health nurses—immunization program.
   Child Development Clinics—diagnoses of various handicaps.

Home care
   Hospice—terminal illness care.
   Visiting Nurses Association—home nursing assistance.
   Homemakers, Inc.—housekeeping assistance.
   Medical equipment and supply companies—home oxygen and sick care items.
   Manpower Health Care Services.
   Home Intravenous Therapy Team.
   Occupational therapist.
   Others listed in Yellow Pages under "nurses" or "health."

Social services
   Department of Public Assistance.
   ADC (Aid to Dependent Children).
   GAU (General Assistance to Unemployed).
   Food Stamp Program—food assistance.
   Medicaid—financial aid for medical services.
   Child Welfare Services—foster care, child abuse.
   Lutheran Social Services—social and psychological services.
   Hill-Burton Funds—free or reduced hospital services provided by some hospitals.

Continued.

TABLE 1–12.—Continued

Psychological services
   Community mental health services.
   Pastoral care through local churches.
   Crisis center—all types of emotional problems.
   Rape crisis center—sexual assault.
   Marriage and family service.
   Association for Retarded Citizens.
   Alcohol and substance abuse programs.

Disease-related associations and general information services
   American Cancer Society
   Birthright
   American Diabetes Association
   Multiple Sclerosis Association
   Muscular Dystrophy Association
   American Lung Association
   American Heart Association
   United Way
   Easter Seals
   Senior Citizens Center
   Social Security Office
   Volunteer Groups

Short-term emergency assistance
   Community Food Pantry
   American Red Cross
   Salvation Army
   Community churches
   REACT and Civil Defense

HOME VISITS

TABLE 1–13.—Indications for Home Visits

The proportion of elderly and home-bound patients is increasing. Rising medical costs have led to earlier discharge from hospitals and pressure on the family to give home care. Reasonable guidelines for home care include:

Initial assessment/management of an acute illness when:
Patient is too elderly to come to office (no transportation capabilities).
Patient is too ill (acute back injury, severe influenza).
Pain is exacerbated by movement (febrile hospice patient with malignancy).
Ambulation is impaired (elderly person with casted leg).
Patient would be infectious to other patients (chicken pox).
Patient's problem needs treatment before transport to hospital can be effected
(acute asthma in elderly single patient, CPR, relief of pain).
Need to assess indications for admission to the hospital.

When patient needs follow-up after release from the hospital:
Assess rehabilitation progress and adaptation to illness.
Assess coping abilities of family members to deal with chronic disease.
To help patients who need more time to recover from disfiguring trauma or
surgery.

Patients with chronic diseases:
Patients confined to the home (severe arthritis, multiple sclerosis, COPD,
CHF).
Patients with a dementing illness or problems with toileting control.
Patients with terminal illness.

When disturbed home situation or family dysfunction is suspected:
Assess financial capabilities, hygiene, family's ability to care for patient.
Family counseling to include members who won't come to office.

TABLE 1–14.—On a Home Visit, A Physician Observes*

O—*Outside:*
Type of neighborhood.
Type of house.
Play area for children.
Condition of patient's home and other homes in area.
Environmental hazards.
B—*Behavior of family members:*
How do they relate to one another? (Degree of love and intimacy; strength; nature of nurturing process; character of communication; exchange of looks; verbal exchange; nature of physical contact (warm and supportive; quarrelsome and rejecting); if different ethnic group, don't misinterpret signs).
How do they relate to the children?
How do they relate to the physician? Is the TV on?
Is there a caretaker (hidden patient)? How is caretaker coping?
Cultural or ethnic activities?
S—*Safety:*
High rate of accidents in home?
Is there much clutter around?
Are there exposed wires, fans, hot water vaporizers, poor lighting, flaking paint, smoke detectors?
Is it poison proof? Presence of ipecac?
Medicines?
E—*Eating area: Habits and patterns:*
Where does the family eat? (In kitchen, dining room; in front of TV; at round table or long narrow one?)
Sanitation of the kitchen?
Is garbage disposed of properly?
What about cooking and storage facilities?
What food is available?
R—*Relationships and support groups in wider community:*
Is there extended family nearby?
Do they know neighbors? Are they supportive? Hostile? Indifferent?
Do they have friends they can contact in an emergency?
Do they belong to a church or civic organization?
Do family members work nearby? Who works? Economic background?
When do they shop?
V—*Variations:*
Had you expected the home to be different? More adequately furnished? Less? Does the inside look different from the outside?
Family member or friend present who was not previously mentioned?
Evidence of children's toys, etc.?

E— *Environment within the home setting:*
Furnishings, pets?
Housekeeping?
Bathroom sanitation?
Homey? (Family pictures, mementos, religious artifacts, hobbies, etc.)
Study area? Play area for children?
Family space? Private space? Where does the family congregate? (What people do in a physical setting turns a space into a place. For example, the bathroom may be the library, a think tank, an escape from the family, or a haven for suicides.)
Sleeping arrangements? (The stage of the family in its life cycle; use of space; communal versus private space within the home.)
S— *Sickness:*
Medications?
Provisions for ill persons (bed-bound patient locations; dust-proofing for asthmatics; hand rails for cardiac)? How does the family perceive the illness?

*Courtesy of Antonnette V Graham, RN, LISW, Assistant Professor of Family Medicine, Case Western Reserve University, Cleveland, Ohio.

GERIATRIC CARE

There is an increasing percentage (11%) of elderly in our population, which is projected to reach 12.5% by the year 2000. Family and social support for the elderly may be lacking, so direct your careful attention toward early discover of their common, major problems: (1) impaired intellectual functioning, (2) instability and immobility, and (3) incontinence.

TABLE 1–15.—THE MINI-MENTAL STATUS EXAM

	MAXIMUM SCORE
Orientation	
1. What is the year, season, day, month, date?	5
2. Where are we (state, county, town, hospital, floor?	5
Registration	
3. Name 3 objects, then have the patient name them. Give 1 point per each correct answer, repeat until all 3 are named (record number of tries _____).	3
Attention/calculation	
4. Begin with 100 and serially subtract 7 until stopped. Stop patient after 5 correct responses. or Ask patient to spell "world" backwards.	5

Continued

TABLE 1–15.—Continued

Recall	
5. Ask patient to name the 3 objects named earlier. Give 1 point per correct answer.	3
Language	
6. Have patient identify a pencil (pen) and watch.	2
7. Ask patient to repeat "no ifs, ands, or buts"	1
8. Have patient follow a 3-step command. "Take the paper in your right hand, fold it in half, and put it on the floor."	3
9. Have the patient read this statement and obey it: "Close your eyes."	1
10. Ask patient to write a sentence.	1
11. Have patient copy a design.	1
TOTAL SCORE[†]	30

*Adapted from Folstein MF, Folstein SE, McHugh PR: *J Psychiatr Res* 1975; 12:189–198.
[†]Significant cognitive impairment ≤ 23.

TABLE 1–16.—ASSESSMENT OF FUNCTIONAL STATUS (ADLs)

*Pulses profile**
    Rate each area on a scale of 1 to 4 (none, mild, moderate, or severe impairment).
    P—physical condition, health/illness problems.
    U—upper limb function in self-care activities.
    L—lower limb function in mobility.
    S—sensory (vision, hearing, communication) function.
    E—excretory (bowel/bladder) control.
    S—support by others for psychological, emotional, financial functions.
Activities of daily living[†]
    Rate each area on a scale of 1 to 3 (none, minimal, or moderate assistance required).
    Bathing—either sponge, tub bath, or shower.
    Dressing—gets clothes from closet/drawers, includes underwear; does fasteners.
    Toileting—goes to the "bathroom" and cleans self afterward; rearranges clothes.
    Transfer—movement in and out of bed/chair.
    Continence—bladder and bowel control.
    Feeding—act of feeding self, not cooking.

*Adapted from Granger CV, Albrecht GL, Hamilton BB: *Arch Phys Med Rehabil* 1979; 60:145.
[†]Adapted from Katz S, Ford AB, Moskowitz BA, et al: *JAMA* 1963; 185:94.

TIME MANAGEMENT

TABLE 1–17.—TIME MANAGEMENT FOR THE FAMILY PHYSICIAN

1. Do not interrupt patient care for phone calls except in cases of emergencies or long-distance calls that would be expensive to return. No phones in exam rooms.
2. Have clearly stated, written protocols for handling telephone calls. Instruct receptionist and nurse which patients to bring into office and which ones to instruct by phone. When doubt exists regarding management, have period of day set aside for returning phone calls.
3. When you are running late or called to hospital for emergency, have receptionist notify patients with appointments.
4. Use the first or last hour of the day for extended visit scheduling (e.g., counseling, minor office operations, complete exams).
5. Use preprinted or computerized questionnaires for database collection prior to your visit with patient.
6. Delegate tasks to professional staff (nurses, clinical pharmacist, social worker) and formulate a complete set of written patient instructions for routine care.
7. Schedule weekly time regularly for house visits and nursing home rounds. Make hospital rounds at same time each day.
8. Use three exam rooms per physician for maximum efficiency.
9. Dictate office records and clearly delegate to nurse in "Plans" section what to carry out prior to your next visit with patient (e.g., "patient should be weighed and pulse/BP checked prior to each visit"). Instruct nurse to read "Plans" section of prior office note when placing patient in exam room.
10. Write notes to yourself about patient data other than medical. Place photos and newspaper clippings about your patients in their record.
11. Delay dealing with noncrisis, nonthreatening "second" problems until another visit. Document what needs to be addressed at that next visit.
12. Use flowsheets and preprinted forms to shorten documentation time for routine care (e.g., hypertension, prenatal visits, well child care).
13. Regularly reserve time in schedule for self and family, personal fitness, and continuing education.
14. Develop system to insure all laboratory, x-ray reports, and written communications get your attention and then are properly filed.
15. Have routine period of time set aside to see pharmaceutical representatives; if none visit, use time for office administration.

2 Dermatology

Edward T. Bope, M.D.

COMMON DERMATOLOGIC DISEASES

In the following pages you will find dermatologic diseases organized according to the type of skin lesion they produce. To conserve space, treatments are listed below in broad groups and identified by number where they are indicated.

1. Topical steroids (see Table 2–9)
2. PO steroids (see Table 2–9)
3. Topical antibiotics
4. PO or IM antibiotics
5. Antihistamines
6. Selenium sulfide shampoo
7. Pain medication
8. Treatment of underlying disorder
9. Topical scabicide
10. Excision (see Figs 2–1 and 2–2)
11. Observation
12. Curettage
13. Topical or PO antifungal agents
14. PO or topical acyclovir
15. Drying agent (e.g., calamine lotion)

MACULES

TABLE 2–1.—ANNULAR LESIONS

DISEASE	SITES	LESION	ETIOLOGY	TREATMENT	DIAGNOSTIC AIDS
Erythema annulare centrifugum	Extremities, trunk	Annular lesions with slight peripheral scale	Allergy, sarcoid, TB, fungus	Organism-specific	Biopsy
Erythema multiforme	Palms, soles, generalized	Target lesions	Drug allergy, viral infection	2	Biopsy, immunofluores-cence
Pityriasis rosea	Trunk, extremities, rarely on face	Herald patch, flame-shaped lesions in lines of cleavage	Unknown	5	None
Purpura annularis telangiectodes	Legs	Purpuric with brown pigmentation after involution	Unknown		Biopsy
Seborrheic dermatitis	Scalp, face, chest, midback, genitalia	Oily, yellow scale	Unknown	6, 1	Biopsy
Tinea circinata and other tinea	Generalized	Concentric circles, may have raised border	Fungus	13	Examination of scrapings, culture

Continued.

19

TABLE 2–1.—Continued

DISEASE	SITES	LESION	ETIOLOGY	TREATMENT	DIAGNOSTIC AIDS
Erythema infectiosum (fifth disease)	Arms and face, then to trunk	Erythematous "slapped cheeks"	Virus	11	Clinical appearance
Enterovirus, coxsackievirus echovirus	Generalized	Red macules; vesicles may also be seen	Virus	11	Clinical appearance, history
Adenovirus	Generalized	Red macules	Virus	11	Clinical appearance, history
Rubella	Face, then trunk	Enlarged postauricular nodes; rash less intense than rubeola	Virus	11	Clinical appearance
Rubeola	Ears, forehead, then trunk	Morbilliform rash, Koplik spots	Virus	11	Clinical appearance
Roseola	Trunk	Faint red, appears after fever subsides	Virus	11	Clinical appearance, history of high fever

PAPULES

TABLE 2-2.—ANNULAR LESIONS

DISEASE	SITES	LESION	ETIOLOGY	TREATMENT	DIAGNOSTIC AIDS
Erythema multiforme	Palms, soles, generalized	Target lesions; macules and vesicles may also be present	Drug allergy, viral infection	2, 5	Biopsy, immunofluorescence
Granuloma annulare	Over bony prominences	Palpable, deep, faintly erythematous papules with elevated borders	Unknown	1	Biopsy
Lichen planus	Flexor surfaces of forearms; genitalia; mouth	Linear groups of violaceous polygonal flat lesions; on mucous membrane—white reticulated	Unknown; anxiety	5, 2, 1	Biopsy

Continued.

TABLE 2–2.—Continued

	Location	Description	Etiology	Treatment	Diagnosis
Pityriasis rosea	Trunk, extremities, rarely on face	Herald patch, flame-shaped lesions in lines of cleavage	Unknown	5	Clinical appearance
Psoriasis	Scalp, elbows, knees, trunk; rarely on face	Profuse scale; bleeding points follow removal of scale	Unknown	1, Tar, PUVA	Biopsy
Sarcoid	Nose, mouth, hands	Plaques, papules, or nodules	Unknown	Intralesional steroids	Biopsy, Kveim test
Secondary syphilis	Face, palms, soles	Brownish red with scale at margin	*Treponema pallidum*	4	Darkfield microscopic examination, STS
Urticaria	Generalized	Transitory, branched	Allergy or psychogenic	5	History, clinical appearance
Scarlet fever	Begins on neck and spreads	Scarlet eruption with pinpoint papules	Streptococcal infection	4	History, throat culture, ASO titer
Molluscum contagiosum	Trunk, face, arms, genitalia	Umbilicated, firm waxy papule	Virus	12	Clinical appearance

VESICLES

TABLE 2–3.—Vesicles

DISEASE	SITES	LESION	ETIOLOGY	TREATMENT	DIAGNOSTIC AIDS
Bullous pemphigoid	Trunk, extremities	Pruritic, annular vesicles which are flaccid and break easily	Unknown	5	Biopsy, immunofluorescence
Dermatitis herpetiformis	Trunk, palms, extremities	Pruritic; vesicles and papules	Unknown	5	Biopsy, potassium iodide test, patch test, add IgA before immunofluorescence, small bowel biopsy
Dermatitis venenata	Where exposed to sensitizer	Vesicles on edematous base; pruritic	Contact sensitivity	5	Patch test
Erythema multiforme	Mouth, genitalia, trunk	Occurs with macules and papules	Drug allergy, viral infection	2	Biopsy, immunofluorescence
Herpes simplex	Lips or genitalia	Pruritic groups	Virus	14	Tissue culture, serology, Tzanck test, biopsy
Impetigo contagiosa	Face and other areas	Blood or pus-filled, yellow crust	*Staphylococcus*, *Streptococcus*	3, 4	Culture, Gram stain, serology
Lymphangioma circumscriptum	Generalized	Round or irregular groups of lymph vesicles with hyperkeratotic top	Congenital		Biopsy

Continued.

TABLE 2–3.—Continued

DISEASE	SITES	LESION	ETIOLOGY	TREATMENT	DIAGNOSTIC AIDS
Pemphigus vulgaris	Mucous membranes, any part	Annular vesicles which break easily	Unknown	2	Biopsy, immunofluorescence
Varicella	Starts on trunk and then involves extremities	Lesions in various stages of age	Virus	5	Tzanck test, tissue culture, serology, biopsy
Zoster	Unilateral, follows nerve	Tense vesicles on edematous base; painful	Virus	5, 7	Tissue culture, serology, Tzanck test, biopsy
Acute eczema	Cheeks, diaper area, flexor surfaces	Pruritic, vesicles, excoriation, crusting	Many; atopy	1, 2, 5	Skin test to confirm sensitivity
Burns	Exposed surfaces	Bullae	Thermal agent	1, 2	History
Enteroviruses, Coxsackievirus, Echovirus	Generalized, hand; foot and mouth possible	Vesicle	Virus	11, 5	Tissue culture
Staphylococcal, scalded skin	Face first, then neck, chest, groin	Thin fragile bullae	Staphylococci	4	Culture
Vasculitis*	Dependent parts	Often urticarial, necrotic and ulcerated	Mostly idiopathic	2	Biopsy if needed
Poison ivy	Exposed skin	Pruritic vesicles, linear streaking	Rhus allergy	1, 15, 2	History

*May also be purpuric.

EXCORIATED LESIONS

TABLE 2–4.—Excoriated Lesions

DISEASE	SITES	LESION	ETIOLOGY	TREATMENT	DIAGNOSTIC AIDS
Atopic eczema	Face, trunk, flexor surfaces	Macules, papules, and vesicles progressing to crusting and scaling	Atopy	1, 2, 5	None
Dermatitis herpetiformis	Trunk	Vesicles and papules becoming blood encrusted	Unknown	6	Biopsy, potassium iodide test, patch test, IgA immunofluorescence
Dermatitis venenata	Exposed parts of body	Linear vesicles progressing to blood and serous crusts	Often secondary infection		Patch test
Hodgkin's disease	Generalized	Macular lesions becoming blood encrusted, excoriations	Hodgkin's disease	8	Biopsy of skin lymph nodes or involved tissue
Jaundice	Generalized	Pruritic icterus leading to linear bloody excoriations	Hepatic dysfunction	8	Liver functions studies, serum bilirubin

Continued.

TABLE 2–4.—Continued

DISEASE	SITES	LESION	ETIOLOGY	TREATMENT	DIAGNOSTIC AIDS
Leukemic cutis	Generalized; may be in only one area	Plaques, nodules, or tumors with blood-encrusted excoriations	Leukemia	8	Biopsy of skin, sternal marrow studies, blood count
Neurotic excoriations	Within reach of hands	Deep bloody excoriations	Psychiatric	8	Psychiatric examination
Papular urticaria	Face, trunk, extremities	Papules and vesicles with bloody crusts	Bites—usually fleas	6	Clinical appearance
Pediculosis capitis	Scalp and forehead and back of neck	Blood-encrusted excoriations with pus	Louse	9	Microscopic examination of ova attached to hair
Pediculosis corporis	Trunk	Bloody excoriations, furuncles	Louse	9	Microscopic examination of parasites
Pediculosis pubis	Pubic area	Blood- and pus-encrusted excoriations	Louse	9	Microscopic examination of ova attached to hair
Scabies	Between fingers, palms, wrists, buttock, genitalia; not on face	Linear papule with blood, serous, and pus crusting	Mite	9	Microscopic study of vesicle contents for *Acarus scabiei* or ova and feces

ULCERS

TABLE 2–5.—Ulcers

DISEASE	SITES	LESION	ETIOLOGY	TREATMENT	DIAGNOSTIC AIDS
Blastomycosis	Face, hands, feet	Granulomatous ulcer which spreads peripherally with pustules in margin	*Blastomyces dermatitidis*	Amphotericin B	Biopsy, culture, direct microscopic examination of exudate
Bromoderma	Legs	Granulomatous ulcer	Bromide ingestion	Withdraw offender	Biopsy, blood bromide; rule out blastomycosis by direct examination and culture
Chancroid	Genitalia	Papule or vesicle which becomes a superficial, irregular, soft ulcer with granular base, covered with pus; inguinal adenopathy	*Hemophilus ducreyi*	4	Culture, Gram stain of ulcer
Ecthyma	Legs, buttock, vulva	One or more well-defined ulcers, covered with pus crusts and surrounded by zones of erythema; heals by scar formation	Streptococci, staphylococci	4	Culture, Gram stain, serology

Continued.

TABLE 2–5.—Continued

DISEASE	SITES	LESION	ETIOLOGY	TREATMENT	DIAGNOSTIC AIDS
Epithelioma (basal cell)	Face, ears	Papule or nodule that spreads peripherally; ulcer is shallow and surrounded by pearly rolled margin	Carcinoma	10	Biopsy
Epithelioma (squamous cell)	Face, lips, hands	More rapidly growing than basal cell; superficial or deep ulcer with granulomatous, irregular central portion that bleeds freely	Carcinoma	10	Biopsy
Erythema induratum	Legs, calves	Deep-seated nodules that grow and ulcerate; little discharge	TB	Anti-TB agents	Biopsy
Factitious ulcer	Areas accessible to hands	Single or multiple well-demarcated ulcers; new ones appearing	Self inflicted; psychiatric	8	History, psychiatric examination
Frostbite	Ears, fingers, toes, nose	Erythema, edema, blebs, leading to ulcers	Freezing	Rewarming	History of exposure

Disease	Location	Appearance	Cause		Diagnostic procedures
Granuloma inguinale	Perineum, genital area	Papule that ulcerates and spreads peripherally; granulomatous-based raised, rolled margin	*Donovania granulomatis*	4	Microscopic examination of Wright's or Giemsa-stained smear of marginal tissue for Donovan bodies
Perforating ulcer of the foot	Plantar surface of foot	Begins as callus, which eventually covers a deep ulcer	Multiple pressure		VDRL, spinal fluid examination, neurologic examination, blood sugar
Radiation dermatitis	Irradiated area	Superficial ulcer surrounded by zones of atrophy and telangiectasia	Radiation	None	Biopsy
Sickle cell anemia ulcer	Lateral aspects of lower third of legs	Round or oval punched-out ulcer, with indurated edge; purulent drainage	Sickle cell	8	Hemoglobin electrophoresis
Stasis ulcer	Lower third of legs	Superficial or deep with profuse seropurulent discharge; surrounded by stasis eczema	Multiple venous insufficiency	8	Clinical appearance
Syphilis (ecthymatous)	Trunk, scalp, extremities	Large round, flat pustules with red-brown areola; thick crust over ulcer	*Treponema pallidum*	4	Darkfield microscopic examination, VDRL

Continued.

29

TABLE 2–5.—Continued

DISEASE	SITES	LESION	ETIOLOGY	TREATMENT	DIAGNOSTIC AIDS
Syphilis, chancre	Genitalia, lips, nipples	Single, hard, indurated ulcer with scant discharge, lymph nodes enlarged, hard and painless	*Treponema pallidum*	4	Darkfield microscopic exam, STS
Syphilis, gumma	Legs, forehead, scalp	Subcutaneous nodule with necrosis to form a deep ulcer	*Treponema pallidum*	4	RPR
Thermal burns	Exposed areas	Well-circumscribed that sheds cover to form ulcer with granulomatous base	Burn	Dependent on degree	History
Tubercularis	Face, neck	Round, oval, ulcer that bleeds easily; nodules in margins	TB	Anti-TB drugs	Biopsy, culture
Unusual cutaneous infections: amebic Diphtheria Chromobacteria *Salmonella* *Listeria* Anaerobes	Anywhere	Abscess that ulcerates	Infectious	8	Biopsy, culture on various media

TABLE 2–6.—PIGMENTARY CHANGES AS DIAGNOSTIC SIGNS IN GENERAL MEDICINE*

CHIEF COMPLAINT OR PRESENTING PROBLEM	PIGMENTARY CHANGE	DISEASES	SYSTEMS INVOLVED
	Addisonian Brown Hyperpigmentation		
"Getting dark"	Generalized diffuse brown hypermelanosis	Addison's disease Hemochromatosis ACTH-producing tumors	Adrenal insufficiency Cirrhosis of liver, diabetes Pituitary tumor, primary; metastatic cancer
		Systemic scleroderma	Dysphagia; pulmonary insufficiency
		Porphyria cutanea tarda	Liver: increased iron stores Diabetes mellitus (25%)
	Circumscribed Brown Macules		
"Abdominal pain, brown spots on lips, fingers"	Circumscribed, mostly small dark-brown macules (many)	Peutz-Jegher syndrome	Polyposis of small intestine
"Brown spots all over"	Circumscribed small dark-brown macules	Progressive lentiginosis	Abnormal ECG Pulmonary stenosis
"Birth mark"; hypertension; precocious puberty	Circumscribed, uniformly brown macules, small or large (café au lait) (few or many)	Neurofibromatosis	Neurofibromatosis of skin and peripheral nervous system; pheochromocytoma
		Albright's syndrome	Polyostotic fibrous dysplasia Precocious puberty
		Watson's syndrome	Pulmonary stenosis
"Funny moles"	Circumscribed dark-brown macules or slightly raised papules with irregular borders and variegation of color (few or many)	Dysplastic nevus syndrome	

Continued.

TABLE 2-6.—Continued

CHIEF COMPLAINT OR PRESENTING PROBLEM	PIGMENTARY CHANGE	DISEASES	SYSTEMS INVOLVED
		Circumscribed White Macules	
"White spots"	Circumscribed, mostly large white macules (few or many)	"Vitiligo"	Hypothyroidism Thyrotoxicosis Pernicious anemia Adrenal insufficiency Diabetes mellitus
"Convulsions"; mental retardation	Congenital circumscribed small (1–3 cm) white macules (more than 3)	Tuberous sclerosis	Mental retardation, abnormal EEG Abnormal CT scan Rhabdomyoma of heart
"Eye trouble"; deafness	Circumscribed white macules, poliosis	Vogt-Koyanagi-Harada disease	Uveitis, dysacousia
"Deafness"	White forelock, congenital circumscribed large white macules	Waardenburg's syndrome	Nerve deafness, heterochromia
		Universal Hypomelanosis	
"Sun sensitivity"; decreased vision	Universal hypomelanosis of skin, hair, and uveal tract	Oculocutaneous albinism, recessive	Decreased visual acuity, iris translucency, nystagmus
"Sun sensitivity"; "Poor tanner"	Type I or type II skin	Oculocutaneous albinoidism, dominant	Iris translucency, normal vision, nystagmus (rare)

*From Petersdorf, A, Braunwald, Isselbacher, et al: *Harrison's Principles of Internal Medicine*, ed 10. New York, McGraw-Hill Book Co, 1983. Reproduced by permission.

COMMON PROBLEMS AND TREATMENTS

TABLE 2–7.—COMMON PROBLEMS AND TREATMENTS

Acne
   The following treatments can be used singly or additively and are listed from the mildest to the strongest treatment. A step approach is suggested. Gently wash face twice daily with mild soap, eliminate foods patient has found to aggravate condition, get extra sun or sun lamp exposure.
  Topical preparations
    Use b.i.d. to the point of dryness and mild erythema but not pain. Use antimicrobial benzoyl peroxide 5%–10%, comedolytic retinoic acid.
  Antibiotics
    Topical: Erythromycin, clindamycin, tetracycline.
    Use these b.i.d. on clean face.
    Oral: Tetracycline, erythromycin, trimethoprim-sulfa.
    Use these q.i.d. for 2–4 wk, then taper to qhs.
  Steroids
    Orally or intralesionally (see Table 2–9).
  Accutane
    Rarely is needed; is toxic, teratogenic.
Diaper rash
   A good history and examination may reveal whether the rash is due to an irritant or a yeast infection. Yeast generally affects the skin creases more than irritants do.
  Irritant
    Remove irritant—if urine, leave the baby undiapered several times per day.
    Use very mild topical steroid such as 1% hydrocortisone cream.
  Yeast *(Candida albicans)*
    Use a nystatin or nystatin-steroid compound like Mycolog.
Corns and calluses
   These are acquired areas of thickened skin over areas of repeated, prolonged friction or pressure. These areas are very painful, but pain is eradicated on removal of thickened skin.
  Surgical debridement
    Use no. 15 blade and 1% xylocaine for anesthesia, if needed.
  Intermittent debridement
    40% salicylic acid plaster, applied with tape, for 1–7 days and then removed. Soak foot and debride dead tissue. Repeat as needed to keep the lesion flat.
Warts (nongenital)
  Destructive
    Electrodesiccation and curettage
    Cryosurgery
  Keratolytic
    10% salicylic acid, 10% lactic acid in flexible collodion, applied daily. May be prescribed as above or as Duofilm.
    Cantharone, cantharone plus.
Warts (plantar)
  Keratolytic
    40% salicylic acid plaster; apply daily and trim away dead tissue.

TABLE 2–8.—Disorders of the Hair and Scalp

DISEASE	DESCRIPTION	ETIOLOGY	TREATMENT
Alopecia areata	Well-defined single or multiple patches of balding	Probably autoimmune	Reassurance, intralesional steroids
Dandruff	Noninflammatory scaling occurring on scalp	Physiological desquamation	Selenium sulfide 2.5%
Seborrheic dermatitis	Inflammatory scaling in sebaceous areas: scalp, face and trunk	Sebum as irritant	Selenium sulfide 2.5%, corticosteroid cream
Psoriasis	Chronic proliferative epidermal disease	Unclear	Tar shampoo, intralesional steroids
Fungal infection	Superficial epidermis infections	Dermatophytes	Antifungal agents topically and rarely orally
Hair loss	Loss of hair in front or crown	Male pattern baldness	Minoxidil topically for crown balding
Folliculitis	Infection around hair follicles	Staphylococcus	Antibiotics

STEROID USAGE

TABLE 2–9.—STEROIDS

Oral

For a burst of steroids with a taper lasting a total of 20 days, prescribe prednisone, 5 mg #100. For a 10- to 14-day course of steroids, tapering is unnecessary.

Prescription: Days 1–3, take 12 in A.M. (total, 60 mg)
Days 4–6, take 8 in A.M. (total, 40 mg)
Days 7–9, take 4 in A.M. (total, 20 mg)
Then 2 in A.M. until finished

Indications: severe poison ivy, sunburn, acne

Steroid Preparation	Equivalent Dosage (mg)
Prednisone	5
Prednisolone	5
Methylprednisolone	4
Triamcinolone	4
Cortisone	25
Hydrocortisone	20
Betamethasone	0.6
Dexamethasone	0.75

Intralesional

Provides high local concentration with minimal systemic side effects and a prolonged depot effect.

Use a 1:4 dilution of one of the following with saline or lidocaine:
Betamethasone acetate suspension
Triamcinolone acetonide
Triamcinolone diacetate
Triamcinolone hexacetonide
Methylprednisolone

Indications: acne cysts, psoriatic plaques, circumscribed neurodermatitis, keloids

Topical steroids

The most potent topical steroids are flourinated and should be used only for a short time. In general, ointment and gel vehicles are superior to cream or lotion vehicles.

Topical Steroids Ranked by Potency
(Group 1 most potent, group 6 least potent)

Group 1:	Diprosone ointment	0.05%
	Florone ointment	0.05%
	Halog cream	0.1%
	Lidex cream	0.05%
	Lidex ointment	0.05%
	Topicort ointment	0.25%
	Topsyn gel	0.05%

Continued.

TABLE 2–9.—Continued

Topical Steroids Ranked by Potency

Group 2:	Aristocort cream	0.5%
	Diprosone cream	0.05%
	Florone cream	0.05%
	Benisone gel	0.025%
	Topicort cream	0.25%
	Valisone lotion	0.1%
	Valisone ointment	0.1%
Group 3:	Aristocort ointment	0.1%
	Cordran ointment	0.05%
	Cyclocort cream	0.1%
	Kenalog ointment	0.1%
	Synalar-HP cream	0.2%
	Synalar ointment	0.025%
Group 4:	Cordran cream	0.05%
	Kenalog cream	0.1%
	Kenalog lotion	0.025%
	Synalar cream	0.025%
	Valisone cream	0.1%
Group 5:	Locorten cream	0.03%
	Tridesilon cream	0.05%
Group 6:	Topicals with hydrocortisone (e.g., Carmol HCl cream, Cort-Dome cream, Hytone cream, Synacort cream), dexamethasone, flumethasone, prednisolone, and methylprednisolone	

TABLE 2–10.—MUCOCUTANEOUS MANIFESTATIONS OF HIV DISEASE

Often skin and oral changes are presenting signs of HIV disease. Careful inspection may lead to early detection of infection.

Herpes Simplex	Bacterial skin infections
Herpes Zoster	Seborrhea
Warts, common and venereal	Psoriasis
Molluscum contagiosum	Telangiectasias and angiomas
Fungal infections	Aphthous stomatitis
Periodontal disease and gingivitis	Kaposi's sarcoma

TABLE 2–11.—Characteristics of Malignant and Benign Pigmented Skin Lesions*

FEATURE	MELANOMA	BENIGN SKIN LESION
Size	Over 1 cm, increasing in size	Less than 1 cm, stable size
Color	Varied, resembling an autumn maple leaf, "flag sign"[†]	Brown, often becomes pale with increasing age
Surface (palpable)	Hard elevated area, scaling, oozing, bleeding	Macule progresses to soft papule with increasing age
Surrounding skin	Fingers of pigment penetrate, erythematous	Unremarkable or white, halo
Patient-reported sensations	Itchiness, tenderness	None
Location	Back most common	Over entire body but more common on sun-exposed surfaces
Precursors	Family history, dysplastic nevi, congenital nevi, giant hairy nevus, excess sun exposure, type I/II (easily burned) skin	Excess sun exposure in youth; family history of similar lesions at same or mirror-image site
Skin marking[‡]	Absent	Often present

*From Love RR: *Principles of Oncology.* Monogr ed 125, *Home Study Self-Assessment Program.* Kansas City, Mo, American Academy of Family Physicians, October 1989. Reproduced by permission.
[†]The "flag sign" is the appearance of red, white, and blue colors in a pigmented lesion.
[‡]With a magnifying glass, normal skin has crisscrosses of grooves. These normal lines are obliterated by the disordered malignant growth of melanomas.

PROCEDURES

TABLE 2–12.—Wood's Light Examination

A Wood's light produces an invisible longwave ultraviolet radiation that will induce visible fluorescence that can aid in differential diagnosis. It is very safe.
Technique
Wood's lamp must be on for several minutes to get to optimum intensity.
Securely seat the patient so that he/she does not fall in the dark.
Turn off room lights and allow the patient's eyes to adjust.
Hold Wood's lamp 4–5 inches from area being inspected.

Continued.

TABLE 2–12.—Continued

Findings*	
Condition	Fluorescent Color
Tinea capitis	
Microsporum audouini	Bright yellow-green
Microsporum canis	Bright yellow-green
Trichophyton schoenleini	Pale green
Erythrasma	Coral-red or pink[†]
Pigmentary alterations	
Depigmentation	Cold bright white
Hypopigmentation	Blue-white
Hyperpigmentation	Purple-brown
Vitiligo	Cold bright white and blue-white
Albinism	Cold bright white
Leprosy	Blue-white
Ash-leaf spot of tuberous sclerosis	Blue-white
Pseudomonas aeruginosa infections	Aqua-green or white-green (rarely, yellow-green)
Porphyria cutanea tarda (urine)	Pink to pink-orange
Tinea versicolor	Golden yellow

*Adapted from Eaglstein WH, Pariser DM: *Office Techniques for Diagnosing Skin Disease.* Chicago, Year Book Medical Publishers, 1978.
†Patients who bathe shortly before Wood's light examination may show little or no fluorescence.

SKIN BIOPSY TECHNIQUE

Punch Biopsy

Punch biopsy for diagnosis of most inflammatory diseases and tumors.

1. Clean the lesion with 70% alcohol.
2. Use infiltration with 0.5%–1.0% lidocaine for anesthesia.
3. Use a 3–4 mm punch. Simultaneously twist and press the cutting edge into the tissue (Fig 2–1, A).
4. Incise as deeply as possible.
5. Elevate the specimen, handling the edges only and cut the base with scissors or a scalpel (Fig 2–1, B). Put in a specimen container.

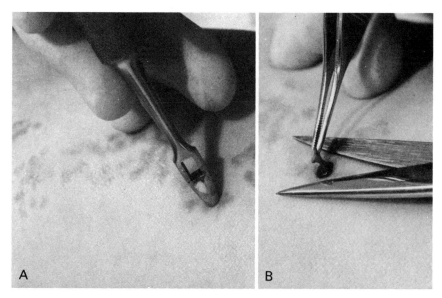

A   B

FIG 2–1.

Shave Biopsy

Parallel incisional (shave) biopsy for removing superficial benign lesions and biopsy of basal cell and squamous cell carcinomas. This procedure is contraindicated in patients with melanoma.

1. Clean the biopsy site with 70% alcohol.
2. Inject 0.5%–1.0% lidocaine beneath or directly into the lesions.
3. With scalpel parallel to the skin, shave the lesion from the skin. Pinching the skin may facilitate this step (Fig 2–2, A and B).
4. Complete the incision and place the thin disk of tissue in a specimen bottle.
5. Achieve hemostasis with either pressure, silver nitrate, or ferric subsulfate solution.

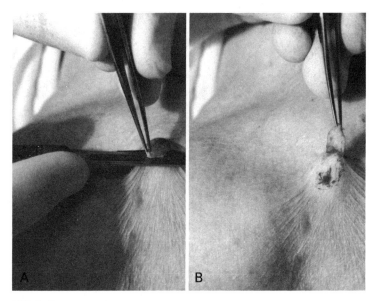

FIG 2–2.

SCABIES DETECTION

Preparing a Scabies Slide

1. Select an unexcoriated papule or tract.
2. Place a drop of immersion oil over the lesion. Scrape off the epidermis over the tract or tease the tract open with a scalpel blade. The mite (Fig 2–3) will grasp the scalpel blade and can be transferred to a slide.

KOH PREP

Potassium Hydroxide (KOH) Examination

KOH causes a destruction of the stratum corneum cells and thus a cleaning of debris so that exogenous materials like hyphae, spores, and fiberglass fibers can be seen (Fig 2–4, A and B).

Indications

1. Scaling disorders.
2. Blisters of the hands and feet.
3. Patches of missing or broken hair.

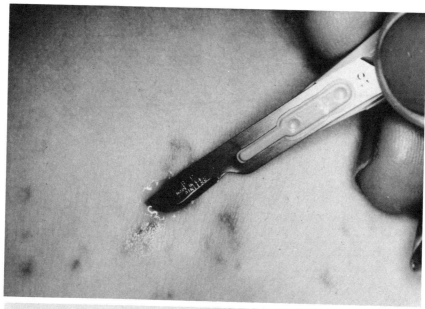

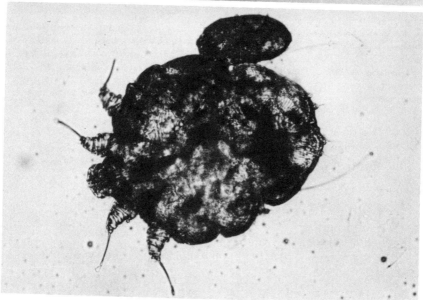

FIG 2–3.
Female mite with four of eight legs in focus. An egg is adjacent to the mite at the top of the picture. (From Eaglstein WH, Pariser DM: *Office Techniques for Diagnosing Skin Disease.* Chicago, Year Book Medical Publishers, 1978. Reproduced by permission.)

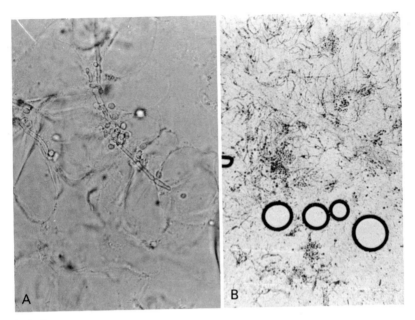

FIG 2–4.
A, spores, budding spores, and hyphae of *Candida* (×400). *Candida* hyphae cross the epidermal cell walls, as do dermatophyte hyphae. **B,** hyphae and spores of tinea versicolor (×100). The findings are often called "spaghetti and meatballs." Short and long hyphae and clusters of spores are seen. In this field, long hyphae predominate. *Large circles* are oil droplets. (From Eaglstein WH, Pariser DM: *Office Techniques for Diagnosing Skin Disease.* Chicago, Year Book Medical Publishers, 1978. Reproduced by permission.)

   4. Disorders of the nails.
   5. Excoriated papules in skin creases.
   6. Warty nodules containing tiny black dots (chromomycosis).

Technique

   1. Remove all powders or creams with acetone or alcohol.
   2. Collect scale on a clean slide by scraping the advancing edge of the lesion with a round-bellied blade.
   3. Place a drop of 10% KOH solution on the material and apply the coverslip.
   4. Gently warm but do not boil the slide over an alcohol burner.
   5. Examine microscopically.

3 Ophthalmology

Edward T. Bope, M.D.

VISION EVALUATIONS

TABLE 3–1.—Percentage of Visual Loss (AMA Method)*

Use best correcting glasses and measure both distance vision by the Snellen chart and near vision by the Jaeger test type. In this method, near and distant vision are weighted equally.

Snellen Chart for Distance Visual Acuity	% Loss
20/20	0
20/25	5
20/40	15
20/50	25
20/80	40
20/100	50
20/160	70
20/200	80
20/400	90

Jaeger Test Type for Near Visual Acuity	% Loss
1	0
2	0
3	10
6	50
7	60
11	85
14	95
(See Fig 3–1)	

$$*\%Vision\ acuity = 100 - \frac{\%\ Near\ loss\ +\ \%\ Distant\ loss}{2}.$$

EXTRAOCULAR MUSCLES

TABLE 3–2.—Extraocular Muscle Innervation

NERVE	CRANIAL NO.	MUSCLE	FUNCTION	RESULTS OF DEFICIT
Oculomotor	III	Medial rectus	Moves eye toward nose	Eye looks downward due to unopposed action of lateral rectus and superior oblique
		Superior rectus	Upward gaze	Weakness of upward gaze
		Inferior rectus	Downward gaze	Weakness of downward gaze
		Inferior oblique	Moves eye up when looking nasally	Vertical diplopia; head remains tilted to compensate
			Rotates eye when looking temporally	
			Moves eye up and out when in forward gaze	
		Levator palpebrae superioris	Elevates upper lid	Severe ptosis
Trochlear	IV	Superior oblique	Moves eye down when looking nasally	Vertical diplopia; head remains tilted to compensate
			Rotates eye when looking temporally	
			Moves eye down and out when in forward gaze	
Abducens	VI	Lateral rectus	Moves eye temporally	Inability to look temporally
Cervical sympathetics		Muller's	Elevates upper lid	Mild ptosis

44

DISEASES OF THE RETINA

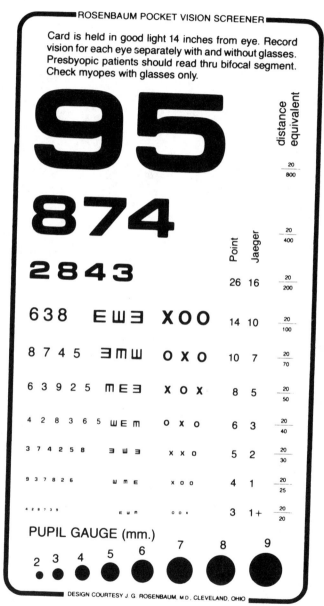

FIG 3–1.
Jaeger test for near visual acuity. (Design courtesy of JG Rosenbaum, MD, Cleveland, Ohio.)

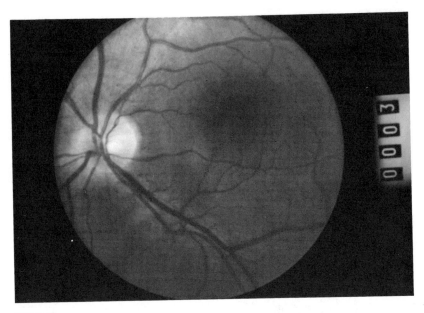

FIG 3–2.
Normal retina.

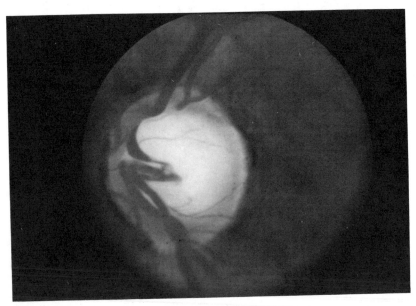

FIG 3–3.
Glaucoma. Cupping due to glaucoma extends to edge of the optic disc.

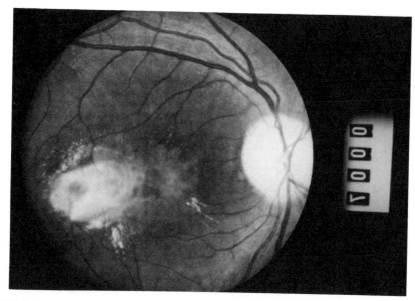

FIG 3–4.
Senile macular degeneration. Note scattered exudates in the macular area and absent foveal light reflex. There may be scattered hemorrhages.

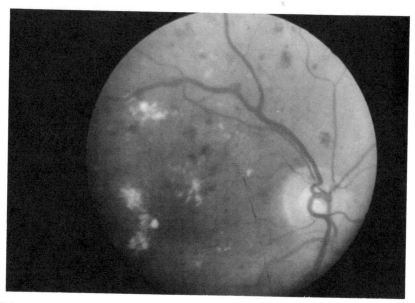

FIG 3–5.
Diabetic retinopathy. Note small hemorrhages and scattered exudates.

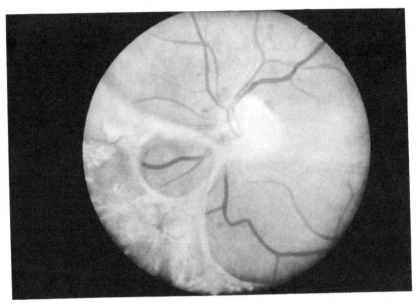

FIG 3–6.
Diabetic retinitis proliferans. Note sheets of connective tissue and new blood vessels near the optic disc.

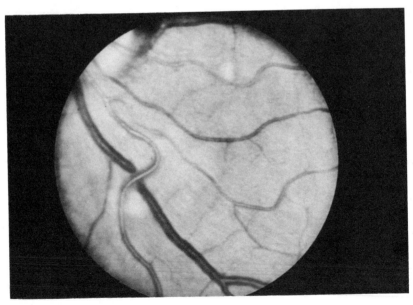

FIG 3–7.
Hypertensive retinopathy. Note AV nicking and hard exudates.

COMMON EYE SYMPTOMS

TABLE 3–3.—Common Eye Symptoms

EYE SYMPTOMS	MOST COMMON DIAGNOSES
Acute spontaneous loss of vision in one eye, transient	Transient ischemic attack involving blood circulation to retina; lasting deficit may indicate central retinal artery occlusion or arteriolar or venous hemorrhage Migraine
Acute spontaneous loss of vision in both eyes, transient	Transient ischemic attack involving blood circulation to visual areas of brain Migraine
Floaters (particles of dust, spots, cobwebs); no other visual difficulties	Vitreous opacities, usually insignificant
Lightning flashes	Migraine (often also manifest as "wavy" appearance of environment); May accompany traction on retina or retinal detachment
Curtain drawn over an eye	Retinal detachment or hemorrhage
Blurred vision—far only	Myopia
Blurred vision—near only	Hyperopia; use of cycloplegic drops; presbyopia
Double vision	Nerve or muscle damage; if monocular, may reflect lens dislocation or cataract
Vertigo (spinning of patient or environment)	Dysfunction of vestibular apparatus or its connection in the brain stem
Loss of central vision in one eye	Macular or optic nerve disease

COMMON EYE SIGNS

TABLE 3–4.—Common Eye Signs

SIGN	DIAGNOSIS	TREATMENT
Tender pimple on lid margin	Hordeolum (sty)	Warm compresses q.i.d. Topical antibiotic Referral for I&D if persistent
Tender nodule in lid away from margin	Chalazion	Warm compresses Antibiotics of little value Referral for excision if persistent

Continued.

TABLE 3–4.—Continued

Ulcerated lesion with pearly border (lower lid)	Basal cell carcinoma	Excision or Referral for excision
Soft, yellow, raised lid lesions	Xanthelasma	Can be cosmetically removed Check for diabetes and hyperlipidemia
Lower conjunctiva exposed and red	Ectropion	Plastic repair
Foreign body sensation; lid margin not seen	Entropion	Plastic repair
Ecchymosis of lid	Black eye	Examine eye for diplopia Ice for 24 hr
Red hemorrhagic sclera	Subconjunctival hemorrhage	No treatment
Warm, tender swelling in superolateral aspect of upper lid	Lacrimal gland inflammation	Treat infection Rule out tumor
Warm, tender swelling of nasal aspect of lower lid	Lacrimal sac inflammation	Antistaph topical antibiotics Warm compresses Massage lacrimal sac
Crusty, sore eyelids with scaling	Blepharitis	Topical antibiotics Dandruff control
Ocular pain—eye injected temporally	Episcleritis	Consultation Steroids
Ocular pain—halos around lights	Glaucoma	Schiøtz tonometry Consultation
Soft yellow patches on sclera at 3 and 9 o'clock	Pinguecula	No treatment
Scleral vascularization extending to nasal cornea	Pterygium	Can be cosmetically removed
Mild ptosis, small pupil and same-sided decreased facial sweating	Horner's syndrome	Consultation, chest x-ray film A large differential, including tumor

RED EYE—DIFFERENTIAL DIAGNOSIS

TABLE 3–5.—Differential Diagnosis of Red Eye

ASPECT	DIAGNOSIS			
	Acute Conjunctivitis	Acute Iritis	Acute Glaucoma	Corneal Ulcer or Trauma
Redness	Diffuse	Circumcorneal	Diffuse	Diffuse
Vision	Normal	Slightly blurred	Markedly blurred	Blurred
Discharge	Large	None	None	Watery or purulent
Pain	None	Moderate	Severe	Moderate to severe
Cornea	Clear	Anterior chamber may be cloudy	Cloudy	Opacity, fluorescein positive
Pupil—size	Normal	Small	Dilated	Normal or small if secondary iritis
Pupil—light response	Normal	Poor	Poor	Normal
Intraocular pressure	Normal	Normal	Increased	Normal
Therapy	Antibiotics	Atropine, Cortisone	Pilocarpine, Diamox, surgery	Antibiotics
Prognosis	3–5 days	Definitive treatment needed to avoid serious complications		

OCULAR MANIFESTATIONS OF SYSTEMIC DISEASE

TABLE 3–6.—Ocular Manifestations of Systemic Disease*

Albinism: Light fundus background (choroidal vessels seen easily with the ophthalmoscope as pigment epithelium is unpigmented; nystagmus; poor vision (high refractive errors and poor macular development); pink-blue iris (iris transilluminates).

Alkaptonuria: Melanin deposits in sclera (at 9 and 3 o'clock positions around the cornea).

Amyloidosis: Weakness of extraocular muscles; vitreous opacities; pupillary abnormalities; amyloid nodules in lids and conjunctiva.

Anemia: Conjunctiva appears pale; retinal hemorrhages and exudates present.

Ankylosing spondylitis: Uveitis; scleritis; scleromalacia perforans (thinning of sclera with exposure of uveal tissue).

Atopic dermatitis: Cataracts; keratoconus.

Behçet's syndrome: Uveitis.

Cystic fibrosis: Papilledema; retinal hemorrhages.

Cystinosis: Deposits of cystine crystals in cornea and conjunctiva.

Cytomegalic inclusion disease (congenital): Chorioretinitis cataracts.

Dermatomyositis: Extraocular muscle palsies; lid edema, scleritis; uveitis; retinal exudates.

Diabetes mellitus: Extraocular muscle palsies; xanthelasmas; retinal microaneurysms; hemorrhages, exudates, and neovascularization of the retina; cataracts; rubeosis iritis (neovascularization of the iris); glaucoma.

Down's syndrome: Up-and-out obliquity to the lids; Brushfield's spots (white speckling of iris); cataracts; myopia; strabismus.

Ehlers-Danlos syndrome: Blue sclera; strabismus; epicanthal folds.

Friedreich's ataxia: Nystagmus; strabismus; retinitis pigmentosa.

Galactosemia: Cataracts.

Glomerulonephritis: Periorbital edema; hypertensive retinopathy.

Gout: Episcleritis, uveitis; deposition of uric acid crystals in cornea.

Hereditary hemorrhagic telangiectasia (Osler-Weber-Rendu disease): Telangiectasias of conjunctiva and retina.

Herpes zoster: Dermatitis along ophthalmic branch of cranial nerve V; uveitis; keratitis.

Histoplasmosis: Chorioretinal scars, retinal hemorrhage.

Homocystinuria: Dislocated lens.

Hyperlipidemia: Xanthelasmas, arcus juvenilis, lipemia retinalis (milky retinal vessels secondary to excessive lipids in the blood).

Hyperparathyroidism: Band keratopathy (gray-white band containing calcium deposits, extending horizontally across the cornea); optic atrophy.

Hyperthyroidism: Proptosis, lid retraction; infrequent blinking (staring); lid lag on downward gaze, weakness of upward gaze; poor convergence; diplopia, corneal erosion (from poor lid closure); papilledema; papillitis.

Hypoparathyroidism: Cataracts; papilledema; optic neuritis.

Hypothyroidism: (congenital cretinism): Strabismus; farsightedness; cataracts; swollen lids with narrow slits between lids; wide-set eyes; retrobulbar neuritis; optic atrophy; loss of outer half of eyebrows.

Impending stroke: Amaurosis fugax (transient blindness from intermittent vascular compromise in arteriosclerotic disease); Hollenhorst plaques (glistening emboli seen at branch points of retinal arterioles).

Kernicterus (erythroblastosis fetalis): Strabismus; nystagmus; retinal hemorrhage.

Lead poisoning: Papilledema; optic atrophy.

Lupus erythematosus: Retinal hemorrhages; cotton wool exudates; papilledema; lid lesions similar to lesions elsewhere; episcleritis; keratitis; uveitis; nystagmus; extraocular muscle palsies; cataracts.

Macroglobulinemia: Venous occlusion (engorged retinal veins with hemorrhages and exudates); papilledema

Marchesani's syndrome: Dislocated lens

Marfan's syndrome: Dislocated lens

Migraine: Throbbing eye pain; transient visual compromise (e.g., flashing lights, waves, hemianopia); miotic (small) pupil (sympathetic axon compromise with carotid artery wall edema).

Mucopolysaccharidoses: Corneal clouding.

Multiple sclerosis: Retrobulbar neuritis; optic atrophy; internuclear ophthalmoplegia; strabismus.

Myasthenia gravis: Ptosis; extraocular muscle paresis.

Myotonia: Cataracts.

Neurofibromatosis: Lid and orbital tumors; optic gliomas.

Osteogenesis imperfecta: Blue sclera (choroid shows through thin sclera).

Polyarteritis nodosa: Episcleritis; corneal ulcers, uveitis; retinal hemorrhages and exudates; papilledema; hypertensive retinopathy; arteriolar occlusion.

Polycythemia: Markedly dilated retinal veins; papilledema.

Pseudoxanthoma elasticum: Angioid streaks (reddish bands radiating from disc region, resembling blood vessels), probably representing defects in the choroidal membrane (Bruch's membrane) just outside the pigment epithelium. Also found in Paget's disease of the bone and sickle cell disease.

Radiation exposure: Cataracts; retinopathy.

Reiter's syndrome: Uveitis; retinal vasculitis.

Rheumatoid arthritis: Uveitis; band keratopathy; scleromalacia perforans (degeneration and thinning of anterior sclera with bulging out of underlying bluish choroid).

Riley-Day syndrome (familial dysautonomia): Decreased tear production; decreased corneal sensation with subsequent exposure keratitis.

Rosacea: Blepharitis; conjunctivitis; keratitis; episcleritis.

Rubella (congenital): Cataracts; microphthalmia; cloudy corneas; uveitis; pigmentary retinopathy.

Sarcoid: Uveitis; whitish perivenous infiltrates in retina band keratopathy.

Sickle cell anemia: Retinal hemorrhages, exudates, microaneurysms, neovascularization (vascular and hemorrhagic changes are worse in sickle C than in sickle S disease); papilledema; angioid streaks.

Sjögren's syndrome: Dry eyes; corneal erosions.

Stevens-Johnson syndrome: Purulent conjunctivitis with scarring of conjunctiva and cornea.

Subacute bacterial endocarditis: Congenital and retinal hemorrhages; Roth spots (retinal hemorrhages with white centers).

Continued.

TABLE 3–6.—Continued

Sturge-Weber disease: Congenital glaucoma on side of facial nevus.

Syphilis: Interstitial keratitis (inflammation, edema, and vascular infiltration of the cornea, particularly the corneal periphery); uveitis; optic neuritis; cataracts; chorioretinitis; lens dislocation; Argyll-Robertson pupil.

Tay-Sachs disease: Cherry red spot (cloudiness of retina, except in fovea region).

Temporal arteritis: Transient or permanent loss of vision from vasculitis affecting the optic nerve.

Toxemia: Hypertensive retinopathy.

Toxoplasmosis: Chorioretinitis.

Trichinosis: Inflammation of extraocular muscles.

Tuberculosis: Uveitis; chorioretinitis.

Tuberous sclerosis: Retinal tumor.

Ulcerative colitis: Uveitis.

Vitamin deficiencies: Vitamin A deficiency.—Night blindness; xerophthalmia (drying of cornea and conjunctiva). *Thiamine deficiency (beriberi).*—Optic neuritis; extraocular muscle weakness. *Niacin deficiency (pellagra).*—Optic neuritis. *Riboflavin deficiency.*—Photophobia; inflammation of conjunctiva and cornea. *Vitamin C deficiency (scurvy).*—Hemorrhages within the outside of the eye. *Vitamin D deficiency.*—Cataracts; papilledema (as in hypoparathyroidism).

Von Hippel-Lindau disease: Retinal hemangiomas.

Wilms' tumor: Aniridia (absence of iris).

Wilson's disease: Copper deposits in Descemet's membrane in the peripheral cornea (Kayser-Fleischer ring) and in the lens (copper cataracts).

*From Goldberg S: *Ophthalmology Made Ridiculously Simple.* Miami, MedMaster, 1982. Reproduced by permission.

TABLE 3–7.—HERPES INFECTIONS OF THE EYE

Simplex—Ulcers on the eyelid may be inoculated into the eye and this forms a dendritic corneal ulcer (a zigzag surface lesion). These are difficult to treat and may cause corneal scarring. N.B.: Topical corticosteroids should not be used because they will encourage corneal spread of this virus.

Zoster—When involving the eye, it is in the typical unilateral trigeminal distribution. The conjunctiva is red and the cornea shows discrete white subepithelial opacities. Fine dendritic ulcers may occur. Mydriatics, antibiotics, and topical corticosteroids should be used.

STRABISMUS AND AMBLYOPIA

TABLE 3–8.—Strabismus and Amblyopia

AMBLYOPIA: Loss of vision in one eye caused by:
  Physical occlusion (e.g., cataract, ptosis)
  Refractive error (unilateral)
  Strabismus
  Mechanism: The brain receives a confusing image from the affected eye and selectively suppresses the image.
STRABISMUS: Deviation of the eye in an inward direction (esotropia, cross-eyed), outward direction (exotropia, wall-eyed) or vertical direction (hypertropia).
  Classification
    Paralytic—due to damage of cranial nerves III, IV, or VI or to a lesion in the extraocular muscle itself. May be caused by brain tumor, encephalitis, intracranial aneurysm, vascular accident, thyrotropic exophthalmos, myasthenia gravis, or orbital cellulitis.
    Nonparalytic—the most common, resulting in suppression amblyopia.
  Detection
    Normal eye position will show a penlight reflected in the exact center of each pupil.
    Alternate cover test:
      Have patient fixate eyes on a penlight.
      Cover one eye.
      Remove cover and observe movement of uncovered eye.
      Alternate eyes in 1-second intervals.
      Interpret movement by table below.
    Cover/uncover test
        To diagnose strabismus, cover the disconjugate eye and then remove the cover. The eye remains deviated.

  Interpretation of alternate cover and cover/uncover tests:

Test	Movement	Meaning
Alternate cover	Inward	Eye rests in outward position (exophoria)
	None	Normal
	Outward	Eye rests in inward position (esophoria)
Cover/uncover	Deviated	Strabismus

Continued.

TABLE 3–8.—Continued

Treatment
Seek consultation soon after age 6 months if not corrected. The ophthalmologist will probably follow this outline:
Nonparalytic
Refractive error:
correct it, remember that if the eye is farsighted it will converge to accommodate, producing esotropia.
No refractive error:
alternately patch the eyes to exercise the extraocular muscles and stimulate vision in both eyes. Consider surgical intervention if the above fails.
Paralytic—specific to neurologic disease.
PSEUDOSTRABISMUS: An optical illusion usually secondary to broad epicanthal folds.

EYE TRAUMA

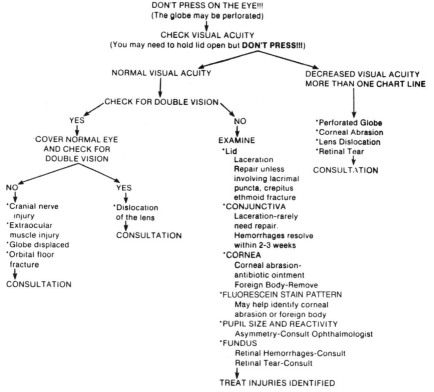

FIG 3–8.
Blunt injury to the eye.

TABLE 3–9.—Treatment for Chemical Burn

Irrigate with water or saline 15–20 minutes.
Clear cornea—Stain with fluorescein to estimate damage.
  Mild to moderate epithelial damage:
    Topical antibiotic
    Patch
    Examine daily until healed (2–3 days)
  Marked epithelial damage:
    Consult ophthalmologist
  Pupillary constriction (indicates intraocular irritation)
    Consult ophthalmologist
    Consider emergency use of cycloplegic drops on recommendation of ophthalmologist
Cloudy cornea—Irreversible damage; consult ophthalmologist

REMOVAL OF A FOREIGN BODY

TABLE 3–10.—Removal of Foreign Body

Persistent pain in the eye suggests presence of a foreign body or corneal abrasion.

Technique
1. Use proparacaine (Ophthaine) or tetracaine (Pontocaine) drops to achieve anesthesia. It will last 10–25 minutes.
2. Inspect globe in all gazes.
3. Inspect conjunctiva by pulling down the lower lid during upward gaze.
4. Evert the upper lid by grasping the upper lid margin and applying pressure over the tarsal plate with a cotton-tipped applicator or tongue blade (see Figs 3–9 and 3–10).
5. Magnifying glasses may be very helpful.

Continued.

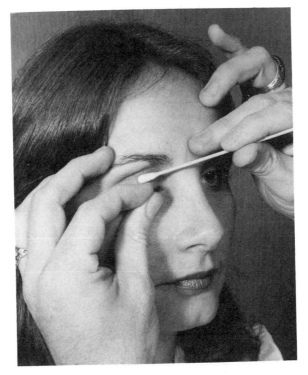

FIG 3–9.

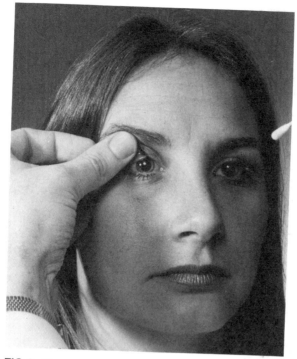

FIG 3–10.

Removal of foreign body
1. Practice on a porcine or bovine globe is essential.
2. Make sure anesthesia is still effective.
3. Attempt irrigation with saline under pressure.
4. Attempt removal by *light* touch of sterile cotton-tipped applicator.
5. Attempt removal with 26-gauge needle on a sterile cotton tip (Fig 3–11) or an eye spud.
6. If unsuccessful, consult an ophthalmologist for slit lamp removal.
7. Prophylactic topical antibiotics should be prescribed for 24–48 hours.
8. Eye patch is optional, depending mostly on patient comfort.

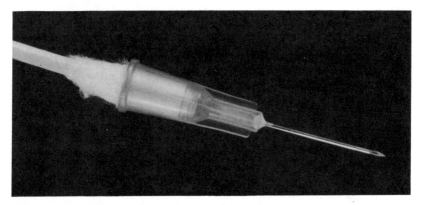

FIG 3–11.

TABLE 3–11.—OCULAR MANIFESTATIONS OF COMMON DRUGS

Amantadine: Visual hallucinations more common in the elderly (reversible).
Antianxiety agents: Diplopia.
Antituberculosis drugs: Optic neuritis and optic atrophy.
Antimalarials: Corneal deposits and edema, ptosis, decreased accommodation.
Contraceptives: Corneal edema (may interfere with contact lens wearing), papilledema, migraine.
Corticosteroids: Cataracts, increased intraocular pressure, retinal edema.
Digitalis: Yellow hue to vision (xanthopsia), conjunctivitis, decreased vision.
Diuretics: Retinal edema, retinal hemorrhages.
Gold: Corneal and lens gold deposits, ptosis.
Haloperidol: Oculogyric crisis.
Metoclopramide: Oculogyric crisis.
Pentazocine (Talwin): Constriction of pupils and visual hallucinations.
Phenothiazines: Posterior corneal deposits, Horner's syndrome, oculogyric crisis.
Phenytoin: Frequent nystagmus, ophthalmoplegia, and resulting diplopia.
Tetracycline: Blurring of vision, diplopia, papilledema (reversible).
Thioridazine (Mellaril): Pigment deposits on retina.
Tricyclics: Increased intraocular pressure in narrow-angle glaucoma.
Tricyclic antidepressants: Angle closure glaucoma.
Vitamin A: Papilledema, nystagmus, diplopia, color vision disturbance.
Vitamin D: Band keratopathy.

SCHIØTZ TONOMETRY AND GLAUCOMA

TABLE 3–12.—SCHIØTZ TONOMETRY AND GLAUCOMA

TONOMETRY

Indication: Routine exam after age 40 since elevated intraocular pressure (glaucoma) is responsible for 12% of cases of blindness in the United States.

Contraindications: Superficial eye infections, corneal edema or damage, uncooperative patients.

Technique (using Schiøtz tonometer):
Place patient in a comfortable position, supine, with the face straight upward. Instill one drop of 0.5% proparacaine.

While waiting 1 minute for anesthesia, check to see that the 7.5-gm weight is in place. Use 5.5-gm weight for very soft eyes and 10-gm weight for hard eyes (Fig 3–12).

Test tonometer accuracy on metal test block. It should read 0.

With patient staring at point on ceiling, gently separate lids with thumb and forefinger applied to orbital rims (Fig 3–13).

Gently place tonometer perpendicularly on center of cornea.

Read scale and interpret from Table 3–13. Pressures of 24 mm Hg or higher suggest glaucoma.

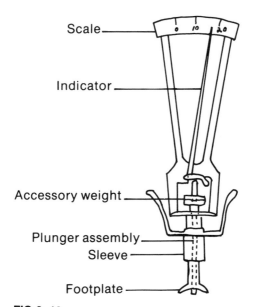

Scale

Indicator

Accessory weight

Plunger assembly

Sleeve

Footplate

FIG 3–12.
Schiøtz tonometer.

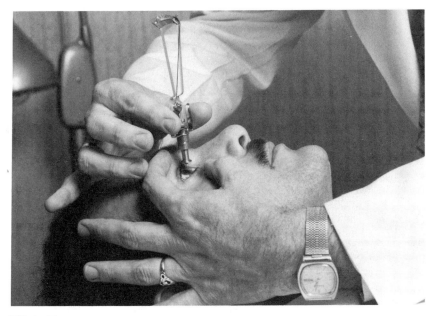

FIG 3–13.
Correct positioning and use of Schiøtz tonometer.

TABLE 3–13.—CALIBRATION SCALE
FOR SCHIØTZ TONOMETER

SCALE READING	5.5	7.5	10.0	15.0
	PLUNGER LOAD (GM)			
0	41	59	82	127
.5	38	54	75	118
1.0	35	50	70	109
1.5	32	46	64	101
2.0	29	42	59	94
2.5	27	39	55	88
3.0	24	36	51	82
3.5	22	33	47	76
4.0	21	30	43	71
4.5	19	28	40	66
5.0	17	26	37	62
5.5	16	24	34	58
6.0	15	22	32	54
6.5	13	20	29	50
7.0	12	19	27	46
7.5	11	17	25	43
8.0	10	16	23	40
8.5	9	14	21	38
9.0	9	13	20	35
9.5	8	12	18	32
10.0	7	11	16	30
10.5	6	10	15	27
11.0	6	9	14	25
11.5	5	8	13	23
12.0		8	11	21
12.5		7	10	20
13.0		6	10	18
13.5		6	9	17
14.0		5	8	15
14.5			7	14
15.0			6	13
15.5			6	11
16.0			5	10
16.5				9
17.0				8
17.5				8
18.0				7

4 Otolaryngology
Charles W. Smith, Jr., M.D.

EXAMINATION TECHNIQUES

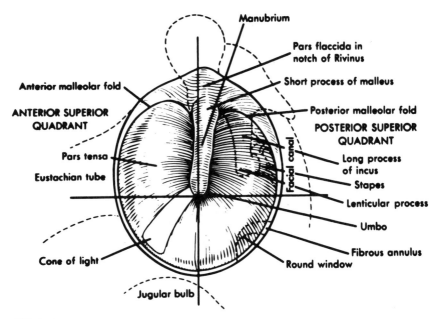

FIG 4–1.
Important middle ear landmarks. (From DeWeese DD, Saunders WH: *Textbook of Otolaryngology*, ed 6. St Louis, CV Mosby Co, 1982. Reproduced by permission.)

TABLE 4–1.—OFFICE HEARING TESTS

TEST	METHOD	INTERPRETATION
Weber test	512-Hz tuning fork placed on top of head; patient asked which ear tone is heard	Conductive loss: sound heard on affected side Neurosensory loss: sound heard on unaffected side
Rinne test	512-Hz tuning fork held against mastoid; when sound is no longer heard, duration of bone conduction is noted; fork transferred to ½ inch from ear; air conduction should be twice as long as bone and louder	Air > bone: normal Bone > air: conductive hearing loss
Whispered voice	Occlude opposite ear; whisper softly, from 2 feet away	Usually indicates 20-dB hearing loss

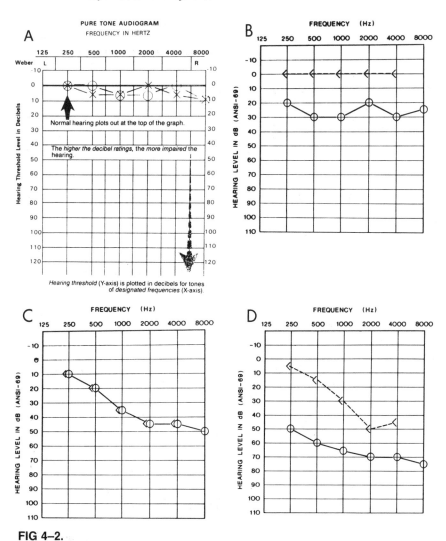

FIG 4–2.
Audiograms. **A,** normal hearing. **B,** conductive hearing loss; **C,** sensorineural hearing loss; **D,** combined sensorineural and conductive hearing loss. Air conduction: *O,* right; *X,* left. Bone conduction: < right; > left. (**A** from Hoffman SR: *Hosp Med* 1984; 20:204. Reproduced by permission.) (**B** to **D** from Adams GL, Boies LR, Paparella M. Audiology, in Boies LR [ed]: *Fundamentals of Otolaryngology,* ed 5. Philadelphia, WB Saunders Co, 1978, pp. 73, 80, 81. Reproduced by permission.)

TABLE 4–2.—TYMPANOMETRY*

Tympanometry records the same movements of the tympanic membrane (TM) elicited during pneumatic otoscopy. It records compliance of the TM with pressures varying from −200 to 200 mm Hg.

TYMPANOGRAM PATTERN	INTERPRETATION
Type A	Normal
Type A_S	Stiff ossicles (tympanosclerosis)
Type A_D	High TM compliance (monomeric TM)
Type B	Middle ear fluid, thickened drum, impacted cerumen
Type C	Retracted TM, eustachian tube dysfunction

*From Jerger JJ, Jerger SJ: Measurements of hearing in adults, in Paparella MM, Shumrick DA (ed): *Otolaryngology,* ed 2. Philadelphia, WB Saunders Co, 1980, vol 2, p 1232. Reproduced by permission.

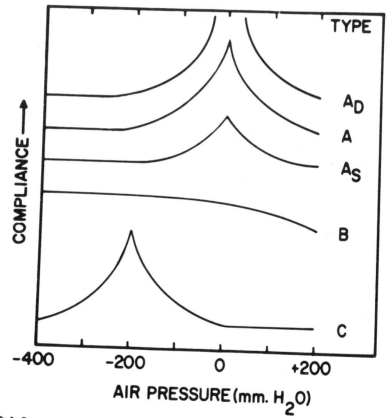

FIG 4–3.

Patterns of tympanograms. See also Table 4–2. (From Jerger JJ, Jerger JS: Measurements of hearing in adults, in Paparella MM, Shumrick DA [eds]: *Otolaryngology,* ed 2. Philadelphia, WB Saunders Co, 1980, vol 2, p 1232. Reproduced by permission.)

TABLE 4–3.—AUDIOMETRIC TESTING

TEST	INDICATION	INTERPRETATION
Pure tone audiometry	Persistent abnormality on office hearing screening tests	Conductive, sensorineural, or combined deficit identified
Speech audiometry	Learning disability; poor school performance; evaluation of need for speech therapy	Shows altered speech reception threshold or diminished speech discrimination
Bekesy audiogram	Sensorineural hearing loss	Helps differentiate between cochlear and 8th nerve hearing loss
Short Increment Sensitivity Index	Sensorineural hearing loss	Positive in early cochlear disease
Threshold tone decay	Sensorineural hearing loss	Positive in cochlear disease

TABLE 4–4.—TECHNIQUE OF INDIRECT MIRROR LARYNGOSCOPY

Approach should be calm but firm.
Topical anesthesia spray, 5% cocaine or 4% lidocaine, best delivered with a bulb-type atomizer.
May use IV Valium, 5–10 mg, over a 2-minute period if patient gags excessively.
Patient should sit erect with chin forward and feet on floor.
Tongue is held with gauze.
Warm mirror over alcohol lamp to prevent fogging. Test on hand for being too hot.
Hold mirror midway on shaft like a pen.
Mirror is placed with back side against the uvula.
Ask patient to breathe regularly; if patient gags, ask him/her to "pant like a dog."
Ask patient to say "EEE" so that approximation of the cords can be seen.

COMMON EAR PROBLEMS

TABLE 4–5.—USUAL BACTERIAL ORGANISMS IN
OTITIS MEDIA*

Pneumococcus (35%–40% of cases)
H. influenza (20% of cases)
B. catarrhalis (<10% of cases)
β-Streptococcus (<10% of cases)
S. aureus (<10% of cases)

*Adapted from Bluestone CD: N Engl J Med 1982;
306:1401.

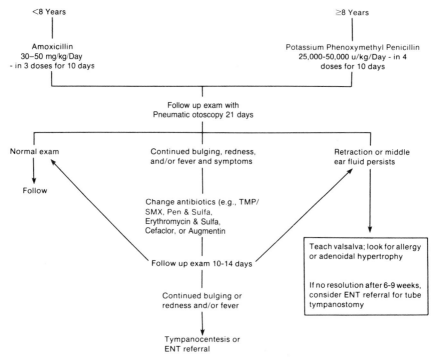

FIG 4–4.
Treatment of otitis media.

TABLE 4–6.—TYMPANOCENTESIS TECHNIQUE

1. Restrain child well.
2. Remove cerumen with irrigation or cerumen spoon.
3. Anesthetize tympanic membrane with 1-2 gtt. of 2% Xylocaine.
4. Use 1-cc syringe with 0.2 cc of nonbacteriostatic saline and an 18-gauge, 3½-inch spinal needle. Make a double bend in the needle so the TM can be visualized.
5. Visualize posteroinferior portion of TM with the otoscope.
6. Perforate TM with the needle and apply brief negative pressure.
7. Send one drop for culture and one drop for Gram stain. Place one drop each on blood and chocolate agar plates. Place remainder in thioglycolate broth.

*Adapted from Rowe PC: *The Harriet Lane Handbook,* ed 10. Chicago, Year Book Medical Publishers, 1984.

TABLE 4–7.—Treatment of Common Ear Problems

EXTERNAL OTITIS

External otitis (swimmer's ear) is seen most often in summer. *Pseudomonas* is the most common organism, but other gram-negative organisms or fungus may be causative.
Treatment:
If pain is severe use oral Codeine, 30–60 mg q4–6h or equivalent.
Polymixin B/Neomycin/Hydrocortisone, e.g. Cortisporin Otic 2-3 gtts. q.i.d. for 7–10 days. (Use solution unless perforation is suspected or present.)
Eardrops may require insertion of a cotton wick with Hartmann forceps if edema is severe.
As inflammation subsides, 70% alcohol may be substituted to keep canal clean and dry.
For recurrent problems use 70% alcohol or 2.5% acetic acid after patient swims and 3 times weekly.
May use systemic antibiotics (e.g., erythromycin or Cefaclor) if fever, marked swelling, and/or lymphadenopathy are present.

FOREIGN BODIES IN EAR

Foreign bodies are most commonly a problem in the external ear canals of children. Methods for removal are:
Apply otologic suction tip to foreign body and attempt to remove with constant suction.
Direct a stream of water (syringe or Water-Pik) superiorly and foreign body may "wash out." Caution: organic material may absorb water and swell.
If larger, place a hook or loop behind object and gently nudge it out.
If animate insect, moisten cotton wick with ether or instill mineral oil for 30 minutes, then irrigate or remove with Hartmann forceps.
If child is uncooperative, care must be taken to avoid trauma to the tympanic membrane. If difficulty is encountered, consider general anesthesia.

DIZZINESS AND VERTIGO

TABLE 4–8.—Dɪᴢᴢɪɴᴇss ᴀɴᴅ Vᴇʀᴛɪɢᴏ

Dizziness must be differentiated from true vertigo.
Dizziness—A disturbed sense of relationship to space.
Vertigo—A sensation of whirling or turning in space.
CAUSES OF DIZZINESS
    Ocular muscle imbalance
    Refractive error
    Glaucoma
    Proprioceptive defect (e.g., tabes dorsalis)
    Mild CNS anoxia (e.g., atherosclerosis, anemia)
    CNS infection
    Trauma
    CNS tumor
    Migraine
    Petit mal epilepsy
    Endocrine lesion (e.g., hypoglycemia)
    Functional
CAUSES OF VERTIGO
    Central (brain, spinal tract, or nuclear lesion)
        CNS infection
        Trauma
        CNS hemorrhage
        Posterior/inferior cerebellar artery thrombus
        CNS tumor
        Multiple sclerosis
    Peripheral (lesion in external, middle, or inner ear, or along 8th nerve)
        Wax or foreign body in canal
        Otitis media or serous otitis
        Labyrinthitis
        Cholesteatoma
        Trauma with middle ear hemorrhage
        Lesion in vestibular vessels
        Ménière's disease
        Motion sickness
        Postural vertigo
        8th nerve infection
        Meningitic involvement of 8th nerve
        Acoustic neuroma
EVALUATION OF VERTIGO
Careful history to distinguish true vertigo from dizziness.
If dizziness, proceed with evaluation of causes listed.
If vertigo, carefully examine ears, including office hearing evaluation.
Perform careful neurologic examination.

Continued.

TABLE 4–8.—Continued

Perform positional test by observing for nystagmus after placing in:
  (a) Upright position.
  (b) Recumbent position with left ear down.
  (c) Recumbent with right ear down.
  (d) Head hanging, pointing at the floor.
Observe for latency of onset of nystagmus, fatigability (sustained or brief), any directional change with positional change, and any unexpected types, considering the position of the patient.
Perform caloric tests (see below for technique).
Refer for audiography, electronystagmography (ENG), and intraauditory canal tomography and/or CT scanning, if indicated.
Refer for otolaryngologic evaluation if cause is still undetermined.
CALORIC TESTING
  Inject 5 cc of ice water over 5 seconds at posteroinferior quadrant of TM.
  Observe for nystagmus, nausea, and vertigo.
  If no response, increase to 10 and then to 20 cc.
  If no response, vestibular apparatus is not functioning.

TABLE 4–9.—Comparative Characteristics of Central and Peripheral Vestibular Disease*

CENTRAL VESTIBULAR DISEASE	PERIPHERAL VESTIBULAR DISEASE
Insidious onset	Sudden onset
Continuous episode	Intermittent episodes
Duration: months	Duration: seconds, minutes, or at most, a few days
Mild disequilibrium	True vertigo and intense disequilibrium during episodes
Little aggravation with head motion	Marked aggravation with head motion
Absence of associated unilateral auditory phenomena	Auditory phenomena (fullness, unilateral hearing loss, and tinnitus)
Presence of other neurologic or vascular signs and symptoms	Absence of other neurologic signs and symptoms
Positional nystagmus: immediate onset, no fatigue, does not adapt, direction changing with different head positions	Positional nystagmus: latent period, fatigue, adapts, direction fixed or changing
Spontaneous nystagmus: horizontal, rotary, or vertical	Spontaneous nystagmus: horizontal, rotary, *not* vertical
Caloric reaction: normal, perverted or dissociated, rarely hypoactive	Caloric reaction: normal or hypoactive, not perverted or dissociated

*From DeWeese DD, Saunders WH: *Textbook of Otolaryngology,* ed 6. St Louis, CV Mosby Co, 1982. Reproduced by permission.

TABLE 4–10.—Comparative Characteristics of Central and Peripheral Spontaneous Nystagmus*

FEATURE	PERIPHERAL	CENTRAL
Form	Horizontal/rotary	Horizontal, vertical, diagonal rotatory, multiple, pendular, alternating
Frequency	0.05 to 6 times/second	Any frequency, usually low or variable, of long intervals (weeks to months)
Intensity	Decreasing intensity	Constant
Direction of fast component	Toward "stimulated" labyrinth or away from "destroyed" labyrinth	Toward side of CNS lesion
Duration	Minutes to weeks	Weeks to months
Dissociation between eyes	None	Possible
Unidirectional	Present	Seldom present
Multidirectional	Seldom present	Present
Past pointing and falling	Direction of slow phase	Direction of fast phase

*From DeWeese DD, Saunders WH: *Textbook of Otolaryngology,* ed 6. St Louis, CV Mosby Co, 1982. Reproduced by permission.

TEMPOROMANDIBULAR JOINT SYNDROME

TABLE 4–11.—Temporomandibular Joint Syndrome

TMJ syndrome is a condition of dysfunction and pain related to the TMJ and its articulating tissues. It is characterized by:
Unilateral dull aching pain
Gradual onset
Worsened by chewing
Crepitation and clicks in the TMJ
Facial muscle tenderness/spasm
Bruxism
Deviation of jaw
Pain on wide opening and on closure
Women affected 4:1
Treatment approaches
Eliminate muscle tenderness and pain with physical therapy measures (heat, ultrasound, cryotherapy, local anesthesia, topical anesthetic)
Eliminate occlusal problems with orthopedic repositioning device (bite block); may require dental referral
Attempt to eliminate bruxism
Exercises designed to stretch and strengthen oral muscles
Attention to associated tension and stress
Systemic therapy if indicated for pain or arthritis

RHINITIS

TABLE 4–12.—DIFFERENTIAL DIAGNOSIS OF RHINITIS

TYPE	DESCRIPTION	TREATMENT
Seasonal allergic rhinitis	Worse in spring and fall; boggy turbinates; nasal polyps; associated with asthma, eczema, and conjunctivitis	Antihistamines; decongestants; nasal beclomethasone, environmental manipulation; systemic steroids; nasal cromolyn
Chronic hypertrophic rhinitis	Mucosal thickening and excessive secretion from recurrent sinus/nasal infections	Antihistamines; decongestants; antibiotics; consider sinus or nasal surgery
Vasomotor rhinitis	Perennial; may be partly psychogenic; nasal secretions are clear and thin	Systemic decongestants; *avoid* decongestant nasal sprays; frequent reassurance may be necessary
Nasal foreign body	Consider in children or in retarded with rhinitis; unilateral chronic purulent discharge	Removal of foreign body

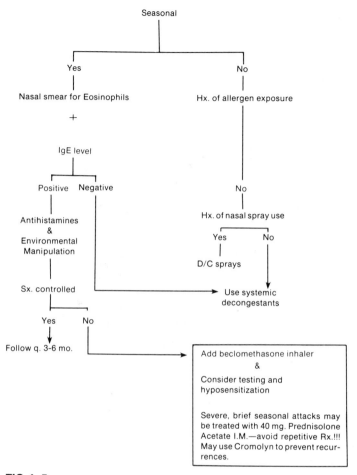

FIG 4–5.
Evaluation and treatment of chronic rhinitis.

EPISTAXIS

The key to successful management is accurate localization of the bleeding site. The most common site is from Kiesselbach's plexus anteriorly. Posterior sites include the posterior ethmoid and septal branch of the spheno-palatine arteries (see Fig 4–6).

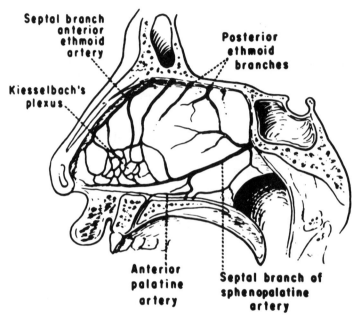

FIG 4–6.
Septal blood supply. (From DeWeese DD, Saunders WH: Nosebleed, in *Textbook of Oto-laryngology,* ed. 6. St Louis, CV Mosby Co, 1982. Reproduced by permission.)

TABLE 4–13.—Technique of Posterior Packing

Insert small rubber catheter through nose, clasp, and pull from nasopharynx through oropharynx with Kelly clamp.

Roll a 4 × 4 and tie two 8-inch and one 3-inch lengths of 3–0 silk suture to the middle of the roll. Apply vaseline to gauze pad.

Attach two of the ties to the catheter.

Pull the catheter and the pad back through the nose, placing the pad, if necessary, with the index finger.

Fix by tying two sutures around another 4 × 4 placed across the nares, as shown.

The third, shorter string hangs from the nasopharynx for removal of the pack in 48 hours.

Anterior pack may then be placed if bleeding continues.

Materials for epistaxis management and nasal packing (see Fig 4–7)
Head mirror
Nasal speculum
Suction equipment
Tongue blades
Cotton balls
Lidocaine with epinephrine (1:1,000)
Bayonet forceps
Silver nitrate sticks
Scissors
Vaseline gauze (½ inch)
Cotton-tipped applicators
Kelly clamp
Posterior packs or Epistat catheter (Xomed, Inc.)
Gauze pads (4 × 4 inches)
Long, 25-gauge needle
5-cc syringe
Cetacaine spray

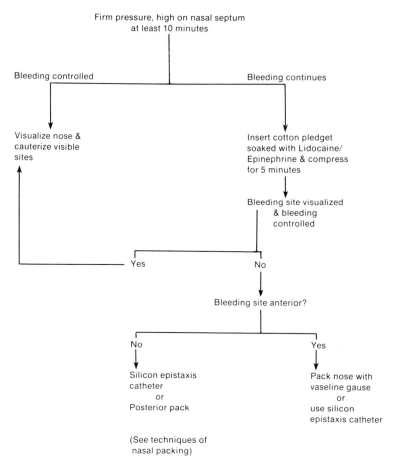

FIG 4–7.
Management of epistaxis.

SINUSITIS

TABLE 4–14.—SINUSITIS

Critical questions to be addressed
  Is it acute or chronic?
  Does it involve the frontal sinus?
  Is it suppurative or allergic?
  Is it related to mechanical obstruction?
Acute suppurative sinusitis
  Usually follows the common cold.
  Pneumococcus and *Hemophilus influenzae* are the most common organisms;
    occasionally *S. aureus,* beta-streptococcus, and anaerobes are causative.
  Leukocytosis and fever are uncommon.
  Maxillary involvement is most common.
  Tenderness over the involved sinus is usual.
  X-rays show cloudiness or air-fluid levels.
Treatment of acute suppurative sinusitis
  Pain medication: aspirin or codeine.
  Moist heat to involved sinuses; cool mist humidifier.
  Local decongestant spray or drops (e.g., Xylometazoline HCl 0.1%, q 3–4 hr.
    Note: limit use to 4 or 5 days).
  Systemic decongestants (e.g., pseudoephedrine HCl 60 mg q.i.d.).
  Antibiotics: amoxicillin or cefaclor 500 mg t.i.d. for 10–14 days.
  If the frontal sinus is involved and drainage does not occur promptly (within 36
    hours of initiating treatment), the risk of spread intracranially demands sur-
    gical drainage.
  Elevate head of bed 20 degrees.
Chronic sinusitis
  Presents as chronic nasal discharge.
  Infection must be differentiated from allergy.
  Treatment usually involves surgery (e.g., Caldwell-Luc procedure).
  If allergy, patient will also have allergic rhinitis.
  May cause chronic headaches.

EMERGENCY AIRWAY

1. Place patient supine with support under shoulders and neck hyperextended.
2. Palpate space between thyroid and cricoid cartilage.
3. Make horizontal incision about 1 inch wide over this space (cricothyroid membrane).
4. Bluntly dissect tissues down to membrane.
5. Make 1-cm incision through CT membrane.
6. Insert flat instrument (e.g., scalpel handle) through incision and rotate 90 degrees to hold incision open.
7. If available, insert small tube through incision.
8. As soon as possible, convert cricothyrotomy to standard tracheostomy.

TONSILLITIS

TABLE 4–15.—INDICATIONS FOR TONSILLECTOMY

ABSOLUTE	RELATIVE	NOT INDICATED OR CONTRAINDICATED
Cor pulmonale secondary to tonsillar airway obstruction	Recurrent tonsillitis documented more than 3 times/year	Colds
		Focal infection
		Fever of unknown origin
	Tonsillar hyperplasia causing some obstruction to swallowing	Cervical adenopathy
Pharyngeal or peritonsillar abscess		Enlarged tonsils (unless there are obstructive symptoms)
Hypertrophy causing dysphagia and weight loss	Residual hyperplasia following mononucleosis	Allergic rhinitis
Suspected malignancy	History of rheumatic fever with heart damage associated with recurrent tonsillitis	Asthma

TABLE 4–16.—Using Clinical Findings to Estimate the Probability of Group A Streptococcal Isolation in Adult Patients*

CLINICAL FINDINGS	PROBABILITY OF + CULTURE (%)	PROBABILITY OF + CULTURE AND ANTIBODY RISE (%)	RECOMMENDED ACTION
Temperature <37.8°C (100°F) *and* no tonsillar exudate *and* no anterior cervical adenitis	3.4	0.4	No culture, no treatment: A false-positive culture could lead to unnecessary and potentially risky treatment.
Temperature >37.8°C (100°F) *or* tonsillar exudate *or* anterior cervical adenitis	13.5	5.6	Culture, and treat patients with positive cultures.
Temperature >37.8°C (100°F) *and* tonsillar exudate *and* anterior cervical adenitis	42.1	16.5	Treat immediately: A false-negative culture could prevent necessary treatment.
SPECIAL "RISK FACTORS"			
Past history of acute rheumatic fever			Treat immediately: Patient is at special risk from strep throat.
Documented strep exposure in past week	*or*		
Known strep epidemic in community	*or*		
Patient is diabetic or otherwise immunocompromised	*or*		
Patient has scarlatiniform rash	*or*		

*From Komaroff AL, Pass TM, Aronson MD, et al: *J Gen Intern Med* 1986; 1:1.

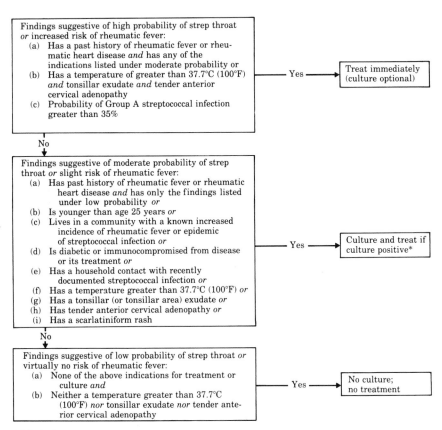

FIG 4–8.

Algorithm describing an evaluation of the probability of Group A streptococcal pharyngitis and the risk of developing acute rheumatic fever. NOTE: Rapid (10-minute) strep test may be substituted for culture. *Immediate treatment is preferred for those individuals whose throat culture results will not be complete for 9 days into the illness (since treatment after that time has not been shown to be protective against rheumatic fever). (From Komaroff AL: Coryza, pharyngitis, and related infections in adults, in Branch WT [ed]: *Office Practice of Medicine*, ed 2. Philadelphia, WB Saunders Co, 1987, p 238. Reproduced by permission.)

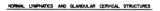

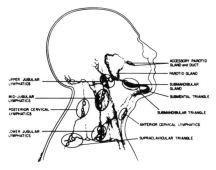

FIG 4–9.
Head and neck lymphatics. (From Fried MP: Evaluation of the adult neck mass. *Med Times* 1982; 110(1):101s, 110s. Reproduced by permission.)

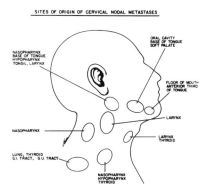

FIG 4–10.
Site of origin of cervical node metastasis. (From Fried MP: Evaluation of the adult neck mass. *Med Times* 1982; 110(1):101s, 110s. Reproduced by permission.)

5 Gynecology
Charles E. Driscoll, M.D.

PEDIATRIC AND ADOLESCENT GYNECOLOGY

TABLE 5–1.—FETAL DEVELOPMENT

Intrauterine sexual development of the fetus is responsible for most early gynecologic disorders in children. Genital structures arise as follows:

Gonad	Derived From	Differentiation
Internal	Genital ridge	6–7 wk
External	Genital tubercle	10–12 wk

The genital system is susceptible to teratogens from 26 to 46 days after conception. Careful exam of the neonate is necessary before the parents are informed of the child's sex. If ambiguity exists, tell parents: "Like a cleft lip, the external sex organ is unfinished. The child will need further laboratory testing to decide what is needed to finish the development." Assign sex only after genetic studies and surgical planning have been completed.

TABLE 5–2.—GYNECOLOGIC EXAM OF NEWBORN AND INFANT

Inspect external genitalia and palpate inguinal areas of abdomen.
Pass soft, neonate feeding catheter through introitus to check patency.
Rectal exam for adnexal mass and palpation of uterus (4 cm length of newborn is larger than at 9 years old 2° estrogen stimulation in utero).
To visualize vagina and cervix, a veterinarian's otoscope speculum may be used (vagina 4 cm at birth).

TABLE 5-3.—GYNECOLOGIC CONDITIONS OF THE INFANT

CONDITION	ETIOLOGY	DIAGNOSIS	TREATMENT	PROGNOSIS
Labial agglutination	Congenital or inflammatory process with adhesions	Visible adhesion of labia, thin livid line; vaginal orifice usually partially patent	Topical estrogen cream b.i.d. for 7–14 days	Normal, may recur
Vaginal bleeding age 3–5 days	Withdrawal of placental estrogens	Normal exam; bleeding stops spontaneously	None; reassurance	Normal
Urethral prolapse	?	Painful, friable mass at vaginal orifice; catheter inserted in center of mass enters bladder	Topically applied estrogen and antibiotic creams; surgical excision if medical therapy fails	Fertile
Adrenal virilization (pseudohermaphroditism)	Inborn error of cortisol metabolism (1/15,000 births)	Labial fusion, clitoral enlargement, uterus palpable; buccal chromatin-positive; elevated urinary 17-ketosteroids and pregnanetriol; check electrolytes	Cortisone; surgical excision of large clitoris, reconstruct vagina; estrogens at puberty	Sterile
Nonadrenal virilization	Maternal progestins taken before 12 wk and to 16 wk	Labial fusion, clitoral enlargement, uterus palpable, buccal chromatin-positive; normal urinary 17-ketosteroids and pregnanetriol, history of progestins to mother	Reassurance, surgical correction of fused labia and clitoral enlargement before age 3; no hormone therapy	Fertile

Continued.

TABLE 5–3.—Continued

Vaginal atresia	Dysplasia or aplasia of müllerian ducts	Absent uterus on palpation, no vaginal orifice, may have associated urinary tract anomaly.	Emergency urinary drainage, surgical vaginal construction	Sterile
Gonadal agenesis	21 different abnormal chromosome complements associated (1/2,500 births)	Edema of hands and feet of newborn; somatic anomalies (low hairline, low-set ears cubitus valgus, growth failure, high palate); abnormal karyotype	Surgical removal of ovarian streaks if Y chromosome present to prevent malignancy; estrogens to develop secondary sex characteristics	Sterile
Testicular feminization	Congenital insensitivity to androgens, familial tendency	Girl with inguinal "hernias," blind vaginal pouch, absent uterus; buccal chromatin-negative; 46 XY; primary amenorrhea	Surgical removal of testes, hormone therapy with estrogens, female sex assigned	Sterile
True hermaphroditism	Ovotestis develops often in absence of Y chromosome (rare)	Hypospadic, small phallus; small vagina; gonads may be palpable in labial or scrotal folds; buccal chromatin-positive	Gonads excised to prevent dysgerminoma, surgical sex assignment carried out, hormones for secondary sex characteristics	Sterile

TABLE 5–4.—PEDIATRIC VULVOVAGINITIS

Perhaps the most common gynecologic problem in childhood (85%–90%) is vulvovaginitis. Treatment without exam is dangerous as symptoms are similar to those of urinary tract infections (itching, burning, dysuria, discharge). Trichomonas, gonorrhea, and *Chlamydia* may imply sexual abuse.

General Rules:
Do exam, cultures, vaginal smears, and urinalysis.
Vaginal pH should be 7.0–8.0 in children and 5–5.5 in adolescents.
Foreign bodies cause about 5% of cases.
Teach perineal hygiene, wiping front to back.
About 20% of cases will resolve with sitz baths and good hygiene.
When pus or *Trichomonas* is present, think of gonorrhea and *Chlamydia*.
If a bloody vaginal discharge is present *without* a foreign body, think of β-streptococcal infection (indications may include recent respiratory or skin infection).
Topical estrogen cream for 5–6 days speeds resolution.
Look for pinworms.

TABLE 5–5.—TREATMENT FOR SPECIFIC CAUSES OF PEDIATRIC VAGINITIS

Candida	Miconazole nitrate vaginal cream* nightly for 7–14 nights
Gardnerella vaginalis or *Trichomonas*	Metronidazole, 35–50 mg/kg/day, in 3 doses, for 7 days
Gonorrhea	If less than 45 kg, ceftriaxone 125 mg IM 1 ×. Children ≥ 8 years of age should also receive doxycycline, 100 mg PO b.i.d. × 7 days. Children ≥ 45 kg: use adult regimen.
Pinworms	One mebendazole 100-mg tablet PO
β-*Streptococcus*	Penicillin G, 200,000 units orally q.i.d. for 10 days

*When vaginal infections of children require placement of intravaginal medication (miconazole, estrogen, etc.), use a 10-cc syringe with butterfly IV tubing (needle removed) attached.

TABLE 5–6.—CHICKENPOX VULVITIS

Pain and itching: Cold compresses, Burow's solution soaks, baking soda or oatmeal baths. Hydroxyzine HCl 15 mg PO t.i.d. may be given.
Urinary retention: Sit in tub of warm water to urinate or apply small amounts of Xylocaine jelly topically.
Infection: Topical Betadine solution diluted 1:4 with water.

Tanner

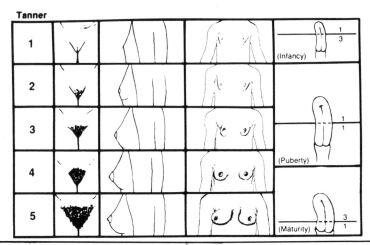

	Pubic Hair	Breast
	1 Infantile pattern. No true pubic hair present, although there may be a fine downy hair distribution.	1 Infantile or childhood pattern.
	2 Sparse growth of lightly pigmented hair, longer than the fine down of the previous stage, appearing on the mons or the labia.	2 Early pubertal breast development, sometimes referred to as a "breast bud." A small mound of breast tissue causes a visible elevation.
	3 The pubic hair becomes darker, coarser, and curlier. Distribution is still minimal.	3 The areola and the breast undergo more definite pronouncement in size, with a continuous rounded contour.
	4 The pubic hair is adult in character, but not yet as widely distributed as in most adults.	4 The areola and nipple enlarge further and form a secondary mound projecting above the contour of the remainder of the breast.
	5 The pubic hair is distributed in the typical adult female pattern, forming an inverse triangle.	5 The adult breast stage. The secondary mound visible in the preceding stage has now blended into a smooth contour of the breast.

FIG 5–1.
Sexual maturation of girl may be assessed using the normal appearance of the external genitalia as described by Tanner and the usual expected sequence and tempo (see Fig 5–2).

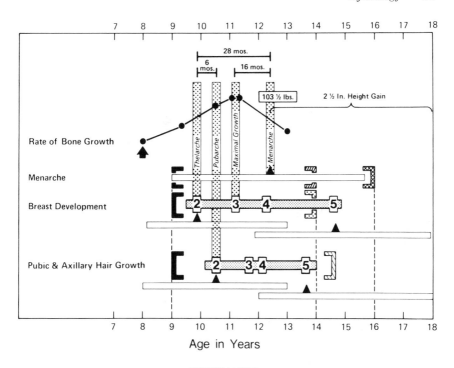

Age in Years

ABNORMAL LIMITS

⌐ Menstruation, breast development or axillary
⌐ or pubic hair growth before age 9.

⌐┐ No breast development by age 14.

⌐╗ No menstruation by age 14 in the absence of growth
╗⌐ or development of secondary sexual characteristics.

⌐┐ No axillary and/or pubic hair growth after breast
⌐┘ development has attained Tanner Stage V.

╗⌐ No menstruation by age 16 regardless of the presence of
╗⌐ normal growth and development with the appearance of
╗⌐ secondary sexual characteristics.

▲ Mean
◻ Mean ± 2 S.D.

▲ Onset of growth spurt

FIG 5–2.

Expected sequence and tempo of sexual development. Numbers in boxes represent Tanner's stages. (From Robie GF Jr: Pediatric gynecology, in Duenholter JH [ed]: *Greenhill's Office Gynecology*, ed 10. Chicago, Year Book Medical Publishers, 1983. Reproduced by permission.)

Infertility - Unable to conceive after 1 year of unprotected intercourse. Of 100 couples attempting conception, 90 will be successful in the first year, 10 will not. Of these 10 subfertile couples, 5 will be successful in the second year and 5 will not. Male factors account for 40% of infertility.

Evaluating the Infertile Couple

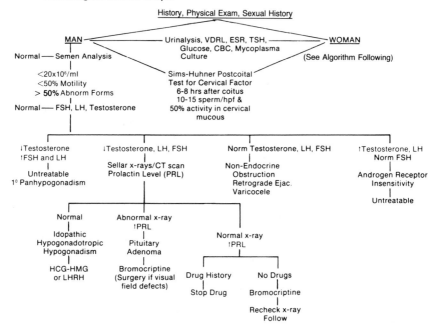

FIG 5–3.
Infertility: evaluating the man.

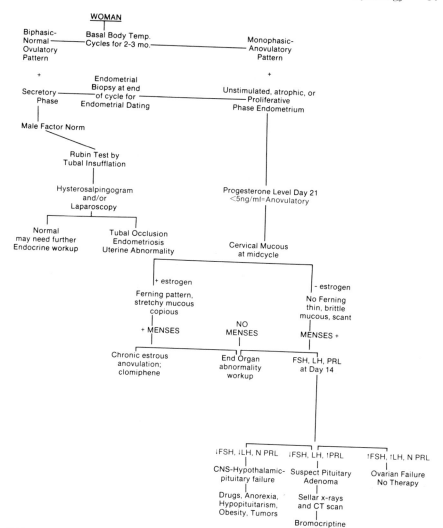

FIG 5–3 (cont.).
Infertility: evaluating the woman.

TABLE 5-7.—Acute Adolescent Menorrhagia*

Bleeding moderate, hemoglobin > 10 gm/dl	Observation and follow-up Oral iron supplements Rule out chronic illness, coagulation disorder, pregnancy, and clear cell adenocarcinoma
Bleeding severe, hemoglobin ≤ 10 gm/dl	Admit to hospital 1. Initial hemostasis Conjugated estrogens, 40 mg IV q4h (maximum 6 doses) Progestin (norethindrone acetate), 5 mg q6h orally If still bleeding heavily after 24 hr, examine under anesthesia and perform D & C. 2. Cyclic regulation of menses Concurrent oral administration of estrogen-progestin (norethynodrel/mestranol 5 mg), 2 tablets stat and 1 q6h, tapered over next month to usual dose of 1 tablet daily Follow with 3 months of cyclic therapy with conventional low-dose combination oral contraceptive (35–50 μg of estrogen) 3. Long-term observation 5% of patients will never ovulate.

*Adapted from Altchek A: *Med Aspects Hum Sexuality* 1988; 22:82.

TABLE 5-8.—Signs of Sexual Abuse in the Prepubertal Girl*

FINDINGS IN ACUTE SEXUAL ABUSE	FINDINGS IN CHRONIC SEXUAL ABUSE
Perineal contusions	Multiple healed hymenal transections
Perihymenal erythema, swelling, petechiae	Rounded hymenal remnants, synechiae
	Spacious introitus ≥ 4 mm (≥ age 5 years)
Abrasions, avulsions, lacerations	Fourchette-hymenal lacerations, scarring, neovascularization
Spasm of pubococcygeus muscle	Capacity to relax pubococcygeus muscle
	Leukorrhea, vaginitis, cervicitis
Seminal products	Anal fissures, scarring, skin tags, pigmentation
Tense rectal sphincter	
Anal fissures	Reflex relaxation of the anal sphincter
Rectal-perianal contusions or ecchymoses	Laxity of vaginal-pubococcygeal muscles
Perianal edema	

*From Abrams ME, Shah RZ, Keenan-Allyn S: *Female Patient* 1988; 13:17–33. Reproduced by permission.

TABLE 5-9.—RELATIVE EFFECTIVENESS OF VARIOUS METHODS OF CONTRACEPTION*

METHOD	USE EFFECTIVENESS[†]
Hysterectomy	0.0001
Abortion	0.01
Vasectomy	0.02
Tubal ligation	0.13
Oral contraceptives[‡]	0.25
Progestin alone	1.2
Intrauterine device	1.4
Foam and condom	1.5
Diaphragm and jelly	1.9
Cervical cap	3–5
Condom	3.6
Foam or jelly alone	11.9
Symptothermal method	22
Coitus interruptus	15–23
Calendar rhythm method	25–40
Chance	80

*Adapted from Romney SL, Gray MJ, Little AB, et al: *Gynecology and Obstetrics: The Health Care of Women,* ed 2. New York, McGraw-Hill Book Co, 1981, p 820, and Mishell DR: *N Engl J Med* 1989; 320:777
[†]Expressed as pregnancy rate per 100 woman-years.
[‡]Medications may interfere with oral contraceptive effectiveness. Patients taking anticonvulsants, antibiotics, and tranquillizers should consider using additional contraceptive protection (e.g., condoms or spermicide).

TABLE 5-10.—CONTRAINDICATIONS TO ORAL CONTRACEPTIVE USE

Absolute contraindications
    Pregnancy
    Breast cancer
    Undiagnosed vaginal bleeding
    Estrogen-dependent neoplasia
    History of or active thromboembolic disorder
    History of or active cardiovascular or cerebrovascular disease
    Acute or chronic liver disease
Relative contraindications
    Hypertension
    Hyperlipidemia
    Diabetes mellitus
    Lactation
    Epilepsy
    Pituitary dysfunction
    Smoking > 15 cigarettes/day
    Age > 35 yr
    Sickle cell disease
    Migraine headaches
    Raynaud's disease

Continued.

TABLE 5–10.—Continued

Collagen vascular disease
Porphyria
Bleeding diatheses
Retinal disease
Active inflammatory bowel disease
Dermatologic disorders (erythema nodosum, melasma, etc.)
Cholelithiasis

TABLE 5–11.—LABORATORY TESTS AFFECTED BY ORAL CONTRACEPTIVES*

A. Values which are increased (serum values, unless otherwise stated)
  1. Erythrocyte sedimentation rate (sometimes the hematocrit, white blood count, and platelets)
  2. Serum iron and iron-binding capacity
  3. Sulfobromophthalein and sometimes bilirubin
  4. Serum glutamic oxaloacetic transaminase, serum glutamic pyruvic transaminase, and serum γ-glutamyl transpeptidase
  5. Alkaline phosphatase
  6. Clotting factors I, II, VII, VIII, IX, X and XII; also: increased antiplasmins and antiactivators of fibrinolysis
  7. Triglycerides, phospholipids, and high-density lipoproteins (sometimes serum cholesterol)
  8. Serum copper and ceruloplasmin
  9. Increase in various binding proteins (transferrin, transcortin, thyroxine-binding globulin)
  10. Renin, angiotensin, angiotensinogin, and aldosterone
  11. Insulin, growth hormone, and blood glucose
  12. C-reactive protein
  13. Globulins (α_1 and α_2)
  14. α_1-antitrypsin
  15. Total estrogens (urine)
  16. Coproporphyrin (feces and urine) and porphobilinogen (urine)
  17. Vitamin A
  18. Xanthuric acid (urine)
  19. Positive antinuclear antibody test and LE preparation
  20. Total T-4
B. Values which are decreased
  1. Antithrombin II
  2. LH and FSH
  3. Pregnanediol and 17-ketosteroids
  4. Folate and vitamin B_{12}
  5. Glucose tolerance
  6. Ascorbic acid
  7. Zinc and magnesium
  8. T-3 resin uptake
  9. Fibrinolytic activity
  10. Haptoglobulin
  11. Cholinesterase
  12. T-3 resin uptake

*From Greydanus DE: Semin Perinatol 1981; 5:53–90. Reproduced by permission.

TABLE 5–12.—RELATION OF SIDE EFFECTS TO HORMONE CONTENT

ESTROGEN EXCESS	PROGESTIN EXCESS	
	Progestational	*Androgenic*

General Symptoms
Chloasma
Chronic nasal pharyngitis
Gastric influenza and varicella
Hay fever and allergic rhinitis
Urinary tract infections
Premenstrual Syndrome
Bloating
Dizziness—syncope
Edema
Headaches (cyclic)
Irritability
Leg cramps
Nausea and vomiting
Visual changes (cyclic)
Weight gain (cyclic)
 	
Reproductive System
Breast cystic changes
Cervical extrophy
Dysmenorrhea, menstrual cramps
Hypermenorrhea, menorrhagia,
  heavy flow and clots
Increase in breast size
Mucorrhea
Uterine enlargment
Uterine fibroid growth
Cardiovascular System
Capillary fragility
Cerebrovascular accident
Deep vein thrombosis hemiparesis
  (unilateral weakness and
  numbness)
Telangiectasias
Thromboembolic disease
Vascular headaches (migraine)
	General Symptoms
	Appetite increased
	Depression
	Fatigability
	Hypoglycemia symptoms
	Libido decreased
	Neurodermatitis
	Tiredness
	Weight gain (noncyclic)
	Cardiovascular System
	Hypertension
	Leg veins dilated
	Hyperlipidemia
	Reproductive System
	Cervicitis
	Flow length decreased
	Moniliasis
		**Androgenic
		Symptoms**
		Acne
		Cholestatic jaundice
		Hirsutism
		Libido increased
		Oily skin and scalp
		Rash and pruritus

ESTROGEN DEFICIENCY	PROGESTIN DEFICIENCY	

Bleeding and spotting continuous
Bleeding and spotting early (pill day 1 to 9)
Flow decreased, hypomenorrhea
Nervousness
Pelvic relaxation symptoms
Vaginitis atrophic
Vasomotor symptoms
Withdrawal bleeding none
	Breakthrough bleeding and spotting late (pill day 10
	  to 21)
	Dysmenorrhea (also estrogen excess)
	Heavy flow and clots (also estrogen excess),
	  hypermenorrhea, menorrhagia
	Withdrawal bleeding delayed	

*From Dickey R: *Managing Contraceptive Pill Patients*, ed 4. Durant, Oklahoma, Creative Infomatics, 1984, pp 104–105. Reproduced by permission.

MENSTRUATION AND ABNORMAL UTERINE BLEEDING

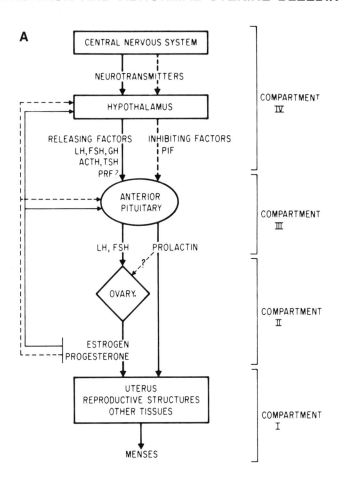

FIG 5–4.
A, coordinated interactions among the CNS, hypothalamus, pituitary, and ovaries required for normal menstruation. **B,** office workup for amenorrhea. Compartments I–IV are defined in **A.** (From Pelosi MA: *J Med Soc NJ* 1981; 78:195–200. Reproduced by permission.)

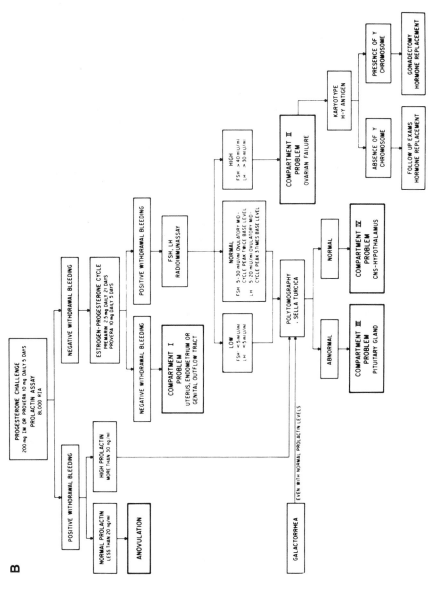

FIG 5–4 (cont.).

TABLE 5–13.—PREMENSTRUAL SYNDROME

Symptoms (occur cyclically beginning 7–14 days before menses)
Anxiety, depression, emotional lability, weight gain, edema, abdominal bloat-
ing, breast tenderness, headache, food craving, painful cramping
Therapy
Aerobic exercise; reduce salt, sugar, and caffeine intake; pyridoxine (B_6), 100–
300 mg/day; spironolactone, 25 mg t.i.d.; oral contraceptives; prostaglandin
synthetase inhibitors (ibuprofen 600 mg PO q.i.d.); progesterone, 200 mg,
vaginal or rectal suppositories; supportive counseling; family education

TABLE 5–14.—CAUSES OF ABNORMAL UTERINE BLEEDING

DISORDER	DIAGNOSTIC STRATEGY
Pregnancy disorders	Serum or urine HCG, U.S.
Thyroid disorder	Thyroid function tests
Synthetic sex steroids	Hx of estrogen/progestin use
Intrauterine device	Look for string, x-ray, infection
Carcinoma of cervix or endometrium	Inspection, PAP, Hx of D.E.S., endometrial aspiration, D&C
Coagulation disorder	Platelets, PT, PTT, bleeding time
Dysfunctional uterine bleeding	
polycystic ovary syndrome	Hirsutism, acne, testosterone and androstenedione
Liver disease and obesity	Excessive estrone production
Ovarian neoplasm	Androgen excess
Theca cell tumor of ovary	↑ Estradiol-17β
Transient disruption of hypothalamic-pituitary-ovarian axis	Environmental stresses
Organic lesions of uterus	Polyps, leiomyomas
Endometritis	Plasma cell infiltrates in endometrial tissue and GC culture positive
Atrophic vaginitis	Inspect vagina, estrogen index of vaginal smear

TABLE 5–15.—COMMON CAUSES OF HYPERPROLACTINEMIA*

Drugs
  Amoxapine, phenothiazines, butyrophenones, thioxanthenes, methyldopa, reserpine, metoclopramide
Hypothyroidism
Prolactinoma
Neural stimulation
  Chest wall and intrathoracic disease (e.g., herpes zoster, chest wall burns, thoracoplasty)
  Nipple stimulation
Hypothalamic disease
  Craniopharyngioma
  Hypothalamic and/or pineal tumors
  Pseudotumor cerebri
  Inflammation (e.g., sarcoidosis, encephalitis)

*From Veldhuis JD: *Hosp Pract* Nov 30, 1988, pp 40–56. Reproduced by permission.

GYNECOLOGIC INFECTIONS

TABLE 5–16.—CASE DEFINITION OF TOXIC SHOCK SYNDROME*

Major symptoms and signs
  Fever: Temperature ≥ 38.9° C (102° F).
  Rash: Diffuse macular erythroderma. Desquamation usually occurs 1–2 wk after onset of illness, most prominently on the palms and soles.
  Hypotension: Systolic blood pressure ≤ 90 mm Hg for adults or below 5th percentile by age for children less than 16 years of age, or orthostatic syncope.
Multisystem involvement—3 or more of the following:
  Gastrointestinal: Vomiting or diarrhea at onset of illness.
  Muscular: Severe myalgia or creatine phosphokinase (CPK) level ≥ 2 × ULN.†
  Mucus membrane: Vaginal, oropharyngeal, or conjunctival hyperemia.
  Hepatic: Total bilirubin, SGOT, or SGPT ≥ 2 × ULN.
  Renal: BUN or creatinine ≥ 2 × ULN or pyuria (≥ 5 white blood cells per high power field) in the absence of a urinary tract infection.
  Hematologic: Platelets ≤ 100,000/mm³.
  CNS: Disorientation or alterations in consciousness without focal neurologic signs when fever and hypotension are absent.
Reasonable evidence for absence of other etiologies:
  Negative results on the following tests, if performed:
  blood, throat (group A, β-hemolytic streptococci), or cerebrospinal fluid cultures. Rises in serologic titers to Rocky Mountain spotted fever, leptospirosis, or measles.

*From Dan BB, Shands KN: *Pediatr Ann* 1981; 10:29–34. Reproduced by permission.
†Two times upper limit of normal for laboratory.

TABLE 5–17.—MANAGEMENT OF TOXIC SHOCK SYNDROME

Primary treatment
Remove inciting focus, obtain culture and sensitivity
Fluid resuscitation
    Crystaloids and colloids to support blood pressure (may take $\geq$ 10 L/24 hr)
    Swan-Ganz catheterization indicated
Ancillary treatment
Corticosteroids controversial, probably useful
Discontinue future tampon use
β-Lactamase-resistant antistaphylococcal antibiotics (lowers recurrence rate with subsequent menses from 40% to 10%)

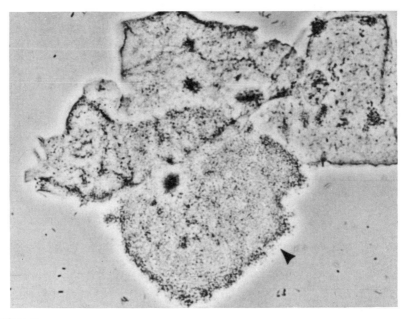

FIG 5–5.
Clue cell *(arrowhead)*. Vaginal epithelial cell with organisms stippling the surface and border. (From Eschenbach D: Vaginal discharge, in Duenhoelter JH [ed]: *Greenhill's Office Gynecology,* ed 10. Chicago, Year Book Medical Publishers, 1983, p 91. Reproduced by permission.)

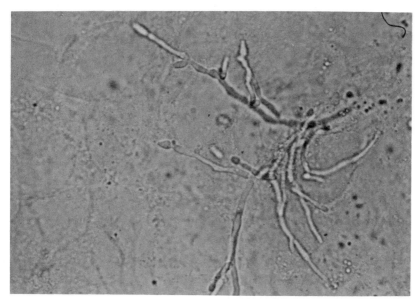

FIG 5–6.
Candida. Branching mycelia and spores are seen with 10% KOH smear. (From Eschenbach D: Vaginal discharge, in Duenhoelter JH [ed]: *Greenhill's Office Gynecology,* ed 10. Chicago, Year Book Medical Publishers, 1983, p 92. Reproduced by permission.)

TABLE 5–18.—GYNECOLOGIC INFECTIONS*

TYPE	SYMPTOMS	CLINICAL FEATURES
Trichomonas vaginalis	Itching, swollen vagina; odor; discharge	Petechiae; "strawberry vagina"; malodorous, frothy yellow-green discharge
Candida albicans	Discharge; itching; dyspareunia	Red, edematous vulva and vagina; scant to thick creamy discharge adherent to vagina
Gardnerella vaginalis	Mild pruritis or burning; odor	Grayish, homogeneous thin discharge gives "fishy" amine odor when mixed with a drop of 10% KOH
Chlamydia trachomatis	Discharge, spotting after coitus	Cervicitis; acute PID; mucopurulent discharge
Neisseria gonorrhea	Discharge, abdominal pain, urethritis	Profuse yellow discharge; cervicitis; PID
Herpes genitalis	Painful ulcers, dysuria, pelvic pain	Shallow ulcers; clear or serous discharge without odor
Syphilis—*T. pallidum*	Painless sores, swollen glands	Chancre with lymphadenopathy
Condyloma acuminatum—HPV	Warts, mild irritation	Vulvar/perineal and anal location
Atrophic vaginitis	Vaginal bleeding, pruritus, dyspareunia	Postmenopausal; thin epithelium; scant serous discharge

*Normal vaginal pH, 3.8–4.2.

LABORATORY	TREATMENT	COMMENTS
Motile trichomonads on saline prep; pH 5.5–5.8	Metronidazole, 2-gm single dose or 250 mg PO t.i.d. × 7d	Sexually transmitted in postmenstrual phase; avoid alcohol intake while taking metronidazole; also treat male sexual partner.
10% KOH prep reveals spores and hyphae and pH 4.0–4.5 (see Fig 5–7)	Butoconazole, Clotrimazole or Miconazole vaginal cream nightly for 7d (terconazole may cause less irritation)	Nickerson's media culture may be confirmatory; exacerbated by pregnancy and diabetes.
Dark, stippled epithelial cells (clue cells) on saline prep (see Fig 5–6); pH 5.0–5.5	Metronidazole, 500 mg b.i.d. × 7d (or clindamycin 300 mg PO b.i.d. × 7d)	Probably sexually transmitted, also treat male sexual partner.
Many WBCs, no organisms on saline prep; pH of mucus 7+	Tetracycline or erythromycin, 500 mg PO q.i.d. × 14d	Associated with gonorrhea in 30%–60% of cases; may cause LGV.
Intracellular gram-negative diplococci; Thayer Martin	Ceftriaxone 250 mg IM 1 × plus doxycycline 100 mg PO b.i.d. × 7d	Usually effective for incubating syphilis, repeat VDRL in 6 weeks; C. trachomatis, M. hominis, U. urealyticum may coexist.
Pos. Tzank smear; multinucleated giant cells	Acyclovir 200 mg PO 5×/d for 7–10d and tub soaks	Primary infection most symptomatic.
Pos. VDRL; FTABS	Benzothine penicillin G, 2.4 million units IM	21-day incubation period tetracycline 500 mg PO q.i.d. for 15d in penicillin allergy.
Acetowhite change with 4% acetic acid	10% podophyllin on for 6–8 hours, then wash off, or trichloroacetic acid	Sexually transmitted virus, long-term follow-up for types 6/11 and 16/18.
No abnormal organisms; pH 6.7–7.0	Topical estrogen cream once daily × 14d, then q.o.d. × 14d	Usually only 4 weeks of therapy needed.

TABLE 5-19.—HIV Infection in Women*

Women with HIV/AIDS account for 20% of cases; majority are black or Hispanic. Transmission is by IV drug use (51%), heterosexual contact (29%), blood transfusion (11%), unknown (9%).
Maternal-fetal transmission rate during pregnancy is 65%.
Opportunistic infections seen in women
   Pneumocystis carinii, cryptococcal meningitis, toxoplasmosis, nonpulmonary tuberculosis, atypical tuberculosis *(Mycobacterium avium-intracellulare),* esophageal candidiasis, enteric pathogens, herpes viral infections.
AIDS symptoms
   Diarrheal syndromes, weight loss, anorexia, dementia, amenorrhea and dysfunctional uterine bleeding (30%).
High-risk women who should be screened
   Women receiving blood transfusion before 1985; prostitutes; IV drug users; sexual partner is HIV+ or high risk.
Patient counseling
   Sexual monogamy with seronegative partner, limit number of partners. Use condoms during *all* sexual contacts, use nonoxynol-9 spermicide.
   Oral-genital sex and anal intercourse increase risk.
   There are no physical or behavioral characteristics of HIV+ persons.
   Never share needles.
Telephone numbers for information
   AIDS Hotline   1-800-342-AIDS
   Retrovir (AZT) Hotline   1-800-843-9388
   CDC
      Printed info.   1-404-329-3534
      Recorded info.   1-404-329-1290

*Adapted from Holmes VF, Fernandez F: *Female Patient* 1988; 13:47–54, and Kapila R, Kloser P: *Med Aspects Hum Sexuality* July 1988, pp 92–94.

SEXUAL DYSFUNCTION

TABLE 5-20.—Assessment for Sexual Dysfunction

Routine sexual history taking should include:
   "How satisfactory is your sexual functioning?"
   "At sometime in their lives most people experience a sexual problem. What type of sexual problems have you experienced?"
   "Many people have unanswered questions or need information about sexual functioning. What questions do you have?"
A modified sexological exam includes:
   Sensitivity of vulva to touch.
   Clitoris is free from adhesions to prepuce.
   Bulbocavernosus contractions are normal.
   Urethra and vagina have normal sensitivity.
   Absence of infection, masses, mucosal lesions.
   Valsalva negative for pelvic relaxation.
   Uterus palpation is normal.
   Breast and nipple exam normal.

TABLE 5–21.—PHASE-SPECIFIC SEXUAL DISORDERS

PHASE OF SEXUAL CYCLE	COMMENT/MANAGEMENT
Desire	Most common clinical problem
	Primary (upbringing) vs. secondary (depression, disappointment, pain, fear, anger, drugs)
	Unless secondary treatable form, refer for sex therapy
Excitement/plateau	Sexual anesthesia from drugs or disease
	General dysfunction with lack of lubrication
	Lack pleasure in sexual experiences
	Try ban on intercourse and sensate focus therapy
	Referral
Orgasm	Primary, secondary, or situational
	Directed masturbation exercises, guided caress, fantasy
	Assume responsibility for own orgasm
	Deal with negative body image and provide education
	Increase awareness of foreplay and clitoral stimulation
Resolution	Delay causes pelvic congestion; more common during pregnancy
	Enhance stimulation to shorten excitement/plateau phases by teaching Kegel's pubococcygeus muscle exercises (see Table 5–34)
Vaginismus	Not easily classified, involuntary vaginal muscle spasms
	Primary (upbringing) vs. secondary (after rape, trauma, vaginitis)
	"No sex life" most common complaint
	Increase stimulation to increase lubrication
	Kegel exercises and progressive vaginal dilators
	Have sexual activity to orgasm other than intercourse

TABLE 5–22.—MANAGEMENT OF THE RAPE VICTIM*

Introduce self and assure patient of safety; never leave patient alone
Empathetic listening about her ordeal; encourage reporting of crime
Give patient total control; involve her in decision-making
    Patient determines rate of questioning and exam
    Inform patient of each procedure and obtain permission
    Patient decides when to contact family
Perform methodical history, physical exam, and collection of well-documented
    evidence according to written protocol
    History of assault, violence, use of weapon, number of attackers
    Type of assault (vaginal, oral, anal, instrument, other)
    Penetration, ejaculation
    Bathed, douched, defecated, brushed teeth, or used mouthwash?
    OB/gyn and general medical history, LMP, contraception
Place collected evidence in sealed, documentation envelopes
    Wood's light exam of pelvic area—semen has bright bluish-white fluorescence
    Vaginal pool aspirate (acid phosphatase, ABH group antigens, motile sperma-
        tozoa, wet mount, dry smear slide, DNA typing)
    Urine for pregnancy test
    Rectal, oral specimens if indicated
    Vulva (pubic hair combing for foreign material, patient's pubic hair clipped for
        sample)
    Fingernail scrapings
    Clothing she wore at the time of attack
    Blood typing, VDRL, serum or urine HCG, HIV, HBSAg
    Cultures for *N. gonorrhoeae, C. trachomatis*
    Pap smear with water-moistened speculum, bimanual exam
Exam of vulva may be done with colposcope, toluidine blue staining
A vaginal washing may be done by irrigating the vaginal vault (avoid the cervix)
    with 10 ml of NaCl. Aspirate the fluid and place in a test tube, which is then
    sealed and labeled. Aspirate can be examined for motile sperm, acid phospha-
    tase, blood group antigens, and sperm precipitins.
Nongynecologic exam for bruises, abrasions, contusions, penetrating injuries,
    fractures (photography of wounds)
Discuss the usual psychological sequelae of rape; alleviate guilt and self-re-
    proach
Provide patient advocate skilled in rape crisis intervention
Arrange for supportive follow-up care of patient's choice
If patient chooses, VD prophylaxis (probenecid, 1 gm, with ampicillin, 3.5 gm
    orally) and pregnancy prophylaxis (DES, 25 mg PO b.i.d. × 5d)
Tetanus toxoid if indicated

*Useful reference: Hicks DJ: The patient who's been raped. *Emerg Med* 1988;
20:106–122.

PAP SMEARS AND COLPOSCOPY

Conduct Pap testing on two specimens, one from the ectocervix obtained by spatula scraping and the second from the endocervix by means of a cytobrush. Cytobrush usage yields endocervical cells in nearly 100% of samples. Smear both specimens together on the same slide and fix immediately. If no endocervical cells are present, the smear is inadequate and must be repeated. If atypical endometrial cells are reported, endometrial aspiration or D&C is needed.

TABLE 5–23.—CLASSIFICATION AND MANAGEMENT OF CERVICAL PAP SMEARS*

CLASS	FINDINGS	COURSE OF ACTION
I	Normal smear; no abnormal cells	Repeat smear in 1 year.
II	Atypical cells present, inflammatory	Treat infection and cervical trauma Repeat smear in 3–6 months. If repeat is Class II, do colposcopy.
III	Smear contains abnormal cells consistent with dysplasia Mild dysplasia = CIN1 Moderate dysplasia = CIN2	Colposcopy, endocervical curettage, directed biopsies, HPV/DNA Pap. Microinvasion or CIN = excisional cone biopsy of cervix, cryotherapy, laser, or hysterectomy Invasion = radical surgery or radiation
IV	Smear contains abnormal cells consistent with carcinoma in situ Severe dysplasia = CIN3 CIS	As above in Class III.
V	Smear contains abnormal cells consistent with squamous cell carcinoma	Metastatic survey, radical surgery or radiation.

*Adapted from Nelson JH, Averette HE, Richart RM: *CA* 1989; 39:157–178.

TABLE 5–24.—Colposcopy: Technique and Findings

Nonresolving Class II and all higher PAP smears require colposcopy to confirm the abnormal cytology. There are no contraindications to the procedure.
Materials needed
  Colposcope, 3%–5% acetic acid, Kervokian-Younge biopsy forceps, vaginal speculum, endocervical curette, endocervical speculum, ferric subsulfate solution, cotton-tipped swabs (large and small), specimen jars with 10% formalin.
Procedure
  1. Explain procedure to patient.
  2. Patient in lithomy position, vaginal speculum in place.
  3. Green filter exam to enhance vascular pattern identification.
  4. White light exam of vulva, vagina and cervix.
  5. Visualize entire squamocolumnar junction under magnification.
  6. Enhance visualization of abnormalities with 3%–5% acetic acid (clears away mucus and causes transient vasoconstriction). Schiller's or Lugal's solution may be used as alternatives (see Table 5–25 for findings).
  7. Perform endocervical curettage and submit as separate specimen.
  8. Biopsy abnormal patterns (anesthesia seldom needed), achieve hemostasis with ferric subsulfate.
  9. No special aftercare.

TABLE 5–25.—Localization of cervical Abnormalities*

Schiller's iodine test is a simple method of detecting abnormal cervical cells by revealing the absence of glycogen. Schiller's (0.3%) or Lugol's (5%) iodine solution is painted onto the cervix. (Toluidine blue 1% aqueous solution is also effective.) Scars, eversion, endocervical glandular epithelium, erosions, reepithelialization, nonmalignant leukoplakia, and CIN appear pale. Acetic acid 3% to 5% cause dysplastic and neoplastic areas to briefly appear white in the acetowhite reaction. Green-filtered light enhances the vascular pattern identification.

Iodine-stained appearance	INTERPRETATION	ACTION
Mahogany brown, all surfaces	Normal	None
Iodine pale (glycogen-neg.)		
From os to squamocolumnar junction	Erosion	Limit trauma, treat infection, follow
Flame-shaped areas contiguous with but outside squamocolumnar junction	Dysplasia	Punch biopsy
Very pale (white) within or contiguous with iodine-pale areas	Leukoplakia	Punch biopsy
Punctate areas	*Trichomonas*	Treat infection

Acetic acid appearance
Well-demarcated areas of:

Epithelium that appears white "chicken wire" pattern	White dysplasia with mosaic pattern, CIN 1–3	Biopsy
Arboreal, fungating, exophytic white lesion	Hyperkeratinized cervical condylomata	Biopsy, cryotherapy, laser or TCA

Green-filtered light

Abnormal vessels with nonarboreal branching, "commas," "squiggles"	Atypical blood vessels, possible invasive carcinoma	Biopsy
Segments of avascular pathologic epithelium outlined by capillaries	Mosaic mucosal pattern, CIN 1–3	Biopsy
Dilated, elongated hairpin capillaries, often irregular and slightly twisted. Punctation (fine red stippling)	Punctate lesions, CIN 1–3	Biopsy

*Useful reference: Felmar E, Payton CE, Gobbo R, et al: Colposcopy: A necessary adjunct to Pap smears. *Fam Pract Recertification* 1988; 10(11):21–32.

TUMORS AND MALIGNANT DISEASE

TABLE 5–26.—CLINICAL FINDINGS SUGGESTIVE OF
BENIGN OR MALIGNANT ADNEXAL MASSES*

BENIGN	MALIGNANT
Unilateral	Bilateral
Cystic	Solid
Mobile	Fixed
Smooth	Irregular
No ascites	Ascites
Slow growth	Rapid growth
Young patient	Older patient

*From Hall DJ, Hurt WG: *J Fam Pract* 1982; 14:135–140.
Reproduced by permission.

TABLE 5–27.—STAGING CLASSIFICATION FOR CARCINOMA OF THE CERVIX
AS ADOPTED BY THE INTERNATIONAL FEDERATION OF GYNECOLOGY
AND OBSTETRICS (FIGO)

	Preinvasive carcinoma
Stage 0	Carcinoma in situ, intraepithelial carcinoma. Stage 0 cases should not be included in any therapeutic statistics for invasive carcinoma.
	Invasive carcinoma
Stage I	Carcinoma strictly confined to the cervix (extension to the corpus should be disregarded).
Ia	Microinvasive carcinoma (early stromal invasion).
Ib	All other cases of stage I. Occult cancer should be marked "occ."
Stage II	The carcinoma extends beyond the cervix but has not extended onto the pelvic wall. The carcinoma involves the vagina, but not the lower third.
IIa	No obvious parametrial involvement.
IIb	Obvious parametrial involvement.
Stage III	The carcinoma has extended onto the pelvic wall. On rectal examination there is no cancer-free space between the tumor and the pelvic wall. The tumor involves the lower third of the vagina. All cases with a hydronephrosis or nonfunctioning kidney should be included, unless they are known to be due to other cause.
IIIa	No extension onto the pelvic wall.
IIIb	Extension onto the pelvic wall and/or hydronephrosis or nonfunctioning kidney.
Stage IV	The carcinoma has extended beyond the true pelvis or has clinically involved the mucosa of the bladder or rectum. A bullous edema as such does not permit assignation of stage IV.
IVa	Spread of the growth to adjacent organs.
IVb	Spread to distant organs.

Risk factors for cervical carcinoma include HPV infection with DNA types 16/18, 31, 33, 35, 52, and 56; early onset of sexual activity with multiple partners, cigarette smoking, early pregnancy, history of any STD, and low socioeconomic status.

TABLE 5–28.—INTERNATIONAL FEDERATION OF GYNECOLOGY AND OBSTETRICS
(FIGO) STAGING SYSTEM FOR ENDOMETRIAL CANCER

Stage 0	Carcinoma in situ. Histologic findings are suspicious of malignancy. Cases should not be included in any therapeutic statistics.
Stage I	Carcinoma is confined to the uterine corpus.
Ia	Length of the uterine cavity is 8 cm or less.
Ib	Length of the uterine cavity is more than 8 cm.

Cases should be subgrouped with regard to the histologic type of the adenocarcinoma, as follows:

G1: Highly differentiated adenomatous carcinomas.
G2: Differentiated adenomatous carcinomas with partly solid areas.
G3: Predominantly solid or entirely undifferentiated carcinomas.

Stage II	Carcinoma involves corpus and cervix.
Stage III	Carcinoma extends outside the uterus but not outside the true pelvis.
Stage IVa	Carcinoma extends outside the true pelvis or obviously involves the mucosa of the bladder or rectum. As such, bullous edema does not permit assignation of stage IV.
IVb	Spread to distant organs.

Risk factors for endometrial carcinoma include unopposed exogenous estrogens, white race, early menarche, nulliparity, obesity, high fat diet, diabetes, and hypertension.

TABLE 5–29.—INTERNATIONAL FEDERATION OF GYNECOLOGY AND OBSTETRICS (FIGO) STAGING SYSTEM FOR CARCINOMA OF THE OVARY

Stage I	Growth limited to the ovaries.
Ia	Growth limited to one ovary; no ascites.
	(i) No tumor on the external surface; capsule intact.
	(ii) Tumor present on the external surface and/or capsule ruptured.
Ib	Growth limited to both ovaries; no ascites.
	(i) No tumor on the external surface; capsule intact.
	(ii) Tumor present on the external surface and/or capsule(s) ruptured.
Ic	Tumor either stage Ia or stage Ib, but with ascites* present or positive peritoneal washings.
Stage II	Growth involving one or both ovaries with pelvic extension.
IIa	Extension and/or metastases to the uterus and/or tubes.
IIb	Extension to other pelvic tissues.
IIc	Tumor either stage IIa or stage IIb, but with ascites* present or positive peritoneal washings.
Stage III	Growth involving one or both ovaries with intraperitoneal metastases outside the pelvis and/or positive retroperitoneal nodes. Tumor limited to the true pelvis with histologically proved malignant extension to small bowel or omentum.
Stage IV	Growth involving one or both ovaries with distant metastases. If pleural effusion is present, there must be positive cytology to allot a case to stage IV. Liver metastasis equals stage IV.
Special category	Unexplored cases thought to be ovarian carcinoma.

*Ascites is peritoneal effusion, which, in the opinion of the surgeon, is pathologic and/or clearly exceeds normal amounts.

Risk factors for ovarian carcinoma include use of talcum powder on vulva, nulliparity, late menarche, and early menopause.

TABLE 5–30.—ENDOMETRIOSIS*

Endometriosis usually slowly pregressive over a number of years, invasive but nonmalignant, and regresses at the menopause.
Symptoms
1. Progressive, acquired severe pelvic pain with or just prior to menses
2. Dyspareunia
3. Premenstrual staining and hypermenorrhea
4. Painful defecation
5. Suprapubic pain, dysuria, hematuria
6. Infertility
Signs
1. Tender uterosacral ligaments
2. Thickened, nodular uterosacral ligaments
3. Thickened, rectovaginal septum; fullness in cul-de-sac
4. Fixed ovarian or adnexal masses
Diagnosis
Laparotomy, laparoscopy, pelvic ultrasound
Treatment

Mild	Observe, analgesics, nonsteroidals (e.g., ibuprofen 600 mg PO q.i.d.).
Moderate/ severe	Low-estrogen/high-androgen hormone therapy; danozol 200–400 mg PO/day when patient desires fertility.
	A total abdominal hysterectomy with bilateral oophorectomy (TAH-BSO) for patient finished with childbearing.
	Wait 3–6 months before estrogen replacement therapy.

Recurrence rate
20% per year recurrence after hormone therapy.
50% failure rate if one ovary left behind at time of hysterectomy.
< 10% recurrence if TAH-BSO done and FSH allowed to rise to menopausal level before estrogen replacement.

*Adapted from Barbieri RL (ed): *Curr Probl Obstet Gynecol Fert* 1989; 12:1–31.

TABLE 5–31.—DIAGNOSIS AND MANAGEMENT OF MENOPAUSE

Definition
Perimenopausal (climacteric)—ovarian function waxes and wanes.
Menopause—last menses occurred ≥ 12 months ago.
Diagnosis
Cyclic menstrual function ceases.
Estrogen index obtained from upper 1/3 lateral vaginal wall.
Estratrophy = 0/100/0* with slight variability.
Teleatrophy = 100/0/0* with moderate variability.
NOTE: Digitalis therapy shifts maturation index to right.

Asymptomatic patient
Progesterone in oil 100 mg IM or provera 10 mg PO b.i.d. × 5d produces no withdrawal bleeding. (If withdrawal occurs, give cyclic progesterone challenge.)
Serum FSH values are twice normal.
Elective estrogen replacement therapy (ERT).
Symptomatic patient
Conjugated estrogens 0.625 mg PO days 1–25 each month plus provera 5–10 mg PO days 16–25 each month.
Withdrawal should occur after day 25 or not at all.
Continue estrogen-progestin cyclic therapy.
Indications for ERT
1. Vasomotor symptoms
2. Genitourinary atrophy
3. Osteoporosis prophylaxis
Contraindications to ERT
1. Breast or endometrial cancer
2. Impaired liver function, acute liver disease
3. Gallbladder disease
4. Thromboembolism or thrombophlebitis
5. Unexplained vaginal bleeding
Aftercare and counseling
Supplement calcium intake to achieve 1,200 mg daily.
Regular exercise is beneficial.
Serum lipids should be rechecked periodically.
Report unexplained vaginal bleeding at once.
Endometrial cytology is recommended every 1–2 years.

*% parabasal cells/% intermediate cells/% superficial cells.

TABLE 5–32.—TECHNIQUE FOR IN-OFFICE ENDOMETRIAL SAMPLING

Pretreat 1 hour with ibuprofen 600 mg PO.
Patient in lithotomy position, cervix cleansed with povidone-iodine solution.
Anesthesia usually unnecessary.
Tenaculum on anterior lip of cervix with gentle traction.
Uterus sounded and depth recorded in centimeters.
Sampling device passed into endometrial cavity.
    Cell sampling may be cytological via Endocyte, EndoPap, Isaacs, or Mi-Mark samplers or histological via biopsy with vacuum curettage cannula, Novak or Randall curette, or Pipelle.
Sample in all quadrants; aspirate tissue and place in formalin. If cytology, smear on glass slide and fix immediately.
With cervical stenosis and office procedure not possible, do D&C.

PELVIC RELAXATION AND INCONTINENCE

TABLE 5–33.—PELVIC RELAXATION AND INCONTINENCE: TREATMENT
OF URINARY INCONTINENCE

TREATMENT	COMMENT
Kegel exercises	See Table 5–34
Diapers	Up to 500-cc capacity
Diet	Weight reduction, control obesity
Estrogens	Topical or systemic
Drugs	
Bethanechol	Increase tone in hypotonic bladder
Propantheline	Decrease tone in hypertonic bladder (urge incont.)
Phenylpropanolamine, imipramine	Stimulates urethral sphincter tone (stress incont.)
Phenoxybenzamine	Reduce urethral sphincter tone (overflow incont.)
Propranolol	Increase outlet resistance (stress incont.)
Electric devices	Implantable, intravaginal, external
Occlusive devices	Inflatable Bonnar balloon, pessary, implantable Scott artificial sphincter
Surgery	Marshall-Marchetti; Krantz

TABLE 5–34.—KEGEL'S PUBOCOCCYGEAL MUSCLE EXERCISES

The patient locates the correct muscle by sitting on the toilet with knees as far apart as possible and begins urination, contracting perineum only (not bringing legs together) to stop urine flow. Exercises are to be practiced three times daily and do not require urination after muscle control has been learned. Begin with 10 and work up to 30.

1. Contract the muscle and hold for count of 3, then relax muscle.
2. Contract and release rapidly in a flicking motion.
3. Breathe deeply imagining that air is being drawn into the vagina, tightening the muscle as you inhale. Begin with 5, work up to 15.

Practice over a period of months may be necessary before results are noted.

DISEASES OF THE BREAST

TABLE 5–35.—BENIGN BREAST DISEASES*

DISORDER	CLINICAL FINDINGS	TREATMENT
Fibrocystic disease	Often multiple lesions, generally mobile, commonly tender and cycle with menses; most common between ages 30 and 55 years; commonly associated with multiple cysts	Symptomatic; rarely diuretics, rarely multiple aspirations
Sclerosing adenosis	Lump that is commonly irregular nodularity	Excisional biopsy
Fibroadenoma	Firm mobile mass; may change with menses; *unreliably* distinguishable from cancer	Excisional biopsy
Solitary large cyst ("blue-domed cyst")	Firm mobile mass, not necessarily fluctuant or cystlike	Aspiration and follow-up; excisional biopsy if recurrent or bloody fluid
Intraductal papilloma	Serous or serosanguineous nipple discharge; mass-variable pruritus or nipple pain	Nipple fluid cytology, ductography and possible excision; exclude Paget's disease
Galactocele	Milky or opalescent nipple discharge in the postpartum period; possible mass	Symptomatic and breast pumping; biopsy if resolution does not occur
Duct ectasia	Nipple discharge of any description; possible mass; nipple erythema or pruritus	Nipple fluid cytology, ductography and possible excision; exclude Paget's disease
Fat necrosis	Poorly defined mass; possibly symptomatic; variably associated with trauma	Excisional biopsy

Continued.

TABLE 5–35.—Continued

Acute mastitis with or without evidence of acute abscess	Hot red, swollen breast or any part thereof; more common during lactation	A trial of antibiotics and heat; if *rapid* resolution does not occur, rule out inflammatory breast cancer; I&D if mass present
Mondor's disease (localized thrombophlebitis)	Superficial warm tender cord; most commonly postpartum	Heat, analgesia; biopsy if prompt resolution does not occur.
Cystosarcoma phylloides	One or multiple rapidly growing masses	Wide excision if 10%– 15% are malignant

*From Lippman ME: Approach to the management of breast cancer, in Kelley WN, et al (eds): *Textbook of Internal Medicine,* Philadelphia, JB Lippincott Co, 1988, p 1236. Reproduced by permission.

TABLE 5–36.—RISK FACTORS FOR BREAST CANCER

White woman, > 50 years of age.
Breast cancer in sister, mother, maternal grandmother.
Prior history of endometrial cancer, cancer of the other breast, mammary dysplasia or colon cancer.
Menarche < 12 years of age, menopause > 50 years; more than 30 years of menstrual activity.
Never married, never pregnant or < 3 pregnancies.
First child born after age 30 years.
Palpable breast lump in upper outer quadrant or beneath nipple.

6 *Obstetrics*
Charles E. Driscoll, M.D.

DIAGNOSIS OF PREGNANCY

TABLE 6-1.—Diagnosis of Pregnancy*

The *"pregnancy test"* is a measurement of human chorionic gonadotropin (hCG) (6% is cleared in the urine) secreted by trophoblastic tissue. Clinical applications include:
Confirmation of a clinical diagnosis of pregnancy in the first trimester.
To exclude pregnancy before surgery, drug treatment, radiation, or rubella vaccination.
To detect ectopic pregnancy in women with abdominal pain (see Table 6–19).
To evaluate pregnancy threatened by abortion.
To diagnose and guide treatment of trophoblastic tumors.
Three methods are in general use:
Immunoassay
Hemagglutination inhibition (HAI)
Latex particle agglutination inhibition (LAI)
Direct latex particle agglutination (DAP)
Radioimmunoassay (RIA)
Whole molecule or beta-subunit
Radioreceptor Assay (RRA)
Serum hCG is detectable 24 hours after implantation (0.005 IU/ml). In the case of inevitable abortion, urine hCG levels of < 3,000 IU/24 hr will be seen 50–90 days after the LMP.
False negatives—50% rate (HAI, LAI, DAP)
Caused by low-level hCG in early pregnancy, ectopic pregnancies, or threatened abortion (hCG levels in ectopic pregnancy are in range of 0.14–0.77 IU/ml).
In second and third trimesters, when hCG normal values are 5–10 IU/ml.
False positives (HAI, LAI, DAP)
Caused by increased LH levels; exogenous hCG; phenothiazines; promethazine; methadone; proteinuria of ≥ 1 gm/24 hr; trophoblastic tumor; carcinomas of ovary, lung, tubo-ovarian abscess; deteriorated reagents; occasionally RRA may be false positive due to cross-reactivity of LH.

*Adapted from Krieg A: Pregnancy tests and evaluation of placental function, in Todd, Sanford, Davidsohn, et al (eds): *Clinical Diagnosis and Management by Laboratory Methods.* Philadelphia, WB Saunders Co, 1979.

117

TABLE 6–2.—GESTATIONAL AGE ASSESSMENT

Prolonged pregnancy may have as many adverse effects on the fetus as prematurity. Careful clinical assessment of gestational age should include:
Dating by LMP and LNMP.
Estimation of dates by size of uterus at first prenatal exam.
Appearance of FHTs on Doppler (~10–12 wk).
Quickening (16–20 wk).
Appearance of FHTs with unamplified fetoscope (~20 wk).
Uterine size at 20 wk (at the navel).
When all these parameters coincide, the EDC may be established with reasonable confidence. If discrepancy exists, order ultrasonographic measurement of the biparietal diameter (BPD) at 12–18 weeks. Ultrasonographic measurements are inaccurate predictors of fetal age in the third trimester. Additional accuracy of estimation of EDC can be obtained from a repeat sonogram 4 weeks after the first. Correlate BPDs with clinical assessment.

FIG 6–1.
Assessing gestational age by uterine growth. (From Iffy L: *1982–1983 Modern Medicine Ob-Gyn Pocket Guide.* New York, Harcourt Brace Jovanovich, 1982, p. 66. Reproduced by permission.)

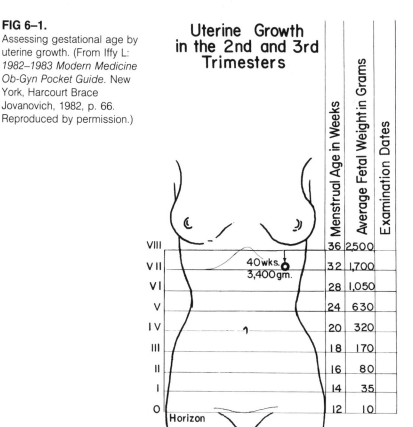

Uterine Growth in the 2nd and 3rd Trimesters

	Menstrual Age in Weeks	Average Fetal Weight in Grams	Examination Dates
VIII	36	2,500	
VII	32	1,700	40 wks. 3,400 gm.
VI	28	1,050	
V	24	630	
IV	20	320	
III	18	170	
II	16	80	
I	14	35	
0	12	10	

Horizon

Pregnancy Table for Expected Date of Delivery

Find the date of the last menstrual period in the top line (light-face type) of the pair of lines. The dark number (bold-face type) in the line below will be the expected day of delivery.

	1	2	3	4	5	6	7	8	9	10	11	12	13	14	15	16	17	18	19	20	21	22	23	24	25	26	27	28	29	30	31	
Jan.	1	2	3	4	5	6	7	8	9	10	11	12	13	14	15	16	17	18	19	20	21	22	23	24	25	26	27	28	29	30	31	
Oct.	8	9	10	11	12	13	14	15	16	17	18	19	20	21	22	23	24	25	26	27	28	29	30	31	(1	2	3	4	5	6	7	**Nov.**
Feb.	1	2	3	4	5	6	7	8	9	10	11	12	13	14	15	16	17	18	19	20	21	22	23	24	25	26	27	28				
Nov.	8	9	10	11	12	13	14	15	16	17	18	19	20	21	22	23	24	25	26	27	28	29	30	(1	2	3	4	5				**Dec.**
Mar.	1	2	3	4	5	6	7	8	9	10	11	12	13	14	15	16	17	18	19	20	21	22	23	24	25	26	27	28	29	30	31	
Dec.	6	7	8	9	10	11	12	13	14	15	16	17	18	19	20	21	22	23	24	25	26	27	28	29	30	31	(1	2	3	4	5	**Jan.**
April	1	2	3	4	5	6	7	8	9	10	11	12	13	14	15	16	17	18	19	20	21	22	23	24	25	26	27	28	29	30		
Jan.	6	7	8	9	10	11	12	13	14	15	16	17	18	19	20	21	22	23	24	25	26	27	28	29	30	31	(1	2	3	4		**Feb.**
May	1	2	3	4	5	6	7	8	9	10	11	12	13	14	15	16	17	18	19	20	21	22	23	24	25	26	27	28	29	30	31	
Feb.	5	6	7	8	9	10	11	12	13	14	15	16	17	18	19	20	21	22	23	24	25	26	27	28	(1	2	3	4	5	6	7	**Mar.**
June	1	2	3	4	5	6	7	8	9	10	11	12	13	14	15	16	17	18	19	20	21	22	23	24	25	26	27	28	29	30		
Mar.	8	9	10	11	12	13	14	15	16	17	18	19	20	21	22	23	24	25	26	27	28	29	30	31	(1	2	3	4	5	6		**April**
July	1	2	3	4	5	6	7	8	9	10	11	12	13	14	15	16	17	18	19	20	21	22	23	24	25	26	27	28	29	30	31	
April	7	8	9	10	11	12	13	14	15	16	17	18	19	20	21	22	23	24	25	26	27	28	29	30	(1	2	3	4	5	6	7	**May**
Aug.	1	2	3	4	5	6	7	8	9	10	11	12	13	14	15	16	17	18	19	20	21	22	23	24	25	26	27	28	29	30	31	
May	8	9	10	11	12	13	14	15	16	17	18	19	20	21	22	23	24	25	26	27	28	29	30	31	(1	2	3	4	5	6	7	**June**
Sept.	1	2	3	4	5	6	7	8	9	10	11	12	13	14	15	16	17	18	19	20	21	22	23	24	25	26	27	28	29	30		
June	8	9	10	11	12	13	14	15	16	17	18	19	20	21	22	23	24	25	26	27	28	29	30	(1	2	3	4	5	6	7		**July**
Oct.	1	2	3	4	5	6	7	8	9	10	11	12	13	14	15	16	17	18	19	20	21	22	23	24	25	26	27	28	29	30	31	
July	8	9	10	11	12	13	14	15	16	17	18	19	20	21	22	23	24	25	26	27	28	29	30	31	(1	2	3	4	5	6	7	**Aug.**
Nov.	1	2	3	4	5	6	7	8	9	10	11	12	13	14	15	16	17	18	19	20	21	22	23	24	25	26	27	28	29	30		
Aug.	8	9	10	11	12	13	14	15	16	17	18	19	20	21	22	23	24	25	26	27	28	29	30	31	(1	2	3	4	5	6		**Sept.**
Dec.	1	2	3	4	5	6	7	8	9	10	11	12	13	14	15	16	17	18	19	20	21	22	23	24	25	26	27	28	29	30	31	
Sept.	7	8	9	10	11	12	13	14	15	16	17	18	19	20	21	22	23	24	25	26	27	28	29	30	(1	2	3	4	5	6	7	**Oct.**

FIG 6–2.

Pregnancy table for expected date of delivery. (From Thomas CL (ed): *Taber's Cyclopedic Medical Dictionary*, ed 16. Philadelphia, FA Davis Co, 1989, p 1470. Reproduced by permission.)

TABLE 6–3.—Correlations of GA and Fetal
BPD*

WEEK OF GESTATION	CROWN-RUMP LENGTH (CM)	WEIGHT (MG)	BIPARIETAL DIAMETER (CM)
6	0.5		
7	0.8	0.07	
8	1.5	0.22	
9	2.5	0.88	
10	3.5	3.50	
11	4.6	6.00	
12	5.7	11.00	2.1
13	6.8	19.00	2.4
14	8.1	33.00	2.6
15	9.4	55.00	3.0
16	10.7	80.00	3.7
17	12.1	120.00	4.0
18	13.6	170.00	4.3
19	15.3	253.00	4.5
20	16.4	316.00	4.7
21	17.5	385.00	5.0
22	18.6	460.00	5.3
23	19.7	542.00	5.6
24	20.8	630.00	5.9
25	21.8	723.00	6.2
26	22.8	823.00	6.6
27	23.8	930.00	6.9
28	24.7	1,045.00	7.2
29	25.6	1,174.00	7.5
30	26.5	1,323.00	7.8
31	27.4	1,492.00	8.0
32	28.3	1,680.00	8.3
33	29.3	1,876.00	8.5
34	30.2	2,074.00	8.7
35	31.1	2,274.00	8.8
36	32.1	2,478.00	9.0
37	33.1	2,690.00	9.2
38	34.1	2,914.00	9.3
39	35.1	3,150.00	9.4
40	36.2	3,405.00	9.5
41		3,600.00	
42		3,650.00	

*Adapted from Iffy L: Pregnancy, in *1982–1983 Modern Medicine Ob-Gyn Pocket Guide.* New York, Harcourt Brace Jovanovich, 1982, and Hobbins JC, Winsberg F, Berkowitz RL (eds): *Ultrasonography in Obstetrics and Gynecology,* ed 2. Baltimore, Williams & Wilkins Co, 1983.

PRENATAL MATERNAL CARE

TABLE 6–4.—PRENATAL MATERNAL CARE

Complete history
  Risk assessment, genetic history (Tay-Sachs, Down's, muscular dystrophy, mental retardation, CNS anomaly), tobacco and drug use, hepatitis and HIV risk, diet, activity, general medical history, occupational (industrial, chemical, day care, health care).

Physical exam
  Height, weight, BP, general exam, especially of thyroid, dentition, heart and vascular system, reflexes, breasts, genitalia, and rectum.

Laboratory screening
  First visit
    VDRL, PAP, GC culture, CBC, rubella titer, type and RH, irregular antibodies, urinalysis, HBsAg (sickle cell, Tay-Sachs, HIV test, herpes simplex culture, and *Chlamydia* test when indicated).
  16–18 wk
    serum α-fetoprotein; consider need for ultrasound.
  24 wk
    Glucose screen 1 hr after 50 gm PO glucose load; recheck hematocrit.

Clinical assessment of pelvis
  Pelvic angle >90°, diagonal conjugate >11.5 cm, intertuberous >8 cm.

Patient education
  Drugs, diet, activity, costs, plan for care, travel, smoking, alcohol, analysis of risk assessment, weight gain, intercourse, fetal development, danger signals, husband's role, childbirth classes, symptoms of labor, breast care, electronic fetal monitoring, delivery, Cesarean delivery indications, analgesia/anesthesia, baby care, newborn circumcision, postpartum depression, contraception, effects on sibs, postpartum care and follow-up.

For further information see *Caring for Our Future: The Content of Prenatal Care,* A Report of the Public Health Service Expert Panel on the Content of Prenatal Care, 1989, U.S. Public Health Service, Department of Health and Human Services, Washington, D.C.

TABLE 6–5.—IDENTIFICATION OF THE HIGH-RISK PREGNANCY

Risk Assessment

About 70%–80% of perinatal mortality and morbidity is seen in 20%–30% of the obstetric population. Early identification of risk is aided by combined antenatal and intrapartum risk assessment scoring. Carefully applied, these scoring scales will identify better than 80% of pregnancies with problem newborns. Only 20%–30% of problem newborns originate from the low-risk population.

Maternal Child Health Care Index*

The scoring system below is an attempt to categorize the degree of maternal and fetal risk based on the information available at the initial history and physical on registration in our obstetric clinics. Please circle the numbers under each of the 8 categories which you feel apply, and at the bottom of this sheet, add up these numbers and subtract from a perfect score of 100

I. Maternal age (yr)		II. Race and marital status		III. Parity	
<15	20	White	0	0	10
15–19	10	Nonwhite	5	1–3	0
20–29	0	Single	5	4–7	5
30–34	5	Married	0	8+	10
35–39	10				
>40	20				

IV. Past obstetric history

Abortions		Prematures		Fetal death		Neonatal death		Congenital anomaly		Damaged infants	
1	5	1	10	1	10	1	10	1	10	Physical	10
2	15	2+	20	2+	30	2+	30	2+	20	Neurologic	20

V. Medical-obstetric disorders and nutrition

Systemic illness
Acute, mild 5
Acute, serious 15
Chronic nondebilitating 5
Chronic debilitating 20

Specific infections
Urinary:
  Acute 5
  Chronic 25
Syphilis:
  Treated 0
  Untreated 20
  At term 30

Chronic hypertension
Mild 15
Severe 30
Nephritis 30

Diabetes
Pre 20
Overt 30

Heart disease
Class I or II 10
Class III or IV 30
History of prior failure 30

Anemia
Hb, 10–11 gm 5
Hb, 9–10 gm 10
Hb, <9 gm 20

Endocrine disorders
Definite adrenal, pituitary, or thyroid problem 30
Recurrent menstrual dysfunction 10
Involuntary sterility: <2 yr 10
                   >2 yr 20

Rh problem
Sensitized 30
Prior infant affected 30
Prior ABO incompatibility 20

Nutrition
Malnourished 20
Very obese 30
Inadequate diet but not malnourished 10

Continued.

TABLE 6–5.—Continued

Maternal Child Health Care Index*—Continued

VI. Generative tract disorders

Prior fetal malpresentations	20
Prior cesarean section	30
Known anomaly or incompetent cervix	20
Myomas:	
>5 cm	20
Submucous	30
Contracted pelvis:	
Borderline	10
Any contracted plane	30
Ovarian masses:	
>6 cm	20
Endometriosis	5

VII. Emotional survey (grade 0–20, based on):

Fears, attitudes, biases, hostilities, motivations, and behavioral patterns; prior pregnancies without supervision at time of registration; standard of child care and responsibilities; family unit, marital relationship; history of psychiatric illness in family

VIII. Social and economic survey (grade 0–10, based on):

Employment—husband, patient; annual income adequacy, public assistance; education—husband, patient; housing—location, quality, facilities, neighborhood environment

IX. Score

Total score of all 8 categories ‒‒‒‒‒‒‒‒‒‒
100 minus above score equals MCH Care Index
High-risk: score of 70: moderate risk: 71–84: low risk: 85
Perform antenatal risk assessment at initial visit and again at 36 wk.

*From Aubry RH, Pennington JC: *Clin Obstet Gynecol* 1973; 16:6–9. Reproduced by permission.

TABLE 6–6.—LABOR INDEX (LI)*

FACTORS	PENALTY POINTS
Maternal factors	
Prenatal care	
<3 prenatal visits	−10
No prenatal visits	−20
Toxemia	
Mild	−20
Severe	−20
Undetected diabetes	−20
Anemia: Hb < 10 gm	−10
Fever	−20
Placental factors	
Bleeding before 20 wk	−10
Bleeding 20 wk to term	−20
Bleeding with pain and/or hypotension	−30
Ruptured membranes > 24 hr	−20
Fetal factors	
Gestational age	
<34 wk	−30
34–37 wk	−20
>42 wk	−20
Multiple pregnancy	−20
Previously undetected Rh sensitization	−20
Meconium staining	−30
Fetal heart rate abnormality (<115 >165)	−30

Scoring

Labor Index score = 100 − above penalties

Total Index = 200 − (penalties from MCHI + LI)

High-risk group: Total Index (MCHI + LI) ≤ 150

*From Aubry RH, Pennington JC: *Clin Obstet Gynecol* 1973; 16:6–9. Reproduced by permission.

TABLE 6–7.—ESTIMATES FOR DIETARY NEED FOR PREGNANCY AND LACTATION (U.S. RDA)*

	NONPREGNANT BY AGES				FOR PREG. ADD	FOR LACTATION ADD
	11–14 yr	15–18 yr	19–22 yr	23–50 yr		
Kcal	2,200	2,100	2,100	2,000	+300	+500
Protein, gm	46	46	44	44	+30	+20
Vit. A, RE	800	800	800	800	+200	+400
Vit. D, IU	400	400	300	200	+200	+200
Vit. E, α-TE	8	8	8	8	+2	+3
Vit. C, mg	50	60	60	60	+20	+40
Folacin, mg	0.4	0.4	0.4	0.4	0.4	0.1
Niacin, mg NE	15	14	14	13	+2	+5
Riboflavin, mg	1.3	1.3	1.3	1.2	+0.3	+0.5
Thiamin, mg	1.1	1.1	1.1	1.0	+0.4	+0.5

Continued.

TABLE 6-7.—Continued

	NONPREGNANT BY AGES				FOR PREG. ADD	FOR LACTATION ADD
	11–14 yr	15–18 yr	19–22 yr	23–50 yr		
Vit. B_6, mg	1.8	2.0	2.0	2.0	+0.6	+0.5
Vit. B_{12}, µg	3.0	3.0	3.0	3.0	+1.0	+1.0
Calcium, mg	1,200	1,200	800	800	+400	+400
Phosphorus, mg	1,200	1,200	800	800	+400	+400
Iodine, µg	150	150	150	150	+25	+50
Iron, mg	18	18	18	18	+20†	+20†
Magnesium	300	300	300	300	+150	+150
Zinc	15	15	15	15	+5	+10

*Adapted from Food and Nutrition Board, National Academy of Sciences–National Research Council: *Recommended Dietary Allowances,* ed 9, revised 1980.

†The increased requirement for iron cannot be met by ordinary diets and supplementation is needed.

Prenatal vitamin supplements usually contribute more than what is needed to satisfy U.S. RDAs. Iron and folacin are probably necessary even if an ordinary diet is taken. Vegetarians require more careful evaluation.

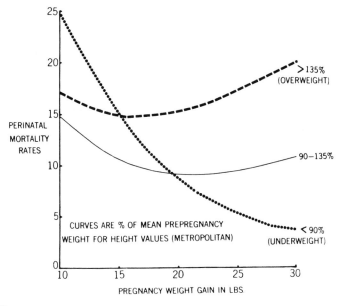

FIG 6–3.
Pregnancy weight gain and perinatal mortality. Overweight mothers had the fewest fetal and neonatal deaths with a 15–16 lb weight gain in term pregnancies. The optimal gain for normally proportioned mothers was 20 lb, and for underweight mothers, 30 lb. With weight gains of more than 20 lb, underweight mothers had significantly lower perinatal mortalities than did mothers who were not underweight ($P<.005$). The underweight mothers in question had fewer losses to amniotic fluid infections, premature rupture of fetal membranes, and major congenital anomalies. (From Naeye RL: *Am J Obstet Gynecol* 1979; 135:3–9. Reproduced by permission.)

TABLE 6–8.—PHYSIOLOGIC NORMS OF PREGNANCY (32–36 WEEKS)*

PARAMETER	NONPREGNANT	PREGNANT
Thyroid		
T_4 (μg/dl)	3.4–6.4	5.5–10.0
T_3 (%)	25–38	12–25
FTI (μg/dl)	1.2–1.6	0.9–1.4
Blood count		
Hb (gm/dl)	12–16	10–14
Hct (%)	37–47	32–42
WBC (total/mm³)	4,500–10,000	5,000–15,000
ESR (mm/hr)	20	30–90
Iron studies		
Serum Fe (μg)	75–150	65–120
TIBC	240–450	300–500
Blood pressure	120/80	114/65
Pulse	70	80
Cardiac output (L/min)	4.5	6.0
ECG	Normal	15° left axis deviation
V_1 and V_2	Normal	Inverted T wave
V_4	Normal	Low T
III	Normal	Q and inverted T
aV_r	Normal	Small Q
Respiratory		
Respirations (rate/min)	15	16
Tidal volume (ml)	475	675
Vital capacity (ml)	3,150	3,300–3,400
Residual volume (ml)	950	750
Pao_2 (mm Hg)	95–100	95–100
$Paco_2$ (mm Hg)	35–40	25–35
Renal		
GFR (creatinine clearance, ml/min)	80–120	110–180
BUN (mg/dl)	10–18	4–12
Creatinine (mg/dl)	0.6–1.2	0.4–0.9
Uric acid (mg/dl)	2.0–6.4	2.0–5.5

*Adapted from Henry JB: *Postgrad Med* 1972; 52:110–114, and 1973; 53:221–226.

GENETIC COUNSELING

TABLE 6–9.—MATERNAL AGE-SPECIFIC RISK ESTIMATES FOR SIGNIFICANT CHROMOSOMAL DISORDER*†

MATERNAL AGE (YR)	DOWN'S SYNDROME PER 1,000 LIVEBORN	OTHER CHROMOSOMAL DISORDERS PER 1,000 LIVEBORN	TOTAL SIGNIFICANT CHROMOSOMAL DISORDERS PER 1,000 LIVEBORN	AS FRACTION‡
15	1.0	1.3	2.3	1/450
16	0.9	1.3	2.2	1/450
17	0.8	1.3	2.1	1/500
18	0.7	1.3	2.0	1/500
19	0.6	1.3	1.9	1/500
20	0.6	1.3	1.9	1/500
21	0.6	1.3	1.9	1/500
22	0.6	1.3	1.9	1/500
23	0.7	1.3	2.0	1/500
24	0.8	1.3	2.1	1/500
25	0.8	1.3	2.1	1/500
26	0.9	1.3	2.2	1/450
27	1.0	1.3	2.3	1/450
28	1.0	1.3	2.3	1/450
29	1.1	1.4	2.5	1/400
30	1.1	1.4	2.5	1/400
31	1.2	1.5	2.7	1/350
32	1.4	1.6	3.0	1/333
33	1.7	1.7	3.4	1/300
34	2.2	1.8	4.0	1/250
35	2.7	2.2	4.9	1/200
36	3.5	2.4	5.9	1/170
37	4.5	2.8	7.3	1/140
38	5.7	3.2	8.9	1/110
39	7.2	3.7	10.9	1/90
40	9.2	4.5	13.7	1/70
41	11.7	5.4	17.1	1/60
42	14.9	6.6	21.5	1/50
43	19.0	8.1	27.1	1/37
44	24.2	10.1	34.3	1/30
45	30.8	12.6	43.4	1/25
46	39.3	16.0	55.3	1/20
47	50.0	20.3	70.3	1/14
48	63.8	26.1	89.9	1/10
49	81.2	33.7	114.9	1/9

*From Iffy L, Kaminetzky H: *Principles and Practice of Obstetrics and Perinatology.* New York, John Wiley & Sons, 1981, vol 1, p 398. Reproduced by permission.
†Numbers are based on various estimates, especially those of Hook and Cross. Clinically significant conditions include Down's syndrome, trisomies 18 and 13, XXY, and XYY, but not XXX.
‡This column provides useful approximations for genetic counseling.

TABLE 6–10.—MATERNAL SERUM α-FETOPROTEIN SCREENING (MSAFP)

Elevations caused by:
Fetus
  Anencephaly, spina bifida, encephalocele, omphalocele,
  gastroschisis, cystic hygroma
Maternal
  Hepatitis, persistent AFP production, hepatocellular carcinoma,
  herpes infection
Pregnancy
  Incorrect estimate of gestation, pre-eclampsia, twins, fetal to maternal
  bleed, abruption, Rh isoimmunization, ataxia-telangiectasia,
  congenital nephrosis, epidermolysis bullosa simplex, severe
  oligohydramnios, spontaneous abortion, stillbirth, prematurity,
  acardiac twin
Depressed levels caused by:
Fetus
  Trisomys 21 and 18
Maternal
  Insulin-dependent diabetes mellitus

    If screening test abnormal, order a level II (high-resolution) sonogram. Consider amniocentesis for amniotic fluid α-fetoprotein (AF-AFP), chromosome analysis, and amniotic fluid acetylcholinesterase assay.

TABLE 6–11.—INDICATIONS FOR MIDTRIMESTER AMNIOCENTESIS
FOR GENETIC DIAGNOSIS*

Clear-cut Indications; High-Risk Situations
Parent is heterozygote for a serious autosomal dominant trait that can be diagnosed in fetus (e.g., achondroplasia; recurrence risk 1 in 2).
Both parents are carriers of a recessively inherited severe metabolic disorder that can be diagnosed in utero (e.g., Tay-Sachs; recurrence risk 1 in 4).
Mother is carrier of severe X-linked recessive disorder that can be diagnosed in utero (recurrence risk 1 in 4). If not diagnosable, determinations of fetal sex with a view to termination of male conceptus can be considered.
Parents are carriers of a recessive or X-linked recessive malformation syndrome that may be diagnosable (e.g., Meckel syndrome; recurrence risk 1 in 4).
One parent is a carrier of a translocation chromosome likely to cause serious chromosomal imbalance in the fetus (e.g., D/G translocation; risk is 1 in 10 when mother is carrier).
Maternal age over 40 (risk of Down's syndrome more than 1 in 100).
Parent or sibling has neural tube defect (recurrence risk 1 in 20).
Previous trisomy, Down's syndrome, or other major chromosome anomaly (risk approximately 1 in 100).
Elevated MSAFP, abnormal level II sonogram
    Indications Less Clear-cut; Moderate or Uncertain Risk
Maternal age 35–39 (risk of Down's syndrome approximately 1 in 200).
Severe maternal anxiety.
    Indication Controversial or Not Accepted
Amniocentesis only to determine sex, with a view to termination of pregnancy of undesired sex.

    *Adapted from Iffy L, Kaminetzky H: Principles and Practice of Obstetrics and Perinatology. New York, John Wiley & Sons, 1981, vol 1, p 397.

TABLE 6–12.—POSSIBLE EFFECTS ON THE FETUS AND NEWBORN
OF MATERNAL DRUG INGESTION*

DRUG	EFFECT
Androgens	Masculinization
Antineoplastics	Congenital anomalies; newborn
Barbiturates	Neonatal withdrawal
Cephalothin	Positive direct Coombs test
Chloramphenicol	"Gray baby" syndrome
Diethylstilbestrol	Vaginal or adenosis adenocarcinoma
Heroin and other narcotics and propoxyphene	Narcotic withdrawal, convulsions, neonatal death; growth retardation
Isotretinoin	Many major fetal abnormalities; wastage
Lithium	Congenital heart disease
Novobiocin	Hyperbilirubinemia
Phenytoin	Cleft lip and palate; congenital height disorder; hydantoin syndrome; skeleton anomalies
Potassium iodide	Goiter; mental retardation
Progestins	Masculinization; septal defects; limb reduction anomalies; hypospadias
Propylthiouracil	Congenital goiter, cretinism
Quinine	Thrombocytopenia
Radioactive iodine	Thyroid ablation
Reserpine	Nasal congestion; drowsiness
Salicylates	Neonatal bleeding; postmaturity; maternal bleeding
Sodium warfarin (Coumadin)	Fetal death; hemorrhage; blindness; mental retardation; and stippled epipheses
Streptomycin	Acoustic nerve damage
Sulfonamides	Hyperbilirubinemia; kernicterus
Tetracyclines	Discoloration of teeth; inhibition of bone growth
Thiazides	Thrombocytopenia
Thiocarbamides	Goiter, hyperthyroidism
Trimethadione	Cleft lip and palate; congenital heart disorder; hydantoin syndrome; skeletal anomalies

*Adapted from Iffy L, Kaminetzky H: *Principles and Practice of Obstetrics and Perinatology.* New York, John Wiley & Sons, 1981, vol 2, p 724.

MEDICAL COMPLICATIONS OF PREGNANCY

TABLE 6–13.—DIABETES IN PREGNANCY

Diabetes in pregnancy.—The perinatal mortality rate in insulin-dependent diabetics is 6.5%. Fluctuating maternal glucose levels and hyperglycemia are largely responsible for morbidity and mortality of the fetus. The classic triad of infant morbidity consists of hyperbilirubinemia, hypoglycemia, and hypocalcemia. The congenital major malformation rate in insulin-dependent diabetics is 9.0%. These rates may approach near normal with tight control.

Diagnosis.—Suspect if woman has prior history of elevated blood sugar, urine glycosuria, strong family history of diabetes, prior delivery of very large infant (>10 lb.), anomalous or still-born infant, hydramnios, habitual abortion, excessive maternal obesity, or fails glucose screen (see Table 6–4).

Diagnosis of diabetes by OGTT (after 100-gm glucose load):

FBS	125 mg/dl
1 hr	185 mg/dl
2 hr	165 mg/dl
3 hr	145 mg/dl

Care during pregnancy should include home glucose monitoring and use of the Hemoglobin A1$_c$ test.

TABLE 6–14.—WHITE CLASSIFICATION OF DIABETES IN PREGNANCY*

CLASS	AGE AT ONSET (YR)	DURATION (YR)	VASCULAR DISEASE	INSULIN
A	Any	Pregnancy	0	0
B	>20	<10	0	+
C	10–19	10–19	0	+
D	<10	20	Benign retinopathy	+
F	Any	Any	Nephropathy	+
R	Any	Any	Proliferative retinopathy	+
H	Any	Any	Heart disease	+

*Adapted from White P: *Am J Med* 1949; 7:609.

TABLE 6–15.—Cardiovascular Disease During Pregnancy

Cardiac disease during pregnancy has a 2% incidence in all pregnant women; 90% is due to rheumatic heart disease (usually mitral stenosis); 1%–3% is due to congenital heart disease. Management is aimed at the prevention of CHF.

Prevention Factors

infection	nutritional deficiencies
anemia	physical stress
venous congestion	fluid retention

Peak cardiac output occurs at 25–32 weeks (30%–50% above nonpregnant levels).

Steps in Management

Diagnose early and classify heart condition according to New York Heart Association criteria.

Auscultate heart frequently; check for anemia often.

Class 1 and 2: frequent rest, housekeeping aid, avoid stairs.

Class 3: greatly reduced activity, bed rest for mild failure.

Class 4: consider therapeutic abortion.

Diet low in salt, lower water intake to 800–1,000 cc/day for failure.

Diuretics for moderate or advanced disease plus edema or venous congestion.

Digitalis for failure apparent by signs and symptoms.

Hospitalize patient prior to EDC to evaluate cardiac status.

Careful monitoring during labor. Avoid hypotension.

Shorten second stage with forceps. Regional block (caudal) recommended.

SBE prophylaxis.

TABLE 6–16.—Differential Diagnosis of the Major Dermatoses Associated With Pregnancy*†

DISEASE PROCESS	ONSET	TYPE AND LOCATION OF LESIONS	SYMPTOMS	ASSOCIATED LABORATORY ABNORMALITIES	THERAPY	MATERNAL/FETAL MORBIDITY-MORTALITY
Herpes gestationis	Second half of pregnancy and postpartum, rare	Erythematous papules, vesicules, bullae on extremities, abdomen, buttocks, mucous membranes (20%) (tendency to symmetry)	Pruritus, few mild systemic manifestations (fever, chills)	Eosinophilia positive immunofluorescence, elevated chorionic gonadotropin level	Systemic corticosteroids	Maternal: none Fetal: reports variable
Papular dermatitis of pregnancy	Anytime during gestation, rare	Erythematous papules (3–5 mm), generalized eruption	Pruritus, no associated systemic symptoms	Elevated urinary chorionic gonadotropin levels, decreased estrogen and cortisol level	Systemic corticosteroids	Maternal: none Fetal: increased mortality

Continued.

TABLE 6–16.—Continued

DISEASE PROCESS	ONSET	TYPE AND LOCATION OF LESIONS	SYMPTOMS	ASSOCIATED LABORATORY ABNORMALITIES	THERAPY	MATERNAL/FETAL MORBIDITY-MORTALITY
Prurigo gestationis	Second half of gestation, 2% of all pregnancies	Small papules (1–2 mm) extensor surface extremities: trunk (tendency to symmetry)	Pruritus, no associated systemic symptoms	None	Antipruritics	Maternal: none Fetal: none
Pruritus gravidarum (idiopathic jaundice of pregnancy)	Last trimester common, 17% of all pregnancies	No primary lesion, localized to abdomen or generalized	Pruritus, no associated systemic symptoms	Elevated bilirubin (in idiopathic jaundice of pregnancy)	Antipruritics	Maternal: none Fetal: increased
Impetigo herpetiformis	Second half of gestation (usually), rare	Small pustules (may coalesce) Groin, inner thighs, extremities, mucous membranes (occasionally)	Pain, severe systemic symptoms common (high fever, chills, vomiting, diarrhea, arthritis, splenomegaly, lymphadenopathy, septicemia)	Hypercalcemia, hyperphosphatemia	Systemic corticosteroids	Maternal: increased mortality Fetal: increased stillbirths

*Adapted from Wade TR, et al: *Obstet Gynecol* 1978; 52:233–242.
†These rashes will be progressive throughout pregnancy and will resolve with delivery; all but impetigo herpetiformis are prone to recurrence with subsequent pregnancies.

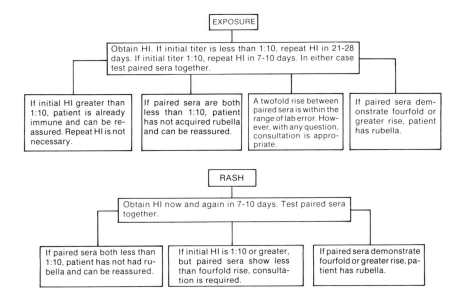

```
                              ┌──────────┐
                              │ EXPOSURE │
                              └──────────┘
        ┌──────────────────────────────────────────────────────┐
        │ Obtain HI. If initial titer is less than 1:10, repeat │
        │ HI in 21-28 days. If initial titer 1:10, repeat HI in │
        │ 7-10 days. In either case test paired sera together.  │
        └──────────────────────────────────────────────────────┘
```

| If initial HI greater than 1:10, patient is already immune and can be reassured. Repeat HI is not necessary. | If paired sera are both less than 1:10, patient has not acquired rubella and can be reassured. | A twofold rise between paired sera is within the range of lab error. However, with any question, consultation is appropriate. | If paired sera demonstrate fourfold or greater rise, patient has rubella. |

```
                              ┌──────┐
                              │ RASH │
                              └──────┘
        ┌──────────────────────────────────────────────────────┐
        │ Obtain HI now and again in 7-10 days. Test paired     │
        │ sera together.                                        │
        └──────────────────────────────────────────────────────┘
```

| If paired sera both less than 1:10, patient has not had rubella and can be reassured. | If initial HI is 1:10 or greater, but paired sera show less than fourfold rise, consultation is required. | If paired sera demonstrate fourfold or greater rise, patient has rubella. |

There are special indications for complement fixation antibody, fluorescent antibody, rubella-specific IgM and other determinations. Consult a specialist in Infectious Disease or the Center for Disease Control if:

1. Exposure has occurred more than two weeks prior to initial consultation.
2. Rash has occurred more than one week prior to initial consultation.
3. Paired sera demonstrate some rise but the rise is less than fourfold.

FIG 6–4.

How to diagnose rubella during pregnancy. (From McCubbin JH, Smith JS: *Am Fam Physician* 1981; 23:205–208. Reproduced by permission.)

OBSTETRIC COMPLICATIONS OF PREGNANCY

TABLE 6–17.—OBSTETRIC COMPLICATIONS OF PREGNANCY: ABORTION

Loss of the products of conception before 20th week of pregnancy.
At least 10% of all pregnancies end in spontaneous abortion.
Most spontaneous abortions occur in first 8 weeks; few occur after 13 weeks.
Abnormalities of ovum in 60% of cases.
Most common causes are polyploidy, trisomy, and sex chromosome aberrations.

Six Types of Abortion

Threatened—70% will go to term; decrease activity and restrict intercourse.
Inevitable—Cervix dilated, conceptus at os; may complete with pitocin.
Incomplete—More common after 10 weeks; remaining material removed by D&C or suction curettage.
Missed—Prolonged retention of nonviable conceptus, uterus does not grow and weight decreases 3–4 lb; check coagulation factors and empty uterus.
Septic—Usually due to induced abortion contaminated by *Streptococcus* or *Staphylococcus* or *E. coli.*
Habitual—Three or more consecutive spontaneous abortions; do CBC, blood sugar, liver and renal function studies, thyroid studies, rubella test, Coomb's test, and TORCH titers; culture for *T. mycoplasma.*

TABLE 6–18.—POSSIBLE CAUSES OF ABORTION*

Chromosomal abnormality of ovum	Age of gametes
	Viruses
Radiation	Hypothyroidism
Chemical exposure	Diabetes
Hyperthyroidism	Chronic renal vascular disease
Chronic infection (*Mycoplasma, toxoplasmosis, parvovirus*)	Septate uterus
	Endometrial polyp
Chronic glomerular nephritis	Incompetent cervix
Bicornuate uterus	Acute illness
Uterine myomas	Parental chromosomal abnormality
Cervical laceration	
Severe mental shock	

*From AAFP Home Study Self-Assessment, Monograph 33: *Complications of Pregnancy.* Kansas City, Mo, American Academy of Family Physicians, 1982, p 12. Reproduced by permission.

Ectopic Pregnancy

TABLE 6–19.—SITES AND INCIDENCE OF ECTOPIC PREGNANCY

SITE	% OF CASES	INCIDENCE
Ampular	47.0	The incidence of ectopic pregnancy is increasing
Isthmic	21.6	and is between 1/100 to 1/200 pregnancies.
Fimbrial	5.8	The typical high-risk patient is older, has a
Interstitial	3.7	higher parity, had prior infertility, and had a
Infundibular	2.5	prior ectopic pregnancy or PID.
Other	19.4	

TABLE 6–20.—PHYSICAL FINDINGS IN ECTOPIC PREGNANCY*

ABDOMINAL	% OF CASES	PELVIC	% OF CASES
Tenderness	83	Adnexal tenderness	72
Rebound	41	Cervix tenderness	43
Guarding	24	Adnexal fullness	35
Distention	29	Adnexal mass (infrequent)	30
Diminished bowel sounds	18	Cul-de-sac fullness	29
Absent bowel sounds	6	Uterine enlargement	26
Mass	3.5	Cervix discoloration	25
		Cervix softness	21

*From AAFP Home Study Self-Assessment, Monograph 33: *Complications of Pregnancy*. Kansas City, Mo, American Academy of Family Physicians, 1982, p 18. Reproduced by permission.

TABLE 6–21.—ULTRASOUND, SERUM HCG AND PROGESTERONE IN THE DIAGNOSIS OF NORMAL AND ABNORMAL PREGNANCIES*

In a normal gestation, the hCG doubling time is 1.98 days.
Abnormal pregnancies are associated with <66% increase in hCG in a 2-day interval.

Ultrasound Findings	Days From LMP	hCG mIU[†]
Sac	32–38	914 ± 106
Fetal pole	37–44	3,783 ± 683
Fetal heart motion	41–53	13,178 ± 2,898

Above 6,000–6,500 mIU of hCG, a normal intrauterine gestation can be visualized with transabdominal ultrasound 94% of the time.
The absence of an intrauterine gestational sac when hCG is >6,000–6,500 mIU is diagnostic of ectopic pregnancy in 86% of cases.
Adnexal masses can be found in ≥ 83% of ectopic pregnancies by ultrasound. (Transvaginal ultrasound is proving to be more accurate earlier than transabdominal ultrasound.)
Serum progesterone(P_4) may be helpful in that most ectopics are associated with <15 ng/mL; intrauterine pregnancies show >20 ng/mL.

*Adapted from Leach RE, Ory SJ: *J Reprod Med* 1989; 34:324–338.
[†]1 ng of hCG = 9.3 mIU (International Reference Preparation).

TABLE 6–22.—TECHNIQUE OF CULDOCENTESIS

Obtain informed consent; risks are hemorrhage and organ puncture.
Swab vagina and cervix with povidine-iodine.
Grasp posterior lip of cervix with tenaculum, and apply gentle traction.
Subcutaneous lidocaine anesthesia may be used in posterior fornix.
Insert spinal needle on a 10-cc Leur-lock syringe into posterior fornix into transitional fold.
Keep parallel to uterus and apply continuous gentle negative pressure while inserting into cul-de-sac.
More than 5 cc of nonclotting blood is 99% diagnostic of ectopic pregnancy.
If bowel is inadvertently punctured, no harm should result; withdraw needle and observe.

TABLE 6–23.—THERAPY OF ECTOPIC PREGNANCY*

Untreated, mortality is 69%.
Surgical therapy
Salpingostomy is used for unruptured ampullary gestations.
Segmental resection preferred for gestations within isthmus (ruptured or unruptured so long as patient is stable).
Fimbrial expression for distal ectopic pregnancies already in process of extrusion.
Salpingectomy for ruptured tubes with overt hemorrhage.
Subsequent intrauterine pregnancy rates range from 23% to 72%; repeat ectopic risk is about 1 in 4.
Nonsurgical therapy
Indications for methotrexate dissolution therapy[†]
  Serum hCG < 1,500 mIU/mL
  Adnexal mass < 3 × 3 cm
  Loss of blood into abdomen <100 mL
Leukovorin rescue may follow methotrexate.
Monitor post-treatment hCG levels to identify persistent trophoblastic tissue.

*Adapted from Leach RE, Ory SJ: *J Reprod Med* 1989; 34:324–338.
[†]Adapted from Ory S, Villanueva A, Sand P, et al: *Am J Obstet Gynecol* 1986; 154:1229.

TABLE 6–24.—MANAGEMENT OF THE INCOMPETENT CERVIX

The incidence of this disorder is about 1% and accounts for 20% of second-trimester abortions. Etiologic factors include congenital, cervical laceration of prior delivery, prior surgery on cervix, overzealous D&C or therapeutic abortion, and exposure to DES in utero. Fetal survival rate ranges from 90% *(if detected early)* to 50% *(with advanced cervical dilation).*
Diagnosis
  History of recurrent second trimester loss
  Painless dilation and effacement of the cervix
  Bulging membranes

Feeling of vaginal pressure with associated discharge
Premature rupture of membranes
Gray scale ultrasound reveals:
  Cervical length <3 cm
  Internal os >2 cm wide
  Bulging of membranes into endocervical canal
Treatment
Referral to obstetrician for either:
Medical therapy—cervical cultures for GC, *Chlamydia,* and β-hemolytic
  strep; bed rest; possibly short-term use of NSAIDs
Surgical therapy—cerclage placement
  (McDonald = purse-string with Mersilene band; or Shirodkar =
  submucosal suture)

Third-Trimester Bleeding

TABLE 6–25.—THIRD-TRIMESTER BLEEDING

Any third-trimester bleeding should be presumed due to the placenta and
the fetus should be considered endangered until proved otherwise. As a general
rule, any third-trimester bleeding should be investigated in the hospital where
surgical care is immediately available. The bleeding may be painful or painless.

Common Causes of Third-Trimester Bleeding

Placenta previa—1 in 125 pregnancies. Maternal mortality is 1%, fetal mortality
  is up to 30%.
Abruptio placenta—1 in 100 pregnancies. Maternal mortality is less than 1%,
  fetal mortality is up to 35%.
Marginal sinus rupture—⅓ to ½ of all cases of third-trimester bleeding. Maternal
  mortality is 0, fetal mortality is 4%.
Velamentous insertion of cord/vasa previa—very rare.
  Maternal mortality is 0, condition may be rapidly fatal for fetus.
Ruptured uterus—rare.
Cervical, vaginal, or vulvar lesions.

General Rules

Do not do a vaginal exam in an unprepared setting; do not insert a finger in the
  cervix.
Have blood for transfusion available.
Surgical team should be alerted and standing by before double setup exam is
  attempted.
Try to distinguish maternal from fetal bleeding using APT test.

APT Test

Mix equal parts of blood from vagina and 0.25% sodium hydroxide.
If bleeding is fetal in origin, no color change (fetal hemoglobin resists alkali).
If maternal in origin, turns light brown (maternal hemoglobin is nonresistant).
Also may look for nucleated RBCs (fetal) by Wright's stain.

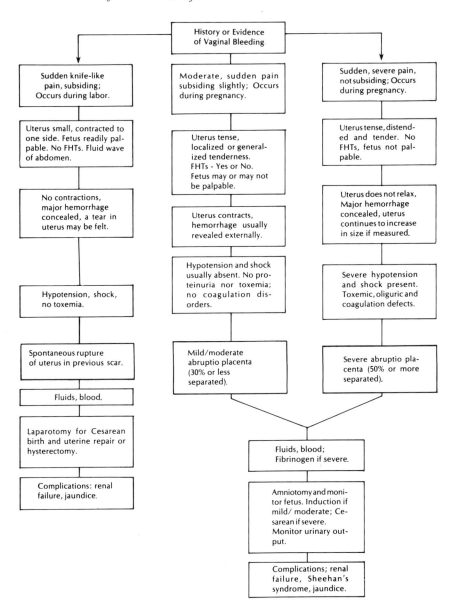

FIG 6–5.
Third-trimester bleeding with pain.

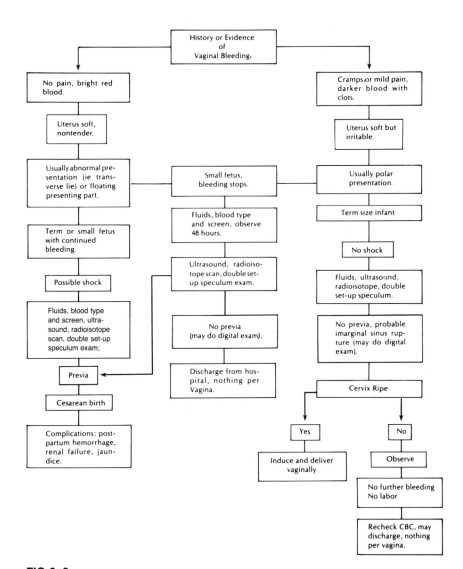

FIG 6–6.
Painless third-trimester bleeding.

TABLE 6–26.—PREMATURE RUPTURE OF MEMBRANES

Spontaneous premature rupture of the membranes (SPROM) usually occurs at or near term and 80% of patients may proceed with labor over the next 24 hours. In some patients SPROM occurs before 38 weeks and may be associated with:
Amniotic bands leading to fetal malformation if <18 weeks.
Chorioamnionitis with maternal and fetal risk for morbidity and mortality.
Premature birth with attendant complications in the infant.

Diagnosis

History of sudden gush of fluid or a continuous leakage.
Palpate uterus for estimation of fetal size and presence of contractions.
Auscultate for FHTs.
Sterile speculum exam to visualize cervix for draining of fluid through os.
Exam of vaginal fluid:
Swab for C&S.
Swab fluid onto glass slide and air dry for fern test—amniotic fluid arborizes and ferns.
Microscopic exam for fetal squamous cells or fat cells which will stain blue with Nile blue sulfate.
Presence of alkaline pH (touching upper ⅓ of vaginal wall in sampling fluid will give false positive).
Meconium staining.
Heat a sample of fluid from external os on a glass slide for 1 minute. Amniotic fluid turns white, endocervical mucus of pregnant patients turns brown.

TABLE 6–27.—OBSERVED MALFORMATIONS USEFUL IN DATING TIMING OF AMNIOTIC RUPTURE*

EVENT IN NORMAL MORPHOGENESIS	DATE BY WHICH STRUCTURE IS DETERMINED	MALFORMATION WHICH RESULTS WHEN PROCESS IS INTERRUPTED
Formation of frontonasal process	28 days	Proboscis
Limb budding	28 days	Absent extremity
Flexion of embryo	28 days	Omphalocele with deficiency of abdominal wall
Fusion of maxillary and medial nasal processes	35 days	Cleft lip
Perforation of nasal passages	45 days	Choanal atresia
Closure of palatal shelves	9 wk	Cleft palate
Return of intestines to abdominal cavity	10 wk	Omphalocele
Eruption of scalp hair	16 wk	Lack of normal hair whorl
Formation of dermal ridges	18 wk	Altered dermal pattern

*From Higginbottom MC: *J Pediatr* 1979; 95:544–549. Reproduced by permission.

TABLE 6–28.—RECOMMENDED MANAGEMENT OF PREMATURE RUPTURE OF
MEMBRANES (PROM) IN PATIENTS WITHOUT EVIDENCE OF AMNIONITIS*

FETUS	MANAGEMENT
<20 wk gestation	Termination of pregnancy
500–749 gm (20–27 wk)	Bed rest; await onset of spontaneous labor; monitor temperature and WBC count
750–1,749 gm (27–33 wk)	Consider corticosteroid induction of pulmonary maturation or nothing per vagina and monitor temperature and WBC count; deliver after 24 hr
1,740–2,249 gm (33–35 wk)	Induction after 16 hr of PROM; do not stop if in labor
2,250 gm (> 35 wk)	Induce within 8–12 hr

*From Iffy L, Kaminetzky H: *Principles and Practice of Obstetrics and Perinatology.* New York, John Wiley & Sons, 1981, vol 2, p 1040. Reproduced by permission.

TABLE 6–29.—DIAGNOSIS OF AMNIONITIS*

CLINICAL	LABORATORY
Fetal tachycardia	Leukocytosis
Maternal tachycardia	Amniotic fluid leukocytes
Maternal fever	Amniotic fluid bacteria (smear)
Uterine tenderness	Amniotic fluid culture (quantitative)
Foul cervical discharge	
Uterine contractions	

*From Iffy L, Kaminetzky H: *Principles and Practice of Obstetrics and Perinatology.* New York, John Wiley & Sons, 1981, vol 2, p 1038. Reproduced by permission.

Premature labor (<36 weeks) resulting in low birth weight is the major cause of neonatal morbidity/mortality. Inhibiting premature labor is possible in 50% of patients with bed rest alone since the supine position increases uterine blood flow, thereby decreasing labor-like activity. When unwanted uterine activity persists, ritodrine may be expected to arrest labor in approximately 60% of patients.

TABLE 6–30.—Recommended Criteria for Selecting Patients for Treatment of Preterm Labor with Ritodrine Hydrochloride*

Qualifying (all)
  Gestation of 20–36 wk
  Fetal weight <2,500 gm
  Regular contractions
  Labor progressing, cervix dilating and/or effacing
Disqualifying
  Active vaginal bleeding
  Eclampsia or severe preeclampsia
  Dead fetus or major fetal malformation incompatible with survival
  Intrauterine infection
  Maternal cardiac disease
  Maternal hyperthyroidism
  Any obstetric or medical condition that contraindicates prolongation of pregnancy
Conditions limiting chances of success
  Incompetent cervix
  Ruptured fetal membranes
  Advanced labor, cervical dilatation more than 4 cm
  Untreated urinary tract infection

  *Adapted from Barden TP, et al: *Obstet Gynecol* 1980; 56:1–6.

TABLE 6–31.—Dosage and Administration of Ritodrine Hydrochloride*

Intravenous infusion
  Monitor maternal heart rate and blood pressure, uterine activity, and fetal heart rate.
  Initial dose, 50–100 µg/min (150 mg diluted in 500 ml of solution gives 300 µg/ml); then increase dose by 50 µg/min every 10 minutes until contractions stop or unacceptable side effects develop.
  Reduce dose if side effects are poorly tolerated. Side effects: maternal tachycardia and hypotension, reduced serum potassium, maternal palpitations, nervousness, nausea, headache.
  Maximum dose: 350 µg/minute.
  Discontinue ritodrine if labor persists at the maximum dose.
  If labor is successfully arrested, continue the infusion for at least 12 hours before beginning oral therapy.
Oral therapy
  Initial dose, 10 mg administered 30 minutes before stopping infusion; then 10 mg every 2 hours, or 20 mg every 4 hours, for 24 hours; then, if the uterus remains quiescent, 10–20 mg every 4–6 hours until further inhibition of labor is not indicated.
  Maximum dose: 120 mg/day.
  If labor recurs during oral administration, infusion may be repeated if the patient is qualified.

  *Adapted from Barden TP, et al: *Obstet Gynecol* 1980; 56:1–6.

TABLE 6-32.—DIAGNOSIS OF HYPERTENSION IN PREGNANCY*

| PARAMETER | PRE-ECLAMPSIA | | ECLAMPSIA |
	MILD	SEVERE	
Blood pressure (on ≥ 2 consecutive readings)	≥ 140/90, or systolic rise of 30 mm Hg or diastolic rise of 15 mm Hg; Mean Arterial Pressure >95 during the second trimester (MAP = diastolic pressure + [systolic − diastolic pressure]/3)	≥ 160/110	Usually elevated
Proteinuria	1–2+ (>300 mg/24 hr)	3–4+ (>5 gm/24 hr)	3–4+
Edema	1–2+ (1 kg or more weight gain)	3–4+	3–4+
Reflexes	Hyperreactive	Markedly hyperreactive with clonus	Convulsions
Other	Headache	Oliguria (<500 ml/24 hr); visual blurring; right upper quadrant or epigastric pain; elevated serum creatinine, ALT, AST levels, uric acid, and thrombocytopenia.	Coma

When these signs appear before the 20th week, consider hydatidiform mole.

From 7% to 10% of all pregnancies are complicated by hypertension; of these, half are due to pre-eclampsia, and half are the result of chronic hypertension.

Many of those who will later develop pre-eclampsia may be predicted by observing blood pressures between 28 and 32 weeks. After 10 to 15 minutes of stabilization in the lateral recumbent position, check blood pressure, then roll patient to the supine position and recheck. This is the Gant rollover test. A rise of 20 mm Hg or more in diastolic pressure has approximately 90% predictive accuracy. Adequate dietary protein intake during pregnancy is perhaps the only preventive measure that can be taken. Some evidence exists for the use of low-dose aspirin therapy.

*Adapted from Carroll J, et al: Complications of Pregnancy. AAFP Home Study Self-Assessment, Monograph 120, Kansas City, Mo, American Academy of Family Physicians, 1989.

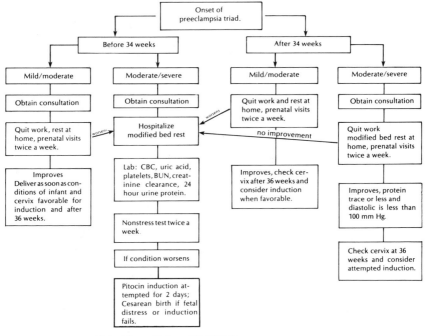

FIG 6–7.
Pre-eclampsia.

During Labor and Delivery of Pre-Eclampsia

* Artificial rupture of membranes as soon as safe and possible
  (unless malpresentation or CPD)
* IV oxytocin induction (see oxytocin induction protocol)
* IV Magnesium Sulfate if hyperreflexic (see magnesium sulfate protocol)
* IV Apresoline if diastolic BP greater than 110 (see apresoline protocol)
* Monitor I & O—output should average 100 cc/3 hrs

TABLE 6–33.—Bishop Scoring of Inducibility of Labor*

	SCORE‡			
FACTOR	0	1	2	3
Dilation (cm)	Closed	1–2	3–4	≥ 5
Effacement (%)	0–30	40–50	60–70	≥ 80
or length (cm)†	4	2–4	1–2	< 1
Station of head from spines (cm)	−3	−2	−1.0	+1, +2
Consistency	Firm	Medium	Soft	
Position of os	Posterior	Mild	Anterior	

*Modified from Romney et al: *The Health Care of Women.* New York, McGraw-Hill Book Co, 1981.
†Use either effacement or length but not both.
‡A score from 0 to 13 indicates increasing ease of inducibility.

TABLE 6–34.—Drug Management Protocols for Pre-eclampsia
and Eclampsia

Magnesium sulfate protocol *(for anticonvulsant and sedation)*
Begin IV infusion of 5% dextrose.
Give 2–4 gm of MgSO$_4$ (10% solution) IV, not to exceed 1.5 ml (150 mg) per min.
Maintain MgSO$_4$ by infusion pump, using 20 gm in 1,000 cc of IV fluid (2% solution).
Usual maintenance dose is 1 gm/hr max. dose 7.5 ml (150 mg) per min. depending on 30-min assessments of reflexes and respirations. Watch urinary output, and if <30 cc/hr, decrease infusion rate.
Have 10% calcium gluconate for IV use at hand to counteract MgSO$_4$ if respiratory depression occurs.
Continue MgSO$_4$ for 24–48 hr after delivery.
Therapeutic serum magnesium up to 7 mg/dl. Higher doses are toxic.
Hydralazine (Apresoline) protocol *(for diastolic BP > 110)*
Give 20 mg of hydralazine diluted in 20 ml of 5% dextrose (1 mg/cc).
Give 5-cc IV bolus over 2–4 min and observe BP for 30 min.
If no decline of BP in 30 min, give 15 cc IV slowly.
Repeat 20-cc dose every 1–2 hr as needed.
Keep diastolic BP around 90 mm Hg.

TABLE 6–35.—Oxytocin Induction Protocol (to Stimulate Onset of Labor)

Begin IV infusion with 5% dextrose.
Monitor externally if cervix is unfavorable for internal monitoring.
Perform amniotomy and attach fetal scalp monitor electrode as soon as presentation is safe/favorable.
A second IV of 1,000 cc of 5% dextrose with 1 ml (10 IU) of oxytocin is connected through an infusion pump and attached piggyback to the first IV tubing. Each 1 cc contains 10 mU of oxytocin.
Start infusion at 0.5 mU/min and increase by 1 mU every 20 min until labor is satisfactory (contractions every 2–3 minutes lasting 60–90 sec).
If infusion pump is unavailable, add 2.5 units to 1,000 cc, giving 2.5 mU/cc; if the apparatus delivers 1 ml every 15 drops, 3 drops/min will equal 0.5 mU/min.
Antidiuretic effect (increase renal tubular absorption of water) may begin around 15 mU/min and reach maximum at 45 mU/min. This may produce water intoxication and convulsions.
The half-life of IV oxytocin is less than 4 minutes, so if overstimulation (uterine contractions with less than 1 minute between) occurs, stop infusion.
Labor induction may also be aided by the prior use of prostaglandin E$_2$ or F$_2$ vaginal suppositories.
Contraindications to induction: Abnormal fetal presentation, absolute fetopelvic disproportion, uterine scar from prior surgery, women of high parity.

TABLE 6–36.—CT PELVIMETRY

Radiation dose is reduced over conventional plain film pelvimetry.
Computer enhancement precludes repeat films because of underexposure or overexposure.
Efficient and highly accurate measurements.
Measurements taken during suspended respiration
>11.0 cm = True conjugate/pelvic inlet (from horizontal pilot scan). Measure from prominence of S_1 to upper region of pubic symphysis.
>12.0 cm = Transverse diameter/widest point of true pelvis (from vertical pilot scan). Measure below ischial spines at widest diameter.
>10.0 cm = Interspinous distance/mid-pelvic diameter (from axial image). Measure between points of ischial spines.

TABLE 6–37.—USE OF THE VACUUM EXTRACTOR FOR PROLONGED SECOND STAGE OF LABOR*

Use of Mityvac device or Silastic cup:
Indications:
    Fetal distress (if delivery imminent)
    Prolonged second stage of labor
    Maternal exhaustion, weak uterine expulsive force
Contraindications:
    Malpresentation (breech, face, brow); must be vertex
    Premature infant
    Intact membranes
    Incomplete cervical dilation; head not engaged
    Presenting part requires rotation
    Cephalopelvic disproportion
    Prior fetal scalp sampling
Technique:
    Connect cup to pump.
    Ascertain fetal head in normal vertex position and well engaged.
    Spread labia, fold cup, and insert into position over posterior fontanelle.
    Sweep finger around edge to check for entrapped maternal tissue.
    Reduce pressure to negative −100 mm Hg.
    With next contraction rapidly reduce pressure to −380–580 mm Hg and begin traction in line with the pelvic axis.
    When contraction subsides, take pressure up to −100 mm Hg.
    Recheck with finger sweep.
    Episiotomy may be needed.
    Once head delivered, remove cup.
Discontinue if:
    Delivery not accomplished after 10 min at maximum pressure or 30 min from start of procedure
    Cup disengages 3 times
    No progress after 3 consecutive pulls
    Fetal scalp traumatized by extractor

Complications:
Injury to maternal tissue (cervix, vaginal wall)
Fourth-degree extension of episiotomy
Cephalhematoma (red or blue circular scalp discoloration)
Skin swelling, petechiae, or injury of fetal scalp
Failure to extract promptly

*Adapted from Epperly TD, Breitinger ER: *Am Fam Physician* 1988; 38:205–210.

TABLE 6–38.—VAGINAL BIRTH AFTER CESAREAN (VBAC) SECTION*

Advantages
Lower maternal morbidity and mortality; shorter hospital stay
Increased maternal satisfaction
Better immediate bonding with the newborn
Less blood loss
Less costly
Disadvantages
Sense of failure if repeat C-section required after labor
Potential for uterine rupture (7% with classical incision/0.5% with low
transverse)
Less safe if 3 or more prior C-sections
Management guidelines for lowering the risk
1. Accurate documentation of number (<3) and type of prior C-sections.
2. Prior incision was low transverse or low vertical not extending into active myometrium.
3. No recurrent indications (e.g., fetal-pelvic disproportion, maternal herpes, hemorrhage, fetal distress, maternal systemic disease, hypertension, uncorrectable uterine inertia, malpresentation).
4. No new indication in current pregnancy (e.g., IUGR, previa, abruption, nonvertex presentation).
5. Patient counseled carefully for informed consent and patient motivation high.
6. Admit patient as soon as signs of active labor appear.
7. Type and screen for 2 units of packed cells.
8. Intravenous line in place during labor.
9. Electronic fetal monitoring during labor's progress.
10. Patient must follow normal course of labor; failure to progress requires repeat C-section.
11. Emergency C-section can be done within 30 minutes of decision and primary physician in constant attendance during labor. Alert surgeon when patient admitted.

*Adapted from Beguin EA: *Female Patient* 1989; 14:119–132, and ACOG Committee on Obstetrics: *Maternal and Fetal Medicine: Guidelines for Vaginal Delivery After Cesarean Birth,* Washington, DC, 1985.

ANTEPARTUM FETAL SURVEILLANCE

TABLE 6–39.—Monitoring Fetal Well-Being

A number of serial antepartum assessments may be used to ensure that the fetus is not adversely affected by the pregnancy.

Indications for assessment
  High-risk pregnancy; SGA; LGA; postdatism; trauma; decrease in fetal movements; prior poor obstetrical performance; diabetes, hypertension, or other chronic maternal condition; antepartum bleeding; suspected fetal abnormality.

Biochemical assessments
  Estriols; minimum urinary value at term is 12 mg/24 hr. Obtain weekly (30–33 wk), then biweekly (34–35 wk), then every 2 days beginning at 36 wks. Norm may be approximated:

$$\text{Minimum} = \left(\frac{\text{Weeks of gestation}}{10}\right)^2 - 4$$

Amniocentesis
  Fluid analyses for meconium or fetal blood and to assess fetal maturity
  Alkaline pH; 98% water + 2% solids
  L/S ratio: 2:1 or more indicates fetal lung maturity (use 2.5:1 for diabetic patients)
  Creatinine: 2 mg/100 ml indicates maturity
  Cells: $\geq$ 25% anuclear cells or $\geq$ 20% fat cells; fetus should weigh > 2,500 gm.
  Foam test: 0.5 cc of normal saline + 1 cc of amniotic fluid + 1 cc 95% ethanol; shake vigorously for 15 sec. Complete bubble ring is positive and indicates maturity; L/S ratio unnecessary.
  Genetic screening may be performed.
  Bilirubin concentration (Rh sensitization)
    Zone I: None to mild fetal effects
    Zone II: Moderate fetal effects
    Zone III: Severe fetal effects

Fetoscopy
  Most accurate for direct exam of fetus and genetic studies. Cannula and trocar placed under ultrasound guidance and sampling of fetal skin and fetal blood taken under direct fiberoptic visualization. Risk of fetal mortality is 7.5%–9.0%. Can lead to premature labor.

Biophysical profile
  Combines five parameters to give score of 0–10 (0 is worst). A score of 8 or 10 indicates fetal well-being. Requires ultrasound.

	Parameter	Score 2	Score 0
Hypoxia/acute stress	Conventional NST*	Reactive	Nonreactive[†]
	Fetal breathing	Sustained for 30 sec	Not sustained for 30 sec.
	Fetal movement	$\geq$ 2 gross body movements (axial rotation) in 20 min	<2 gross body movements

		≥ 1 episode of flex-ion/extension	No flexion/ex-tension
Fetal tone			
Chronic stress	Amniotic fluid volume	≥ 1 pocket 1 × 1 cm	No pocket > 1 cm

*NST = non-stress test.
†NST may be nonreactive if infant sleeping. Try retest after giving orange juice to mother and tapping on her abdomen to interrupt fetal sleep period. See Table 6–40 for interpretation of NST.

Fetal movement counts

Fetus should be noted to move by mother at least 10 times/12 hr period. Have mother count number of movements felt during a 60-min recumbent period 2 hr after main meal. Three to 10 or more movements is normal. Excess movement is not alarming.

TABLE 6–40.—INTERPRETATION OF OXYTOCIN CHALLENGE TEST (OCT) AND NST*

TEST RESULT	INTERPRETATION
OCT	
Negative	No late deceleration of FHR†
Positive	Late decelerations of FHR occurring with 90% of contractions‡
Equivocal	Late decelerations of FHR occurring with <90% of contractions
Unsatisfactory	Unable to interpret
NST	
Reactive	2 or more accelerations of FHR in 30-min period; acceleration defined as increase above baseline FHR of at least 15 bpm, lasting at least 30 sec
Nonreactive	No accelerations of FHR in 30-min period
Equivocal	Only 1 acceleration of FHR in 30-min period
Unsatisfactory	Unable to interpret

*Adapted from Pratt D, et al: *Obstet Gynecol* 1979; 54:419–423.
†FHR = fetal heart rate.
‡Fetal respirations in utero can aid interpretation of the OCT—30–70 breaths/min, episodic, 55%–90% of time. If OCT is positive and fetal breathing movements are normal, there is an 87% chance that OCT is false positive. If there is no fetal breathing, OCT is probably a true positive.

TABLE 6–41.—FETAL HEART RATE MONITORING

Baseline features (between contractions)
Rate
　120–160 bpm (normal)
　<120 bradycardia (heart block, drugs, hypothermia, hypoxia)
　>160 tachycardia (catecholamines, asphyxia, infection, fever, drugs, tachy-
　　dysrhythmia, thyrotoxicosis, prematurity)
Variability
　Short-term or beat-to-beat type, differing serial or adjacent beats.
　Requires fetal scalp lead for reliable interpretation.
　Long-term or sine wave type, > 6 bpm of wavy oscillation;
　3–6 cycles/min.
　Variability normal or decreased (hypoxia, anencephaly, drugs, complete
　　heart block)
Periodic changes
Acceleration (normal with contractions)
Decelerations (see Fig 6–8)
　Early
　　Transient hypoxia, noncompromised fetus.
　Late
　　Maternal hypotension if normal FHR variability. With absent FHR variabil-
　　ity, suspect hypoxia and decompensation.
　Variables
　　Abrupt drop of 60 bpm with quick recovery. Usually reassuring to see
　　"shoulders" of acceleration at onset and end.
　Ominous severe variables
　　>60 bpm drop, >60 bpm baseline, >60 sec long.
　"W" wave type of deceleration
　　Nuchal cord with compression.
Patterns
Reassuring
　All parameters normal
Acute stress
　Normal or abnormal rate, > 6 bpm variability, late or variable decelerations
Prolonged stress
　Normal or abnormal note, < 6 bpm variability, late or variable decelerations
　or absent periodicity
Sinister
　Normal or abnormal rate, absent variability, severe late or variable deceler-
　ations or absent periodicity
Sinusoidal
　Monotonously regular, smooth, sine wave baseline with frequency of
　3–6/min and range of amplitude up to 30 bpm (Rh-isoimmunized fetus,
　acid-base abnormality)
Saltatory
　Excessive variability, bizarre pattern like venous tachycardia in appearance
　(drug use, brief hypoxia)

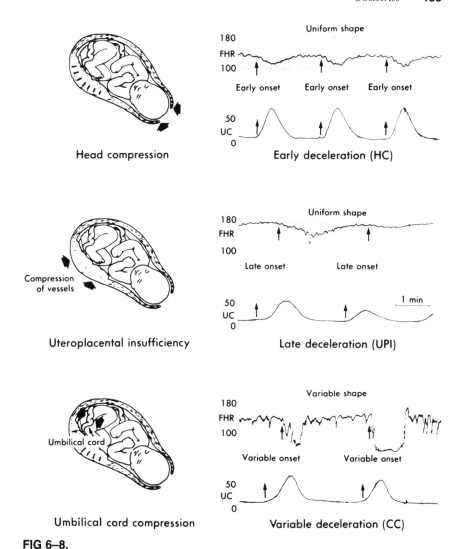

FIG 6–8.
Changes in fetal heart rate patterns due to various causes. (From Hon EH: *An Atlas of Fetal Heart Rate Patterns.* New Haven, Conn, Harty Press, 1968. Reproduced by permission.)

TABLE 6–42.—FETAL SCALP BLOOD SAMPLING

When an abnormal FHR pattern is detected, fetal scalp blood should be sampled:
Cervix is dilated to at least 2 cm with the patient in the dorsal lithotomy position. Contraindications: bleeding disorder, amnionitis.
Endoscope is passed through the cervix and the fetal scalp visualized.
Fetal scalp is swabbed with ethyl chloride to achieve reactive hyperemia, and then with silicon to facilitate blood collection.
A deep puncture, 2–3 mm, is made with a small scalp blade.
Blood is drawn into heparinized pipette or capillary tube. Analyze immediately.
pH requires 50 μl, base deficit 120 μl.
Scalp pH of 7.25–7.35 is acceptable; a progressive decline, or scalp pH <7.2 is ominous.
A difference of 0.15 to 0.19 in maternal-fetal pH is preacidemic.
A pH difference of >0.2 indicates fetal acidemia.
Fetal P_{O_2} is normally 20–25 torr, indicating 50% saturation.
Fetal P_{CO_2} is normally 41–51 torr.

TABLE 6–43.—INTRAUTERINE RESUSCITATION OF DISTRESSED INFANT

Place patient in lateral decubitus position.
Start O_2 by mask.
Start IV with D5W solution; infuse at rate of 125 cc/hr after 200-cc bolus.
Do vaginal exam to check for prolapse of cord, and if found, decompress cord if possible.
Arrest labor if possible; administer a single 250-μg dose of terbutaline by bolus IV injection. If oxytocin is being administered, discontinue it.
Place intrauterine pressure catheter and fetal scalp electrode; discontinue external Doppler tracing.
Administer amnioinfusion 250–500 cc of sterile saline through intrauterine catheter.

LABOR AND DELIVERY

TABLE 6–44.—ASSESSMENT AT ONSET OF LABOR

History: Bleeding; membranes ruptured; green color to fluid; recent illness; headache; nausea or epigastric pain; recent weight gain.
Physical exam: Maternal BP, pulse, temperature; FHTs; breasts; heart sounds; lungs; reflexes; edema; veins of the legs; abdominal exam; costovertebral percussion. Vaginal exam: presenting part; dilation of cervix; descent; BOW.
Laboratory: If prenatal care, none needed. Otherwise, do CBC, VDRL, typing and Rh sensitivity, catheterized urinalysis. Consider fetal vital signs.

TABLE 6–45.—Cervical Dilation: Translating Fingers into Centimeters*

FINGERS	CENTIMETERS
1 (tight)	
1 (loose)	1
2 (tight)	2
2 (loose to slightly spread)	3
2 (spread)	4
1 fingerbreadth of lateral cervix	5–7
½ fingerbreadth of lateral cervix remaining on each side	8
	9
Only anterior cervix palpable	
No palpable cervix	9+ (anterior lip)
	10 (complete dilation)

*From Iffy L, Kaminetzky H: *Principles and Practice of Obstetrics and Perinatology.* New York, John Wiley & Sons, 1981, vol 2, p 818. Reproduced by permission.

TABLE 6–46.—Stages of Labor*

PHASE OF LABOR	DEFINITION	DURATION/RATE	
		Nulliparas	Multiparas
First stage (onset of labor to complete dilation)			
Latent	Slow dilation	21 hr., ≤ 0.5 cm/hr	14 hr., ≤ 0.5 cm/hr
Active			
Acceleration	Usually begins at 4–5 cm	0.6–1.0 cm/hr	0.6–1.0 cm/hr
Maximum slope	Cervix ≥ 5 cm	1.2 cm/hr (ave., 3.0)	1.5 cm/hr (ave., 5.7)
Deceleration	Cervix ≥ 9 cm, but not complete	Descent 1.0 cm/hr (ave., 3.3)	Descent 2.1 cm/hr (ave., 6.6)
Second stage (complete dilation to delivery)		2 hr (ave., 33 min)	45 min (ave., 8.5 min)
Third stage (from delivery of fetus to placenta)		10 min or less	10 min or less
Total labor (onset of labor to delivery of placenta)		25.8 hr (mean, 10.0)	19.5 hr (mean, 6.2)

*Adapted from Iffy L, Kaminetzky H: *Principles and Practice of Obstetrics and Perinatology.* New York, John Wiley & Sons, 1981, vol 2, pp 818–820.

TABLE 6–47.—DYSFUNCTIONAL LABORS: DIAGNOSIS AND MANAGEMENT*

Latent phase disorders (prior to 4 cm of cervical dilation)
Dx: Prolonged latent phase = >20 hr in nulliparas; >14 hr in multiparas
  Etiologies
    Unripe cervix 18%   Sedation 19%   Unknown 17%
    False labor 10%   Anesthesia 7%
    Uterine inertia 9%   CPD rare
  Rx
    False labor observed (10%): Discharge.
    Observed to progress: Expect NSVD or cesarean.
    Fail to progress (5%): Oxytocin stimulation.
Active phase disorders (from ≥4–5 cm of cervical dilation)
Dx: Primary dysfunctional labor = <1.2 cm/hr nullipara; <1.5 cm/hr multipara
  Etiologies
    CPD 28%   Sedation 42%
    Malposition 74%   Anesthesia 14%
  Rx
    CPD: Cesarean delivery.
    Other causes: Observed and 2/3 progress to vaginal delivery.
    If not progressing and suspect uterine inertia, try oxytocin stimulation.
Dx: Secondary arrest of labor = in active phase but without full dilation
  Etiologies
    CPD 45%   Malposition 73%   Exhaustion
    Sedation 63%   Anesthesia 19%
  Rx
    CPD: Cesarean delivery.
    Other causes: Try oxytocin; many will require cesarean.
  Montevideo units can be used to determine the existence of sufficient uterine expulsive forces to accomplish delivery. A minimum of 200–225 Montevideo
units should be sought before cesarean delivery is considered for presumed uterine inertia or cephalopelvic disproportion.
  An intrauterine pressure catheter must be placed:
  1. Count the number of contractions in 10 min.
  2. Determine baseline uterine tone (usually 10–20 mm).
  3. Sum the intensities of all contractions over a 10-min period (to find inten-
     sity, subtract baseline from peak reading of each contraction).
  4. This determination can be repeated several times in an hour and aver-
     aged. For example, 5 contractions occurring over 10 min have a mean
     intensity of 45 mm over baseline and supply 225 Montevideo units.
NOTE: All dysfunctional labors should be monitored with internal fetal scalp electrode and uterine pressure catheter as soon as insertion is possible.

*Adapted from Friedman EA, et al: *Obstet Gynecol* 1965; 25:845.

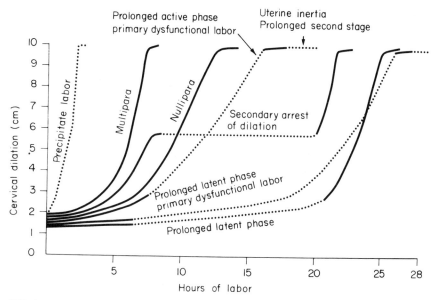

FIG 6–9.
Friedman labor curves typifying various normal and abnormal patterns of cervical dilation. (From Vorherr H: Disorders of uterine function during pregnancy, in Assali NS [ed]: *Pathophysiology of Gestation.* New York, Academic Press, 1972, p 191. Reproduced by permission.)

TABLE 6–48.—PELVIMETRY

X-ray pelvimetry is thought to be rarely indicated: CT pelvimetry is preferable (see Table 6–36), but when it is unavailable and when lack of adequate progress is accompanied by moderate to forceful uterine contractions as documented by electronic monitoring, particularly in a primipara, plainfilm pelvimetry may be indicated.
Mengert's pelvimetry rules:
Inlet: AP ($\sim$11 cm) $\times$ transverse ($\sim$13 cm) = $\sim$145*
Midplane: AP ($\sim$11.5 cm) $\times$ transverse ($\sim$10.5 cm) = $\sim$125*

*Values less than these imply narrow pelvis.

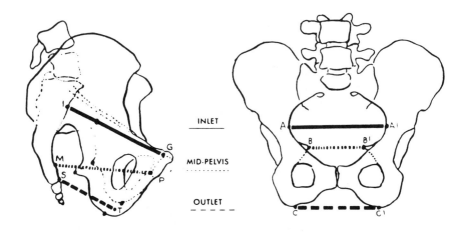

DIAMETERS			AVERAGE NORMAL	AVERAGE TOTAL	LOW NORMAL
ACTUAL INLET	Anteroposterior	1 to G	12.5	25.5	22.0
	Transverse	A to A¹	13.0		
MID-PELVIS	Anteroposterior	M to P	11.5	22.0	20.0
	Transverse (Bispinous)	B to B¹	10.5		
OUTLET	Anteroposterior (Post. Sagittal)	S to T	7.5	18.0	16.0
	Transverse (Bituberal)	C to C¹	10.5		

FIG 6–10.
Standard pelvic diameters. Three levels embody all salient bony landmarks of the true pelvis. (Courtesy of Mercy Hospital X-Ray Department, Iowa City, Ia.)

TABLE 6–49.—GUIDELINES FOR USE OF FORCEPS

Use when:
  Cervix dilated to 10 cm, membranes ruptured
  Fetal head on or just above pelvic floor (below interspinous plane)
  Vertex or face presentation, or after-coming head of breech
Indications
  Obliterated perineal reflex, as with conduction anesthesia
  Maternal heart disease, hypertension, neurologic disorder, vascular anomaly
  Abruptio placenta
  Second stage fails to progress (>2 hr) and head is well into pelvis
  Rotatory arrest
  Some cases of fetal distress
  Breech
Technique
  Forceps selection: Simpson, DeWeese, or Tarnier forceps for primipara with
    fetus with long, molded head
    Elliot (fenestrated) or Tucker-McLane (nonfenestrated) forceps for multipara
      with rounded fetal head

Kielland forceps (no pelvic curve) for rotation
Piper forceps (long blades with deep curve) for breech
Wash genitalia, empty bladder by straight catheterization
Assess position of head, sutures, and fontanelles
Give adequate anesthesia (pudendal, conduction, general)
Insert left blade (lies to your right) first, then right, keeping hand between maternal tissue and blade
Close forceps and check position by palpation of fetal head, maternal vaginal and cervical tissues
Cut generous episiotomy
Gently test pull, then pull for effect in a downward and outward axis moving to almost vertical upward as head emerges, then remove forceps

TABLE 6–50.—APGAR SCORING

PARAMETER	SCORE		
	0	1	2
Heart rate	Absent	Less than 100	100 or greater
Respiratory effort	Absent	Shallow or irregular breathing	Lusty breathing, crying
Reflex irritability*	No response	Little response	Normal response
Muscle tone	Limp	Intermediate	Spontaneously flexed extremities that resist extension
Color	Entirely cyanotic	Partly cyanotic	Entirely pink

*A perfect score is 10. Scores of 6 or less are currently interpreted as significant depression. Any form of stimulation may be used. Commonly, Dr. Apgar evaluated coughing, gagging, or sneezing in response to suctioning of the mouth or nose.

TABLE 6–51.—CLINICAL RESPIRATORY DISTRESS SCORING SYSTEM*

PARAMETER	SCORE		
	0	1	2
Respiratory rate (per minute)	60	60–80	>80 or apneic episodes
Cyanosis	None	In air	In 40% O_2
Retractions	None	Mild	Moderate to severe
Grunting	None	Audible with stethoscope	Audible without stethoscope
Air entry (crying)[a]	Clear	Delayed or decreased	Barely audible

[a]Air entry represents the quality of inspiratory breath sounds as heard in the mid-axillary line. The RDS score is the sum of the individual scores for each of the five observations.
RDS score: 0–3, give oxygen by hood.
4–5, continuous positive pressure breathing.
≥6, Mechanical ventilation required.
*From Downes JJ, Vidyasagar D, Morrow GM, et al.: *Clin Pediatr* 1970; 9:325. Reproduced by permission.

ESTIMATION OF GESTATIONAL AGE BY MATURITY RATING Side 1
Symbols: X - 1st Exam   O - 2nd Exam

Scoring system: Ballard JL, *et al*: A Simplified Assessment of Gestational Age. Pediatr Res 11:374, 1977. Figures adapted from Sweet AY in Care of the High-Risk Infant by MH Klaus and AA Fanaroff, "Classification of the Low-Birth-Weight Infant" by AY Sweet in Care of the High-Risk Infant by MH Klaus and AA Fanaroff, WB Saunders Co, Philadelphia, 1977, p. 47.

NEUROMUSCULAR MATURITY

	0	1	2	3	4	5
Posture						
Square Window (Wrist)	90°	60°	45°	30°	0°	
Arm Recoil	180°		100°-180°	90°-100°	< 90°	
Popliteal Angle	180°	160°	130°	110°	90°	< 90°
Scarf Sign						
Heel to Ear						

PHYSICAL MATURITY

	0	1	2	3	4	5
SKIN	gelatinous red, transparent	smooth pink, visible veins	superficial peeling &/or rash, few veins	cracking pale area, rare veins	parchment, deep cracking, no vessels	leathery, cracked, wrinkled
LANUGO	none	abundant	thinning	bald areas	mostly bald	
PLANTAR CREASES	no crease	faint red marks	anterior transverse crease only	creases 2/3	creases cover entire sole	
BREAST	barely percept.	flat areola, no bud	stippled areola, 1–2 mm bud	raised areola, 3–4 mm bud	full areola, 5–10 mm bud	
EAR	pinna flat, stays folded	sl. curved pinna, soft with slow recoil	well-curv. pinna, soft but ready recoil	formed & firm with instant recoil	thick cartilage, ear stiff	
GENITALS Male	scrotum empty, no rugae		testes descending, few rugae	testes down, good rugae	testes pendulous, deep rugae	
GENITALS Female	prominent clitoris & labia minora		majora & minora equally prominent	majora large, minora small	clitoris & minora completely covered	

Gestation by Dates _____ wks

Birth Date _____ Hour _____ am / pm

APGAR _____ 1 min _____ 5 min

MATURITY RATING

Score	Wks
5	26
10	28
15	30
20	32
25	34
30	36
35	38
40	40
45	42
50	44

SCORING SECTION

	1st Exam=X	2nd Exam=O
Estimating Gest Age by Maturity Rating	____ Weeks	____ Weeks
Time of Exam	Date ____ am Hour ____ pm	Date ____ am Hour ____ pm
Age at Exam	____ Hours	____ Hours
Signature of Examiner	____ M.D.	____ M.D.

FIG 6–11.
Newborn maturity rating and classification. Estimation of gestational age by maturity rating. *X*, first exam; *O*, second exam. (Scoring system from Ballard JL, et al: A simplified assessment of gestational age. *Pediatr Res* 1977; 11:374. Figures adapted from Sweet AY: Classification of the low-birth-weight infant, in Klaus MH, Fanaroff AA: *Care of the High-Risk Infant*. Philadelphia, WB Saunders Co, 1977, p 47.)

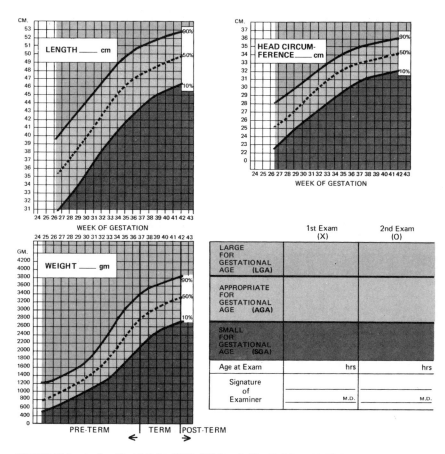

Lubchenco LC, Hansman C, and Boyd E: Pediatr 37:403, 1966; Battaglia FC, and Lubchenco LC: J Pediatr 71:159, 1967.

FIG 6–12.

Classification of newborns based on maturity and intrauterine growth. *X*, first exam; *O*, second exam. (From Lubchenco LC, Hansman C, Boyd E: *Pediatrics* 1966; 37:403, and Battaglia FC, Lubchenco LC: *J Pediatr* 1967; 71:159. Reproduced by permission of CV Mosby Co and the American Academy of Pediatrics, which portion is ©1966, American Academy of Pediatrics.)

TABLE 6–52.—MATERNAL AND FETAL INDICATIONS FOR CESAREAN SECTION*

MATERNAL OR FETAL CONDITION	ABSOLUTE INDICATION	STRONG INDICATION	MODERATE INDICATION	WEAK INDICATION	CONTRAINDICATION
Prolapsed cord	Undeliverable		Deliverable		
High-risk pregnancy (diabetes, etc.)		Positive stress test		Questionable stress test	
Abnormal monitoring patterns		Definite		Equivocal	
Hypertensive disease		Fetal distress	Patient not severely ill		Very ill patient, unfit for immediate surgery
Abruptio placentae	Severe abruption	Severe abruption Fetus undeliverable		Mild abruption (marginal—no indication)	Clotting disorder Fetus deliverable
Cephalopelvic disproportion	Severe	Small pelvis	Mild		
Instead of midforceps delivery				Epidural anesthesia	
Breech	Size-position progress			Frank, average size Good progress	
Multiple birth	Viable triplets, etc.		Twins		
Premature breech		Viable			

Placenta previa	Total or partial	Lateral	Low-lying		
Abnormal presentation of fetus	Transverse Face-posterior	Transverse Face-posterior		Brow Face-anterior	
Maternal infection		Herpes; fetus not infected			Severe infection (special operation)
Cervix unfavorable				Attempt induction	
Dead fetus					No indication
Nonviable fetus					No indication
Obstruction of birth canal	Pelvic mass or tumor				
Vascular disease			Previous cerebral hemorrhage from aneurysm		
Cervical neoplasia	Invasive carcinoma			Noninvasive carcinoma in situ	
Cardiac disease		Obstetric indications only			
Previous pelvic injury					
Fistula	Vesicovaginal				
Cesarean section	Recurring indication (e.g., CPD)		Nonrecurring indication (e.g., previa)		Not indicated per se

*Adapted from Iffy L, Kaminetzky H: *Principles and Practice of Obstetrics and Perinatology.* New York, John Wiley & Sons, 1981, vol 2, pp 1536, 1537.

POSTPARTUM MATERNAL CARE

TABLE 6–53.—POSTPARTUM MATERNAL CARE

General

Control uterine atony.

Estimated blood loss should be 250–500 ml.

Postpartum hemorrhage is defined as 500 ml or more.

Inspect cervix, vagina, and perineum, provide hemostasis and repair (3%–5% incidence of significant lacerations with normal delivery; 10%–15% incidence after forceps use).

Uterine atony

Abdominal uterine massage, repeat every 15 minutes.

Bimanual compression; express clots.

Give oxytocin, 10 units IM (after placenta delivery to avoid entrapment).

Start IV, add 20 units of oxytocin to 1,000 cc and give 20–50 mU/min.

Ergot drugs may be added if no hypertension: ergonovine or methylergonovine, 0.2 mg orally or IM.

If uterine hemorrhage continues, explore uterine cavity under anesthesia for retained placenta and give volume expanders, oxygen, and blood replacement.

MAST trousers may be used on legs for therapy of shock.

Routine postpartum orders

Observe vital signs, fundus, and perineum for hemorrhage every 15 minutes for 2 hours, then every 30 minutes for 2 hours, then every 60 minutes for 4 hours, then every 8 hours if stable. Patient's temperature should be checked at least daily.

Uterine massage every 15 minutes for 2 hours and as needed thereafter.

Patient may ambulate as possible, at first with assistance. Encourage activity.

If patient unable to void in 6 hours following delivery, may be catheterized.

Prescribe general lactating diet (increased protein and fluids).

Prescribe tight breast binder and ice to breasts for engorgement symptoms if patient is not nursing.

If patient is breastfeeding on demand of infant, begin as soon as possible after delivery.

Perineal care: ice bags to perineum for first 12 hours, followed by warm sitz baths as needed. Perineal pads used with Tucks® applied to anal area and perineum.

Stool softener and laxatives used as needed.

Analgesics as needed (acetaminophen with or without codeine). The appearance of fever may be masked.

If mother is Rh negative, check infant cord blood for type, Rh, and direct Coombs test. If infant is Rh positive, administer appropriate dose of RhoGAM to mother.

Recheck hemoglobin and hematocrit on 2d postpartum day; may need to begin iron replacement.

Ensure appropriate bonding and interaction of parents with newborn.

Appointments made for follow-up of infant (2 and 4 wk) and mother (4 wk).

Discharge on 3d postpartum day (or before) if no contraindications; instruct in contraception, infant care, danger signals of puerperium.

TABLE 6–54.—Protocol for Administration of RhoGAM*

OFFICE	BLOOD BANK
Initial Visit	
Draw clotted blood for ABO group, Rh type, and antibody screening test.	If patient is Rh negative and antibody screen is negative for anti-Rh$_o$ (D), report as candidate for RhoGAM at 28 weeks and at delivery
28 Weeks	
If patient Rh negative: Draw clotted blood for antibody screen. Inject RhoGAM, 300 microgram dose	If antibody screen is negative or antibody other than anti-Rh$_o$ (D) is detected, report as candidate for RhoGAM at delivery if infant is not Rh negative.
Following Delivery	
Collect mother's blood and cord blood. Inject RhoGAM, 300-μg dose.	Perform fetal cell screen on maternal sample using micro-D^u procedure. Type cord blood. If not Rh negative (D and D^u negative), issue appropriate amount of RhoGAM.

*Modified from *Advances in Blood Group Antigens and Antibodies: Managing Changes in Rh Immune Globulin Utilization.* Raritan, NJ, Ortho Diagnostic Systems, 1981.

LACTATION

TABLE 6–55.—Lactation

Milk production occurs in stages which may be recognized by the nutritional content of the milk. Colostrum, secreted from 0 to 5 days after birth, contains 55–60 kcal/100 gm. Maturation of the milk occurs through transition milk (5–10 days), immature milk (10–30 days), to mature milk (>30 days), which contains 65–75 kcal/100 gm.

Milk letdown may be encouraged by:
Increased amount of fluid intake
Heat to the breasts
Relaxation exercises (yoga, Lamaze, etc.) and quiet rest
Gentle breast massage or caress
Increased frequency of suckling
Syntocinon® nasal spray (one spray in each nostril, 2–3 min prior to nursing)

TABLE 6–56.—MANAGEMENT OF BREAST-FEEDING IN THE PRESENCE OF MATERNAL INFECTION

ORGANISM	CONDITION	ISOLATE FROM MOTHER
Bacteria	Premature rupture of membranes; >24 hr without fever:	
	Full-term infant	No
	Premature infant	No
	Maternal fever > 38°C twice, 4 hr apart, 24 hr before to 24 hr after delivery, or endometritis; full-term or premature infant	Yes, until mother afebrile for 24 hr
Salmonella, Shigella, Staphylococcus, Group B β- Streptococcus	Mother with possible cervical culture but otherwise negative obstetric history	No No No
	Mother with possible cervical culture and obstetric history of fever, premature rupture of membranes >24 hr, fetal distress, meconium, low Apgar score, any symptoms of prematurity	No
	Infant with surface colonizing:	
	Negative history and physical exam	No
	With PROM or maternal infection	No
Group A Streptococcus	Mother with infection	Yes
Gonorrhea	Mother with positive smear or culture; infant well	No
	Infant with conjunctivitis	No
Syphilis	Mother with positive VDRL or clinical disease not treated	Only if mother has second-degree disease or with skin lesions
	Mother treated	No
Tuberculosis	Mother with inactive disease	No
Hepatitis	Mother had in first trimester, well at delivery	No
	Mother with active hepatitis at delivery or in third trimester	No, may room-in after good handwash technique followed
	Mother is chronic carrier	No
Protozoa		
Toxoplasma	Toxoplasmosis	No

MOTHER CAN VISIT NURSERY	MOTHER CAN BREAST-FEED	IMMEDIATE TREATMENT	CONTACT WITH PREGNANT WOMEN ALLOWED
Yes	Yes	Observe	Yes
Yes	Yes	Treat with ampicillin and kanamycin	Yes
No, until mother afebrile for 24 hr	No, until mother afebrile for 24 hr	Treat with ampicillin and kanamycin	Yes
Yes, if culture negative	Yes, if culture negative	In most cases	Yes
Yes	Yes	Yes	Yes
Yes	Yes		Yes
Yes	Yes, after treatment	Treat with ampicillin and kanamycin	Yes
Yes	Yes	Observe	Yes
Yes	Yes	Treat with penicillin	Yes
Not in acute stage	Not in acute stage, after 24 hr treatment	Prophylactic penicillin for 10 days	Yes
Yes, after treatment	Yes, after treatment	AgNO$_3$ to the eyes, once in delivery room and once in nursery	Yes
Yes, after treatment	Yes, after treatment	Penicillin IM or IV, plus chloramphenicol drops topically	Yes
No, if skin lesions; yes otherwise	Yes	Penicillin IM or IV after workup done; follow-up after discharge	Yes
Yes	Yes		Yes
Yes	Yes	Consider BCG if follow up in doubt	Yes
Yes	Yes		Yes
No	No	Pooled globulin or hyperimmune if available	Yes
Yes, not kiss other infants	Ask for infectious disease opinion		Yes
Yes	Yes		No

TABLE 6–57.—EFFECTS OF DRUGS MOTHERS INGEST ON NURSING INFANTS*

DRUGS	CONTRAINDICATED	EFFECTS ON INFANT	SAFE	UNCERTAIN: USE WITH CAUTION	EFFECTS ON INFANT
Analgesics			Acetaminophen, propoxyphene, morphine, codeine; meperidine; aspirin in small doses	Aspirin in large doses	May cause bleeding problems
Anticoagulants	Ethyl biscoumacetate, phenindione	May cause bleeding problems	Warfarin sodium, heparin (not excreted in breast milk)		
Antidiabetics			Insulin		
Antihistamines			All		
Antihyper-tensives	Reserpine	May cause lethargy, diarrhea, nasal congestion	Guanethidine, propranolol		
Anti-infectives				Antibiotics Sulfonamides, chloramphenicol, nalidixic acid	May cause methemoglobinemia or hypnotic effects May cause hemolytic anemia; may affect infant's bone marrow

Antimicrobials	Isoniazid	May cause peripheral neuropathy, hepatitis, vomiting	Tetracyclines, metronidazole, streptomycin	Could cause teeth staining and bone retardation
Antineoplastics			All	Inconclusive results; experts disagree
Antithyroid drugs	Radioactive iodine	May be destructive to the infant's thyroid synthesis and release	Propylthiouracil	
Autonomic drugs	Atropine, benztropine mesylate, trihexiphenidyl	May cause constipation and inhibit lactation		
Cathartics	Anthroquinone derivatives	May affect GI tracts of mother and infant	Most cathartics are not absorbed	
Diuretics			Chlorothiazide	Could cause thrombocytopenia
Hypnotics			Chloral hydrate, flurazepam	
Oral contraceptives	Estrogens	May reduce lactation; some cause fetal gynecomastia		

Continued.

TABLE 6–57.—Continued

DRUGS	CONTRAINDICATED	EFFECTS ON INFANT	SAFE	UNCERTAIN: USE WITH CAUTION	EFFECTS ON INFANT
Psychotropic agents	Lithium carbonate	May cause hypotonia, hypothermia, and episodes of cyanosis	Chlordiazepoxide, chlorpromazine	Haloperidol Marijuana, theophylline, reserpine	Occasionally causes restlessness
Sedative hypnotics	Diazepam (regular use) Meprobamate	May cause lethargy, weight loss, changes in EEG	Diazepam (occasional use)		
Steroids	All except low doses (see "safe")	May suppress growth and interfere with endogenous corticosteroid production	Prednisone, prednisolone (in low doses)		
Miscellaneous	Dihydrotachysterol Ergot alkaloids (in migraine preparations) Gold thioglucose	May cause renal calcification May cause symptoms of ergotism May cause rashes, nephritis, hepatitis, hematologic alterations			

*Adapted from Guidelines to Professional Pharmacy.

7 Cardiology

Edward T. Bope, M.D.

EVALUATION OF HEART DISEASE

TABLE 7–1.—EVALUATION OF THE PATIENT WITH HEART DISEASE*

A variety of studies have emerged to help in the diagnosis of heart disease. These are not to replace a good history and physical exam, but to complement them. The Criteria Committee of the New York Heart Association suggests that cardiac diagnosis be recorded in the following standardized manner:
Etiology
Anatomy
Physiology
Cardiac status
    Class 1 Uncompromised
    Class 2 Slightly compromised
    Class 3 Moderately compromised
    Class 4 Severely compromised
Prognosis
    Class 1 Good
    Class 2 Good with therapy
    Class 3 Fair with therapy
    Class 4 Guarded despite therapy

*From The Criteria Committee of the New York Heart Association: *Nomenclature and Criteria for Diagnosis of Diseases of the Heart and Great Vessels,* ed 8. New York, New York Heart Association, 1979. Reproduced by permission.

TABLE 7–2.—AUSCULTATION

Each heart sound should be evaluated separately. Begin with S_1 and S_2 and evaluate the splitting of S2. Figure 7–1 illustrates the patterns of splitting and their diagnostic significance.
There are several other diastolic filling sounds with which you should be familiar and be able to identify because of their pathologic significance. The following description refers to Figure 7–2:
a. An atrial sound *(A)* occurs in presystole in patients with hypertension, coronary artery disease, and long P-R intervals.

Continued.

TABLE 7–2.—Continued

b. A filling sound may occur in early diastole in children and young adults, but it disappears with age. This sound is called a normal third heart sound. When it is heard in middle age, it is called a ventricular gallop and indicates myocardial failure or AV valve incompetence.

c. In constrictive pericarditis, a sound occurs in early diastole *(K)* which is earlier, louder, and higher-pitched than the usual ventricular gallop but is, in fact, an accelerated form of this filling sound.

d. If both an atrial *(A)* and ventricular *(V)* gallop are present, a quadruple rhythm results.

e. At faster heart rates these sounds occurring in rapid succession may give the illusion of a mid-diastolic rumble.

f. When the heart rate is sufficiently fast, the two rapid phases of ventricular filling reinforce each other and a very loud summation gallop (SG) may appear. This sound may be louder than the other two heart sounds.

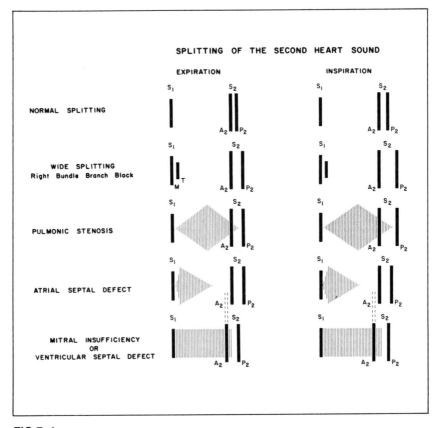

FIG 7–1.
Patterns of splitting of S_2 and their significance. (From *Examination of the Heart,* part 4: Auscultation. Dallas, American Heart Association, 1974. Reproduced by permission.)

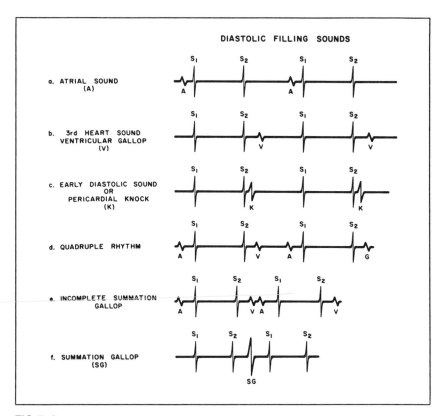

FIG 7–2.
Diastolic filling sounds. See text for explanation. (From Leonard JJ, Kroetz FW: *Examination of the Heart,* part 4. Dallas, American Heart Association, 1967. Reproduced by permission.)

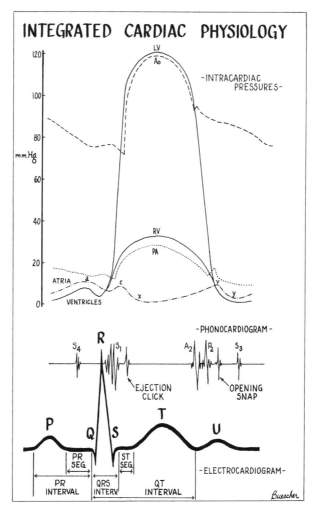

FIG 7–3.
Integrated cardiac physiology. (From Cole CH [ed]: *The Harriet Lane Handbook*, ed 10. Chicago, Year Book Medical Publishers, 1985. Reproduced by permission.)

TABLE 7-3.—HEART MURMURS

Murmurs should be identified by their length, intensity (grade), the area in which they are best heard, and the area toward which they radiate.

Grading of murmurs (classification of Freeman and Levine):

Grade I—Murmur very difficult to hear and not immediately apparent.

II—Faintest murmur immediately heard.

III—Intermediate intensity.

IV—Intermediate intensity with thrill.

V—Loudest murmur heard with rim of stethoscope touching skin.

VI—Murmur audible with stethoscope removed from chest wall.

Nonorganic (Innocent):

Systolic. Usually heard at the pulmonic area, second left interspace or at the left border of the sternum or in the mitral area. It is not transmitted and is unaccompanied by hypertrophy of the heart or any other evidence of abnormality. It is usually heard only in the sitting position and changes with position.

Organic:

Mitral regurgitation: Systolic. Maximum intensity at apex, transmitted to axilla, heard behind at angle of scapula. Accentuation of pulmonic second sound.

Aortic stenosis. Systolic. Maximum intensity at right second interspace close to sternum. Transmitted upward into great vessels of the neck.

Aortic regurgitation. Diastolic. Replaces or follows the second sound. Maximum intensity at second right interspace, radiating to third and downward.

Mitral stenosis. Presystolic, running into snapping first sound. Heart in mitral area. Not transmitted. Usually accompanied by a thrill along left margin of heart area.

TABLE 7–4.—HEART MURMURS AND MANEUVERS TO DIFFERENTIATE THEM

MANEUVER	AS	IHSS	MR	MVP
Isometric—squeeze hands	Decrease	Decrease	Increase	No change
Valsalva—causes decreased ventricular filling	Decrease	Increase	Decrease	Increase
Squatting—increases venous return and arteriolar resistance	No change	Decrease	Increase	Decrease
Standing—decreases heart size	Increase	Increase	Decrease	Increase
Amyl nitrite—decrease in left ventricular volume and pressure	Increase	Increase	Decrease	Increase

ELECTROCARDIOGRAPHY

TABLE 7–5.—Electrocardiography

Electrocardiography (ECG) is a noninvasive procedure that provides information about heart rate, rhythm, state of the myocardium, the presence or absence of hypertrophy, ischemia, necrosis or abnormalities of conduction.
Rate.—The cardiac rate can be determined in two ways: (1) Count the number of dark EKG lines between R waves and divide this number into 300. (2) Many use the method illustrated in Figure 7–4 and memorize the underlined landmarks for quick reference (e.g., 300, 150, 100, 75, 60, 50, 43).
Rhythm.—Is the rhythm regular or irregular?

Rhythm	P Wave
Sinus arrhythmia	Identical
Wandering pacemaker	Different shapes
Atrial fibrillation	No P waves discernible

# of small squares	Rate/min.	# of small squares	Rate/min.	# of small squares	Rate/min.
5	300	**20**	75	**35**	43
6	250	21	71	36	42
7	214	22	68	37	41
8	187	23	65	38	39
9	167	24	62	39	38
10	150	**25**	60	**40**	37
11	136	26	58	41	37
12	125	27	56	42	36
13	175	28	54	43	35
14	107	29	52	44	34
15	100	**30**	50	**45**	33
16	94	31	48	46	33
17	88	32	47	47	32
18	83	33	45	48	31
19	79	34	44	49	31
				50	30

FIG 7–4.
Guide for determining ECG rate. Count the number of small squares between R waves and use this table to convert to heart rate per minute.

TABLE 7–6.—ELECTRICAL EVENTS

Evaluate each electrical component of the ECG using the following tables of normal values.

P wave
Upright in I, II, and aV$_F$
Inverted in III, aV$_R$
Amplitude should not exceed 2 or 3 mm.

PR interval
Becomes shorter as the rate rises.

Age	Average Interval
1 yr	0.11 sec
6 yr	0.13 sec
12 yr	0.14 sec
Adult	0.12–0.20 sec

QRS complex
Normal: 0.04–0.10 sec
Normal variant or conduction delay: 0.10–0.12 sec
Right or left bundle-branch block: 0.12 sec

If the QRS is greater than 0.12 sec and occurs before the expected sinus beat, the following may be helpful in diagnosis:

Feature	RBBB Morphology	QRS	Direction of Initial 0.02 sec of QRS
Ventricular ectopy	60%–70%	Monophasic in V$_1$ or triphasic R > R′	Different from normal beats
Supraventricular beat with aberrancy	90%	Triphasic R < R′	Same as normal beat

PR Prolongations

A delay or interruption in conduction between the atria and ventricles.

● First degree-atrioventricular block
PR interval greater than 0.20 seconds
● Second- and third-degree atrioventricular block
Rate or number of dominant atrial waves is greater than number of QRS complexes

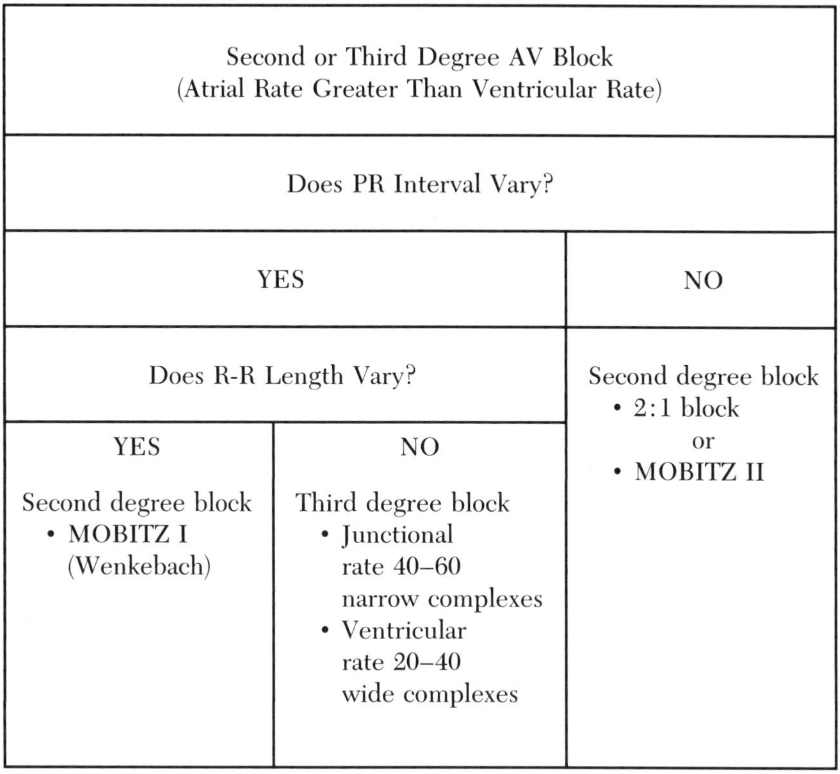

Second or Third Degree AV Block (Atrial Rate Greater Than Ventricular Rate)		
Does PR Interval Vary?		
YES		NO
Does R-R Length Vary?		Second degree block • 2:1 block or • MOBITZ II
YES Second degree block • MOBITZ I (Wenkebach)	NO Third degree block • Junctional rate 40–60 narrow complexes • Ventricular rate 20–40 wide complexes	

FIG 7–5.
AV block.

The T wave

TABLE 7–7.—NORMAL ORIENTATION OF T WAVE*

AGE	V_1, V_2	aV_F	I, V_5, V_6
Birth to 1 day	Either	Positive	Either
1–4 days	Either	Positive	Positive
4 days to 12 yr	Negative	Positive	Positive
Adult	Positive	Positive	Positive

*Adapted from Cole CH (ed): *The Harriet Lane Handbook,* ed 10. Chicago, Year Book Medical Publishers, 1981.

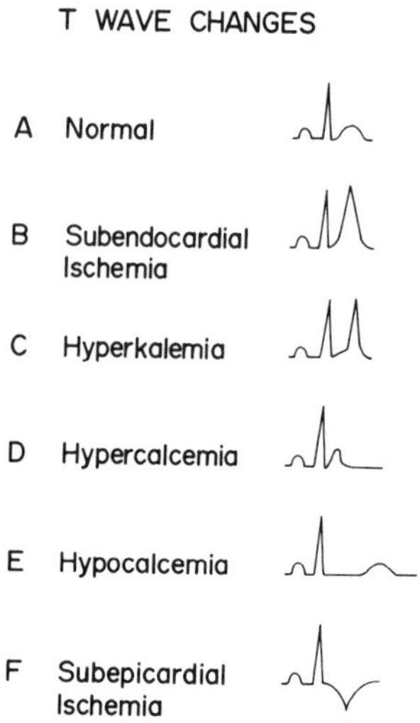

T WAVE CHANGES

A   Normal

B   Subendocardial
    Ischemia

C   Hyperkalemia

D   Hypercalcemia

E   Hypocalcemia

F   Subepicardial
    Ischemia

FIG 7–6.
T wave changes in normal and abnormal conditions.
(From Gazes PC: *Clinical Cardiology: A Bedside
Approach,* ed 2. Chicago, Year Book Medical
Publishers, 1983. Reproduced by permission.)

The S-T Segment

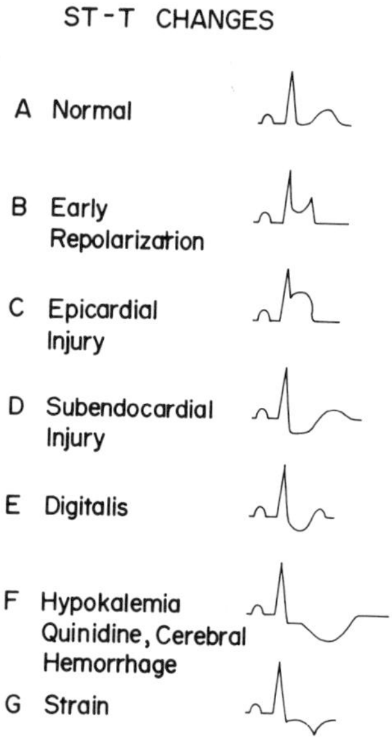

FIG 7–7.
ST-T wave changes in normal and abnormal conditions.
(From Gazes PC: *Clinical Cardiology: A Bedside
Approach,* ed. 2. Chicago, Year Book Medical
Publishers, Inc., 1983. Reproduced by permission.)

ST-T CHANGES

A   Normal

B   Early
    Repolarization

C   Epicardial
    Injury

D   Subendocardial
    Injury

E   Digitalis

F   Hypokalemia
    Quinidine, Cerebral
    Hemorrhage

G   Strain

Normal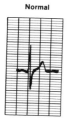

Ischemia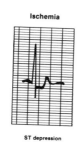

ST depression

Injury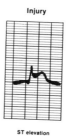

ST elevation

Infarction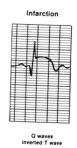

Q waves
inverted T wave

FIG 7–8.
Progression of ST-T wave in infarction.

TABLE 7–8.—QT INTERVAL*

HEART RATE PER MINUTE	MEN AND CHILDREN (sec)	WOMEN (sec)	UPPER LIMITS OF THE NORMAL	
			Men and Children (sec)	Women (sec)
40.0	0.449	0.461	0.491	0.503
43.0	0.438	0.450	0.479	0.491
46.0	0.426	0.438	0.466	0.478
48.0	0.420	0.432	0.460	0.471
50.0	0.414	0.425	0.453	0.464
52.0	0.407	0.418	0.445	0.456
54.5	0.400	0.411	0.438	0.449
57.0	0.393	0.404	0.430	0.441
60.0	0.386	0.396	0.422	0.432
63.0	0.378	0.388	0.413	0.423
66.5	0.370	0.380	0.404	0.414
70.5	0.361	0.371	0.395	0.405
75.0	0.352	0.362	0.384	0.394
80.0	0.342	0.352	0.374	0.384
86.0	0.332	0.341	0.363	0.372
92.5	0.321	0.330	0.351	0.360
100.0	0.310	0.318	0.338	0.347
109.0	0.297	0.305	0.325	0.333
120.0	0.283	0.291	0.310	0.317
133.0	0.268	0.276	0.294	0.301
150.0	0.252	0.258	0.275	0.282
172.0	0.234	0.240	0.255	0.262

*From Ashman R, Hull E: *Essentials of Electrocardiography.* New York, Macmillan Publishing Co, 1945. Reproduced by permission.

TABLE 7–9.—Drugs That Will Affect the ECG

DRUG	EFFECT	TOXICITY
Disopyramide	Prolongation of QT	AV block
	Widened QRS	Ventricular dysrhythmia
Quinidine	Prolonged QT	Intraventricular block
	Widened QRS	Ventricular dysrhythmia
Procainamide	Prolonged QT	Intraventricular block
	Widened QRS	Ventricular dysrhythmia
Digitalis	Depression of ST segment	PVCs, PAT, AV block 1, 2, 3
Tricyclic antidepressants	Prolonged conduction time	Dysrhythmia, tachycardia
Encainide	Widened QRS	Ventricular dysrhythmia
	Unchanged or prolonged QT	AV block
Flecainide	Widened QRS	Ventricular dysrhythmia
	Prolonged PR	1° AV block
	Unchanged or prolonged QT	Intraventricular block
Amiodarone	Prolonged PR	Ventricular dysrhythmia
	Prolonged QT	SA node dysfunction AV block Intraventricular block

TABLE 7–10.—Defects in Conduction: QRS
Prolongation

Right bundle-branch block (RBBB)
   QRS > 0.12 sec
   V_1—Late intrinsicoid, M-shaped QRS
   V_6—Early intrinsicoid
   I—Wide S wave
Incomplete RBBB
   Same as above except QRS < 0.12
Left bundle-branch block (LBBB)
   QRS > 0.12
   V_1—Early intrinsicoid
   V_6—Late intrinsicoid, no Q wave
   I—Monophasic R
Left anterior hemiblock
   Normal QRS duration
   Left axis deviation
   Small Q in I, and R in III

Left posterior hemiblock
Normal QRS duration
Right axis deviation
Small R in I and Q in III
No evidence of right ventricular hypertrophy
Right and left bundle-branch block are associated with:
Coronary artery disease
Hypertensive cardiovascular disease
Rheumatic heart disease
Cardiomyopathy
Myocarditis
Nonspecific fibrosis
Trauma

RBBB Only	LBBB Only
Congenital heart disease	Aortic valvular disease
Pulmonary embolism	Short left main coronary artery
Cor pulmonale	

TABLE 7–11.—Cause of Axis Deviation

RIGHT	LEFT
Normal variation	Normal variation
Mechanical shifts: inspiration, emphysema	Mechanical shifts: expiration, high diaphragm (e.g., pregnancy)
Right bundle-branch block	
Right ventricular hypertrophy	Left anterior hemiblock
Left posterior hemiblock	Left bundle-branch block
Dextrocardia	Congenital lesions
Left ventricular ectopic rhythms	Wolf-Parkinson-White syndrome
Some right ventricular ectopic rhythms	Emphysema, hyperkalemia, right ventricular ectopic beats

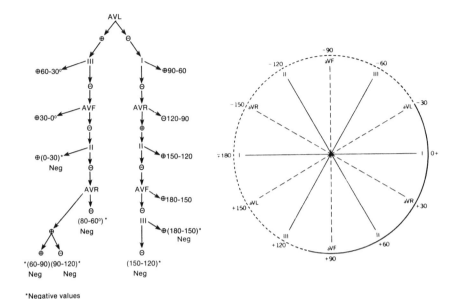

*Negative values

FIG 7–9.
Vector flowsheet and axis diagram.

TABLE 7–12.—DETERMINATION OF AXIS

To determine the axis, proceed through the vector flow sheet shown in Figure 7–9 looking at each QRS complex on the ECG to decide if it is positive or negative. Start with the QRS in aVL. Work through each QRS in the limb of the flowsheet until a range is identified, then go to the axis diagram to find the area of the range you have determined.

Look at each lead on the ECT bounding that range to determine which has the QRS of greatest magnitude. The vector is in the direction closest to that lead.

Example:

Range: −60 to −90

aVF's QRS is greater in magnitude than III's → vector is −90.

Interpretation of axis

−30 to +90	Normal axis
−30 to −90	Left axis deviation
+90 to +180	Right axis deviation
−90 to +180	Marked right axis deviation

MANAGING AMBULATORY ANGINA

TABLE 7–13.—ANTIANGINAL DRUG THERAPY: NITRATES

Treatment of angina usually includes a combination of medications. Nitrates are usually first line.

NITRATES	DOSE	DURATION
NTG		
Sublingual (SL)	0.15–0.6 mg PRN	20–30 min
Transmucosal	1–2 mg t.i.d.	4–5 hr
Ointment	½–2 in. (7.5–30 mg)	q 4–6 hr
Sustained release	6.5–19.5 mg	q 8–12 hr
Transdermal	2.5–15 mg	8–18 hr[†]
Isosorbide		
Oral	10–60 mg	4–5 hr

SL and chewable isosorbide have relatively short action and provide little advantage.

[†]Evidence suggests there should be an 8–10-hr nitrate-free interval to limit tolerance.

TABLE 7–14.—ANTIANGINAL DRUG THERAPY: OTHER*

		Beta-Blockers		
Drug	Receptors Blocked	Dose	Half-Life (hr)	Metabolism
Propranolol	B1, B2	40–480 per day given b.i.d. or q.i.d.	3–6	100% liver
Nadolol[†]	B1, B2	40–240/day	14–45	100% kidney

[†]Reduce dosage with reduced renal function.
See individual beta blockers in chapter 16.

	Calcium Channel Blockers		
Drug	Dose	Half-Life (hr)	Use with Beta-Blockers
Verapamil	80–160 Q8h	3–7	No (or extreme caution)
Nifedipine	10–30 mg q.i.d.	3–5	O.K.
Diltiazem	60–90 mg q.i.d.	2–6	Caution

See Chapter 16 and Table 16–3 for additional information.

*Adapted from Ellrodt G, Chew CYG, Singh BN: Therapeutic implication of slow channel blockade in cardiocirculatory disorders. *Circulation* 1980; 62:669–679.

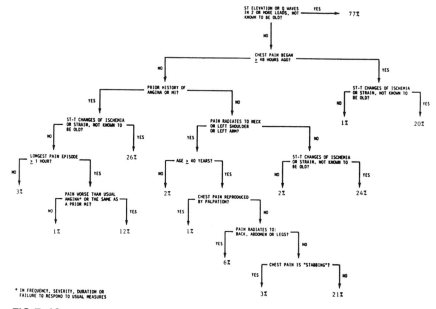

FIG 7–10.
Probability of myocardial infarction in emergency room patients with acute chest pain. (From Lee TH, Lee R: *Cardiology Problems in Primary Care*. Oradell, New Jersey, Medical Economics Books, 1990. Used by permission.)

SILENT MYOCARDIAL ISCHEMIA

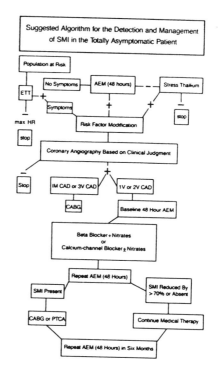

FIG 7–11.

Suggested algorithm for the detection and management of silent myocardial ischemia in the totally asymptomatic patient. *AEM* = ambulatory electrocardiographic monitoring; *MAX HR* = maximum heart rate; *ETT* = exercise thallium testing; *SME* = silent myocardial ischemia. (From Bertolet BD, Hill JA: *Pract Cardiol* January 1989; 15:X. Reproduced by permission.)

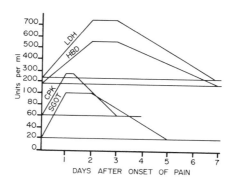

FIG 7–12.

Changes in serum enzyme levels following an acute myocardial infarction. Horizontal lines indicate top normal levels. *HBD* = α-hydroxybutate dehydrogenase. (From Gazes PC: *Clinical Cardiology: A Bedside Approach,* ed 2. Chicago, Year Book Medical Publishers, 1983. Reproduced by permission.)

MYOCARDIAL INFARCTION

TABLE 7–15.—DIAGNOSIS AND MANAGEMENT OF MI

Myocardial infarction (MI) requires an accurate diagnosis and careful management. One of the most important parts of management is the prevention or treatment of complications.
Diagnosis requires at least two of the following:
History of typical chest pain.
ECG changes evolving with Q waves appearing.
Elevated CPK, SGOT, and LDH levels (Fig 7–10).
Other aids in diagnosis: Myocardial imaging (technetium-labeled pyrophosphate) is positive within 24 hours and until 7 days. This test is most useful to establish the diagnosis in a patient a few days after the infarction.
Think about the *differential* for chest pain:
Myocardial infarction
Aneurysm
Pericarditis
Pulmonary embolus
Pneumothorax
Management:
Admit and monitor
Maintain IV
Provide rest; sedate if needed
Control pain:
Morphine 1–4 mg IV
NTG SL or IV and/or beta blocker; see Tables 7–16 and 7–17
Administer oxygen by nasal
cannula at 2–3 L/min. Keep PO_2 above 70 mm Hg.
Restrict diet to low salt, easily chewed and digested foods, no caffeine
Prevent constipation by administering a stool softener
Watch for and treat common complications: premature ventricular contractions, congestive heart failure, dysrhythmias, heart block, papillary muscle dysfunction, VSD, aneurysm, pericarditis
Consider prophylactic lidocaine drip for 1st 48 hr; see Table 7–14
Maintain normal blood pressure
Percutaneous transluminal angioplasty (PCTA)
PCTA (balloon angioplasty) has proven to be an effective new therapeutic modality for patients with single and, in some cases, multivessel coronary artery disease. Stretching of the stenotic coronary artery can be done in patients with unstable angina or early in MI to limit infarct size.
Thrombolytic therapy
There is very good evidence that intracoronary or IV administration of streptokinase within the first 4–6 hr of MI will reduce the infarct size and may also reduce mortality. Tissue plasminogen activation (TPA) is given only intravenously and has been shown to limit both infarct size and mortality. Contraindications include recent trauma (including CPR) and active bleeding in the CNS or GI tract, uncontrolled hypertension, pregnancy, diabetic retinopathy with hemorrhage, recent cardiovascular arrest, or allergy to the medication. They may be used in conjunction with PCTA in the acute MI setting. Most hospitals have a protocol for administration of these medications.

TABLE 7–16.—Lidocaine in Acute MI

Indication: Pathologic ventricular ectopy or prophylactically for the first 48 hr in acute myocardial infarction.
Dosage:
Normal liver and cardiac function:
  100-mg (1–1.5 mg/kg) bolus, then 3–4 boluses of 25–50 mg every 5 min, then infusion at 2–4 mg/min
With liver disease:
  100-mg bolus, followed by infusion at 1–2 mg/min (50% reduction)
With congestive heart failure:
  50-mg bolus (50% reduction), followed by infusion at 1–2 mg/min (50% reduction)
To increase levels when at steady state, give a new bolus of 25–50 mg and increase the infusion rate

TABLE 7–17.—Correlation Between ECG, Location of Ischemic Changes and Area of Myocardium and Coronary Artery Involved*

ISCHEMIC CHANGES	MYOCARDIAL AREA	CORONARY ARTERY
II, III, aV_F	Inferior	Right coronary artery
V_1, V_2 (reciprocal changes)	Posterior	Right coronary artery
V_2–V_4	Anteroseptal	Left anterior descending branch of left coronary artery
V_3–V_5	Anterior	Left anterior descending branch of left coronary artery
I, aV_L	High Lateral	Marginal branch of circumflex artery or diagonal branch of left coronary artery
V_5, V_6	Apical	Usually left anterior descending branch of left coronary artery; may be posterior descending branch of right coronary artery

*Adapted from Rubinstein E, Federman D: *Scientific American Medicine.* New York, Scientific American, 1982.

DYSRHYTHMIAS AND RESUSCITATION

Cardiac Rhythm Review

Normal Sinus Rhythm *(Fig 7–13)*

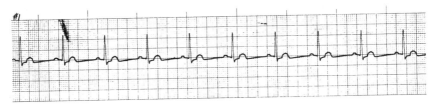

FIG 7–13.
Criteria:
  Rate: 60–100/min
  Rhythm: Regular
  P waves: Upright in leads I, II, aV$_F$

Sinus Bradycardia *(Fig 7–14)*

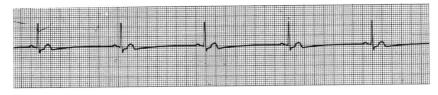

FIG 7–14.
Criteria:
  Rate: <60/min
  Rhythm: Regular
  P waves: Upright in leads I, II, aV$_F$

Sinus Tachycardia *(Fig 7–15)*

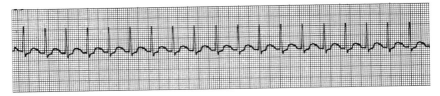

FIG 7–15.
Criteria:
  Rate: >100/min
  Rhythm: Regular
  P waves: Upright in leads I, II, aV$_F$

Premature Atrial Contractions (Fig 7–16)

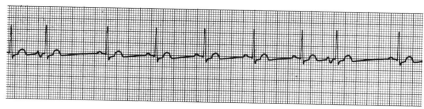

FIG 7–16.
PACs illustrated by 2nd and 8th complexes.
Criteria:
Rhythm: Irregular
P waves: Differ in morphology because they are from different foci. PP interval varies.
PR interval: Normal or prolonged
QRS: Normal or prolonged

Paroxysmal Atrial Tachycardia (Fig 7–17)

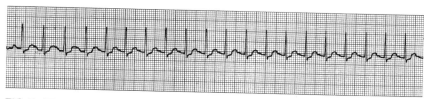

FIG 7–17.
Criteria:
Rate: 160–220/min
Rhythm: atrial—regular; ventricular—may have block (2:1, 3:1, or 4:1)
P waves: Hard to see, different from sinus P waves
PR interval: Normal or prolonged
QRS: Normal or prolonged

Atrial Flutter (Fig 7–18)

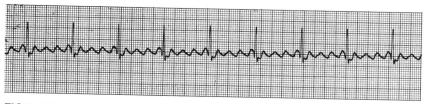

FIG 7–18.
Criteria:
Rate: Usually 300/min (range, 220–350/min)
Rhythm: atrial—regular; ventricular—varying block (2:1, 3:1)
P waves: Sawtoothed pattern seen in II, III, aV$_F$
PR interval: Regular
QRS: Usually normal, perhaps aberrant

Atrial Fibrillation *(Fig 7–19)*

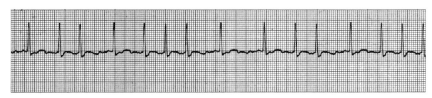

FIG 7–19.
Criteria:
  Rate: atrial—400–700/min; ventricular—160–180/min
  Rhythm: Irregular
  P waves: No P waves
  QRS: Usually normal, perhaps aberrant

Premature Junctional Complexes *(Fig 7–20)*

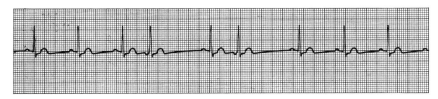

FIG 7–20.
Criteria:
  Rhythm: Irregular
  P waves: Negative in leads II, III, aV$_F$
  PR interval: If P wave is before the QRS the PR interval is less than 0.12 sec. PR interval
    may be prolonged or show complete block.
  QRS: Normal or widened.

Junctional Escape Complexes *(Fig 7–21)*

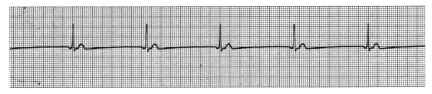

FIG 7–21.
Criteria:
  Rate: 40–60/min
  Rhythm: Complexes may or may not occur regularly
  P waves: Negative in II, III, aV$_F$; may precede, coincide with, or follow QRS
  PR interval: Variable
  QRS: Normal

Premature Ventricular Complexes *(Fig 7–22)*

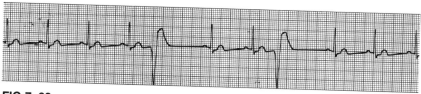

FIG 7–22.
Criteria:
  Rhythm: Irregular
  P waves: Often hidden by QRS of PVC
  QRS: >0.12 sec; bizarre morphology
  ST segment and T wave: Opposite in polarity to the QRS
  Full compensatory pause

Ventricular Tachycardia *(Fig 7–23)*

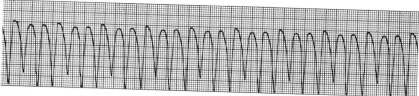

FIG 7–23.
Criteria:
  Rate: 100–220/min
  Rhythm: Usually regular
  P waves: May not be seen
  QRS: Wide
  ST segment and T wave: Opposite in polarity to the QRS

Ventricular Fibrillation *(Fig 7–24)*

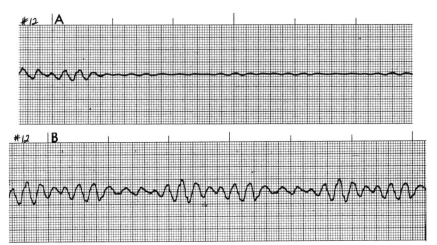

FIG 7–24.
Criteria:
Rate: Very rapid, cannot count
Rhythm: Irregular
No P wave, QRS, ST segment or T wave

First-Degree AV Block *(Fig 7–25)*

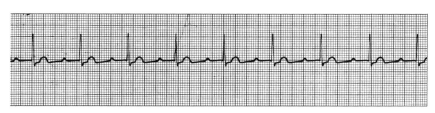

FIG 7–25.
Criteria:
Rhythm: Regular
P waves: Followed by QRS
PR interval: >0.20 sec

Second-Degree AV Block
Mobitz type I (Wenckebach) *(Fig 7–26)*

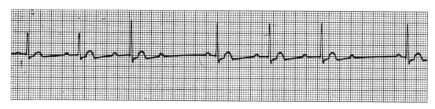

FIG 7–26.

Criteria:

Rate: Atrial—normal; ventricular—less than atrial

Rhythm: Atrial—regular; ventricular—irregular; progressive shortening of RR interval until QRS is dropped

P waves: Normal

PR interval: Progressive increase until one P wave is blocked

QRS: Normal

Mobitz type II *(Fig 7–27)*

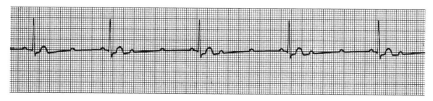

FIG 7–27.

Criteria:

Rate: Atrial—normal; ventricular—less than atrial

Rhythm: Atrial—regular; ventricular—regular or irregular with pauses at nonconducted beats

P waves: Normal except for blocked one

PR interval: Normal or prolonged

QRS: Normal or wide

Third-Degree AV Block *(Fig 7–28)*

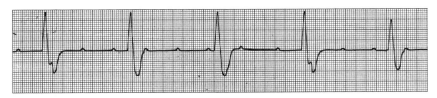

FIG 7–28.
Criteria:
Rate: Atria and ventricles at different rates; ventricles slower than atria
Rhythm: Atria—usually regular; ventricle—regular
P waves: Normal
PR interval: Varies
QRS: Normal or wide
PR Interval: Progressive increase until one P wave is blocked
QRS: Normal

Other Dysrhythmias

Wolff-Parkinson-White *(WPW) Syndrome (Fig 7–29)*

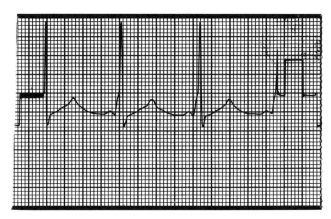

FIG 7–29.
ECG
  PR: 0.12 sec
  QRS: 0.11 sec
  Delta wave
  These changes may be intermittent
Complications: This syndrome may lead to atrial fibrillation or supraventricular tachycardia that resembles ventricular tachycardia due to wide, rapid QRS complexes. Digitalis is not used in atrial fibrillation and WPW syndrome since it may speed conduction and lead to rapid ventricular response. Procainamide and propranolol are indicated. Lidocaine is safe when ventricular tachycardia cannot be distinguished from supraventricular tachycardia with aberrancy.

Torsades de Pointes (Fig 7–30)

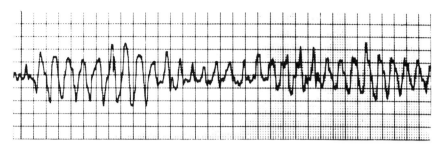

FIG 7–30.
A ventricular dysrhythmia with prolonged QT interval and rapidly changing polarity of QRS.

TABLE 7–18.—Summary of Treatment of Dysrhythmias

DYSRHYTHMIA	CHARACTER	TREATMENT*
Sinus bradycardia	Rate: <60/min	Atropine—treat if pt. is symptomatic; pacemaker may be necessary
Sinus tachycardia	Rate: >100/min Transient slowing with carotid massage	None if stable Treat underlying cause: fever, sepsis, Po_2, volume, pain
Premature atrial	PR intervals Contractions vary; P waves different	None if stable Treat underlying cause
Junctional rhythm	Rate: 40–70/min, or 130–150/min No p waves	None if rate is adequate; consider digitalis toxicity If rapid, treat as PAT
Paroxysmal atrial tachycardia (PAT)	Rate: 160–220/min Normal P waves May have aberrant QRS If block present, consider digitalis toxicity	Carotid massage, verapamil, Valsalva, phenylephrine, edrophonium, cardioversion, digitalization, beta-blockers, procainamide, lidocaine
Tachybrady dysrhythmia	Chaotic atrial rhythm	Pacemaker
Atrial flutter	Rate: 220–350/min "Sawtoothed pattern"	Verapamil or digitalization or cardioversion

Continued.

TABLE 7–18.—Continued

DYSRHYTHMIA	CHARACTER	TREATMENT*
Atrial fibrillation	Atrial rate: 400–700/min; ventricular rate: 160–180/min Irregularly irregular	*Digitalization,* verapamil, cardioversion, consider anticoagulation
PVC and ventricular tachycardia	No P wave Wide QRS Compensatory pause Rate: 100–220/min	*Lidocaine bolus and infusion,* then procainamide or bretylium; treat hypotension and chest pain if present
Ventricular fibrillation	Emergency No organized rhythm	*CPR, defibrillation, lidocaine,* bretylium
Asystole	Emergency condition, no electrical activity	*CPR, epinephrine, atropine* isoproterenol
First-degree AV block	Prolonged PR	*None;* check for digitalis toxicity
Second-degree AV block	Type I Wenckebach Type II Mobitz	*None* *Pacemaker*
Third-degree AV block	Atria, ventricles	*Atropine or pacemaker*

*Treatment of choice is italicized. See Table 7–21 for dosages.

TABLE 7–19.—Drugs for Resuscitation and Dysrhythmias in Adults

DRUG	INITIAL DOSE	THERAPEUTIC LEVEL	FREQUENCY	ACTION	INDICATION	SIDE EFFECTS
Quinidine	200–300 mg	2–8 μg/ml	4 mg/kg/6 hr	Depress phase 0 depolarization, slow conduction, prolongs phases 2 and 3, decrease phase 4	Atrial fibrillation, ventricular ectopy, reentry, WPW, automaticity	Dysrhythmias, tinnitus, increased QT, diarrhea
Procainamide	100 mg over 5 min, up to 1 gm	4–12 μg/ml	7 mg/kg/4 hr			Decreased BP, SLE, dysrhythmias
Disopyramide	200–300 mg	2–7 μg/ml	400–800/day divide q6			Negative inotrope, CHF, increased QT, anticholinergic
Lidocaine	50–100 mg IV	2–6 μg/ml	Bolus and infusion	Speed conduction, decrease resting potential	Acute VT	Paresthesias, seizures, rash, dysrhythmia
Phenytoin	100 mg q 5–10 min, up to 1 gm	10–20 μg/ml	1.5–2 mg/kg/ 6 hr		Digitalis-induced SVT and VT	CNS, rash, sedation
Propranolol	0.1 mg/kg; 1 mg IV over 5 min		10–120 mg qid	Inhibit sympathetic activity	SVT	Negative inotrope, bronchospasm, AV block, hypotension
Metoprolol	50–100 mg		50–200 mg bid			
Nadolol	40 mg		40–240 mg/ day			
Timolol	10–20 mg		10–40 mg/day			
Bretylium	5 mg/kg, up to 30 mg/kg	1.5	5–10 mg/kg/ 6 hr	Prolongs duration of action potential	Resistant VT and ventricular fibrillation	Parotid pain, hypotension, nausea and vomiting, bradydysrhythmia

Continued.

TABLE 7-19.—Continued

DRUG	INITIAL DOSE	THERAPEUTIC LEVEL	FREQUENCY	ACTION	INDICATION	SIDE EFFECTS
Verapamil	5 mg IV over 1–2 min		Give 10 mg in 15–30 min if needed	Slows AV conduction	PAT, SVT	HA, flushing, constipation, hypotension, bradycardia, AV block, asystole
Epinephrine 1:10,000	0.5–1.0 mg	*Dose in ML* (5–10 ml)	q5 min	Adrenergic cardiac stim.	Asystole, fine ventricular fibrillation	Dysrhythmias, hypertension, myocardial ischemia
NaHCO₃	1 mEq/kg	(8–16 ml)	1/2 initial dose q5–10 min	Increases pH	Acidosis	Alkalosis, sodium overload
Atropine	0.5	(5 ml)	q3–5 min	Increases SA and AV nodal conduction	Bradycardia asystole	Anticholinergic, tachycardia
CaCl₂	500 mg	(2.5–50 ml)	q10 min as needed	Improves or stimulates conduction	Electromechanical dissociation, asystole	Arrest if the heart is beating
Morphine	2–5 mg		2–5 mg q5 min	Reduced afterload analgesia, venous capacitance	Acute MI Pulmonary edema	Sedation Respiratory depression

TABLE 7–20.—DRUGS FOR RESUSCITATION IN ADULTS

DRUG	AVAILABLE	INFUSION DOSE	ACTION	INDICATION	SIDE EFFECTS
Dopamine	400 mg/5 ml	400 mg in 250 ml D5W = 1,600 μg/ml; infuse 2–4 μg/kg/min	α and β and dopamine receptor stimulation	Cardiogenic shock	Tachydysrhythmias, ectopy, nausea, vomiting, peripheral ischemia
Dobutamine	250 mg/20 ml	250 mg in 1 L infuse 2.5–10 μg/kg/min	Inotropic β-receptor stimulation	Refractory heart failure	↑ HR, BP, PVCs
Isoproterenol	1 mg	1 mg in 500 ml D5W = 2 μg/ml; infuse 2–10 μg/min	Inotropic, chronotropic	Bradycardia due to heart block	↑ PVCs, cardiac output
Amrinone		0.75 mg/kg dose over 2–3 min, followed by 5–10 μg/kg/min	Inotropic, Vasodilation	CHF	May exacerbate MI
Sodium nitroprusside		0.5–10 μg/kg/min	Peripheral vasodilator, cardiac output	CHF, hypertension	↑ Cardiac output

TABLE 7–21.—DRUGS USED IN PEDIATRIC ADVANCED LIFE SUPPORT*

DRUG	DOSE	HOW SUPPLIED	REMARKS
Atropine sulfate	0.02 mg/kg/dose	0.1 mg/ml	Minimum dose of 0.1 mg (1.0 ml)
Calcium chloride	20 mg/kg/dose	100 mg/ml (10%)	Give slowly
Dopamine hydrochloride	2–20 μg/kg/min	40 mg/ml	α-Adrenergic action dominates at 15–20 μg/kg/min
Dobutamine hydrochloride	5–20 μg/kg/min	250 mg/vial lyophilized	Titrate to desired effect
Epinephrine hydrochloride	0.1 mL/kg (0.01 mg/kg)	1 : 10,000 (0.1 mg/mL)	1 : 1,000 must be diluted
Epinephrine infusion	Start at 0.1 μg/ kg/min	1 : 1,000 (1mg/ml)	Titrate to desired effect (0.1–1.0 μg/kg/min)
Isoproterenol hydrochloride	Start at 0.1 μg/ kg/min	1 mg/5 ml	Titrate to desired effect (0.1–1.0 μg/kg/min)
Lidocaine	1 mg/kg/dose	10 mg/ml (1%), 20 mg/ml (2%)	
Lidocaine infusion	20–50 μg/kg/min	40 mg/ml (4%)	
Norepinephrine infusion	Start at 0.1 μg/ kg/min	1 mg/ml	Titrate to desired effect (0.1–1.0 μg/kg/min)
Sodium bicarbonate	1 mEq/kg/dose or 0.3 × kg × base deficit	1 mEq/ml (8.4%)	Infuse slowly and only if ventilation is adequate

*From JAMA 1986; 255:2966. Reproduced by permission.

TABLE 7–22.—PREPARATION OF INFUSIONS*

DRUG	PREPARATION	DOSE
Isoproterenol, epinephrine, norepinephrine	0.6 × body weight (kg) is mg added to diluent† to make 100 mL	Then 1 ml/hr delivers 0.1 μg/kg/min; titrate to effect
Dopamine, dobutamine	6 × body weight (kg) is mg added to diluent to make 100 mL	Then 1 ml/hr delivers 1.0 μg/kg/min; titrate to effect
Lidocaine	120 mg (3 mL of 4% solution) into 100 ml of 5% dextrose in water, 1,200 μg/ml	Then 1 ml/kg/hr delivers 20 μg/kg/min

*From JAMA 1986; 255:2967. Reproduced by permission.
†Diluent may be 5% dextrose in water, 5% dextrose in half normal saline, normal saline, or Ringer's lactate.

VENTRICULAR TACHYCARDIA

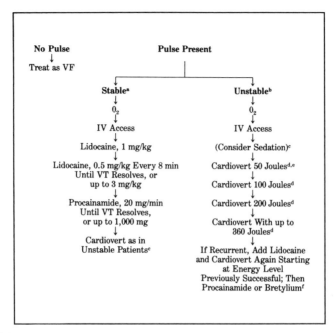

FIG 7–31.

Sustained ventricular tachycardia (VT). This sequence was developed to assist in teaching how to treat a broad range of patients with sustained VT. Some patients may require care not specified herein. This algorithm should not be construed as prohibiting such flexibility. Flow of algorithm presumes that VT is continuing. *VF* = ventricular fibrillation.

[a]If patient becomes unstable (see footnote *b* for definition) at any time, move to "Unstable" arm of algorithm.

[b]Unstable indicates symptoms (e.g., chest pain or dyspnea), hypotension (systolic blood pressure <90 mm Hg), congestive heart failure, ischemia, or infarction.

[c]Sedation should be considered for all patients, including those defined in footnote *b* as unstable, except those who are hemodynamically unstable (e.g., hypotensive, in pulmonary edema, or unconscious).

[d]If hypotension, pulmonary edema, or unconsciousness is present, unsynchronized cardioversion should be done to avoid delay associated with synchronization.

[e]In the absence of hypotension, pulmonary edema, or unconsciousness, a precordial thump may be employed prior to cardioversion.

[f]Once VT has resolved, begin infusion of antiarrhythmic agent that has aided resolution of VT. If hypotension, pulmonary edema, or unconsciousness is present, use lidocaine if cardioversion alone is unsuccessful, followed by bretylium. In all other patients, recommended order of therapy is lidocaine, procainamide, and then bretylium. (From *Textbook of Advanced Cardiac Life Support.* Dallas, American Heart Association, 1989. Reproduced by permission.)

VENTRICULAR FIBRILLATION

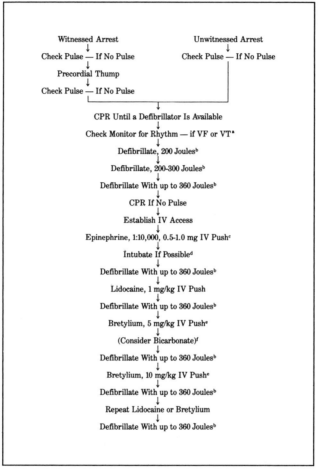

FIG 7–32.

Ventricular fibrillation (and pulseless ventricular tachycardia). This sequence was developed to assist in teaching how to treat a broad range of patients with ventricular fibrillation *(VF)* or pulseless ventricular tachycardia *(VT)*. Some patients may require care not specified herein. This algorithm should not be construed as prohibiting such flexibility. Flow of algorithm presumes that VF is continuing. *CPR* = cardiopulmonary resuscitation.

[a]Pulseless VT should be treated identically to VF.

[b]Check pulse and rhythm after each shock. If VF recurs after transiently converting (rather than persists without ever converting), use whatever energy level has previously been successful for defibrillation.

[c]Epinephrine should be repeated every 5 minutes.

[d]Intubation is preferable. If it can be accomplished simultaneously with other tech-

ASYSTOLE

If Rhythm Is Unclear and Possibly Ventricular
Fibrillation, Defibrillate as for VF. If Asystole is Present[a]
↓
Continue CPR
↓
Establish IV Access
↓
Epinephrine, 1:10,000, 0.5 - 1.0 mg IV Push[b]
↓
Intubate When Possible[c]
↓
Atropine, 1.0 mg IV Push (Repeated in 5 min)
↓
(Consider Bicarbonate)[d]
↓
Consider Pacing

FIG 7–33.
Asystole (cardiac standstill). This sequence was developed to assist in teaching how to treat a broad range of patients with asystole. Some patients may require care not specified herein. This algorithm should not be construed to prohibit such flexibility. Flow of algorithm presumes asystole is continuing. VF = ventricular fibrillation; IV = intravenous.
[a]Asystole should be confirmed in two leads.
[b]Epinephrine should be repeated every 5 minutes.
[c]Intubation is preferable. If it can be accomplished simultaneously with other techniques, then the earlier the better. However, cardiopulmonary resuscitation *(CPR)* and use of epinephrine are more important initially if patient can be ventilated without intubation. (Endotracheal epinephrine may be used.)
[d]Value of sodium bicarbonate is questionable during cardiac arrest, and it is not recommended for the routine cardiac arrest sequence. Consideration of its use in a dose of 1 mEq/kg is appropriate at this point. Half of original dose may be repeated every 10 minutes if it is used. (From *Textbook of Advanced Cardiac Life Support.* Dallas, American Heart Association, 1989. Reproduced by permission.)

←Fig 7–32 (cont.).
niques, then the earlier the better. However, defibrillation and epinephrine are more important initially if the patient can be ventilated without intubation.
[e]Some may prefer repeated doses of lidocaine, which may be given in 0.5-mg/kg boluses every 8 minutes to a total dose of 3 mg/kg.
[f]Value of sodium bicarbonate is questionable during cardiac arrest, and it is not recommended for routine cardiac arrest sequence. Consideration if its use in a dose of 1 mEq/kg is appropriate at this point. Half of original dose may be repeated every 10 minutes if it is used. (From *Textbook of Advanced Cardiac Life Support.* Dallas, American Heart Association, 1989. Reproduced by permission.)

ELECTROMECHANICAL DISSOCIATION

Continue CPR
↓
Establish IV Access
↓
Epinephrine, 1:10,000, 0.5 - 1.0 mg IV Push[a]
↓
Intubate When Possible[b]
↓
(Consider Bicarbonate)[c]
↓
Consider Hypovolemia,
Cardiac Tamponade,
Tension Pneumothorax,
Hypoxemia,
Acidosis,
Pulmonary Embolism

FIG 7–34.
Electromechanical dissociation. This sequence was developed to assist in teaching how to treat a broad range of patients with electromechanical dissociation. Some patients may require care not specified herein. This algorithm should not be construed to prohibit such flexibility. Flow of algorithm presumes that electromechanical dissociation is continuing. *CPR* = cardiopulmonary resuscitation; *IV* = intravenous.
[a]Epinephrine should be repeated every five minutes.
[b]Intubation is preferable. If it can be accomplished simultaneously with other techniques, then the earlier the better. However, epinephrine is more important initially if the patient can be ventilated without intubation.
[c]Value of sodium bicarbonate is questionable during cardiac arrest, and it is not recommended for routine cardiac arrest sequence. Consideration of its use in a dose of 1 mEq/kg is appropriate at this point. Half of original dose may be repeated every 10 minutes if it is used. (From *Textbook of Advanced Cardiac Life Support*. Dallas, American Heart Association, 1989. Reproduced by permission.)

PAROXYSMAL ATRIAL TACHYCARDIA

Unstable	**Stable**
↓	↓
Synchronous Cardioversion 75-100 Joules	Vagal Maneuvers
↓	↓
Synchronous Cardioversion 200 Joules	Verapamil, 5 mg IV
↓	↓
Synchronous Cardioversion 360 Joules	Verapamil, 10 mg IV
↓	(in 15-20 min)
Correct Underlying Abnormalities	↓
↓	Cardioversion, Digoxin,
Pharmacological Therapy + Cardioversion	β-Blockers, Pacing as Indicated
	(See Text)

If conversion occurs but PSVT recurs, repeated electrical cardioversion is *not* indicated. Sedation should be used as time permits.

FIG 7–35.

Paroxysmal supraventricular tachycardia *(PSVT).* This sequence was developed to assist in teaching how to treat a broad range of patients with sustained PSVT. Some patients may require care not specified herein. This algorithm should not be construed as prohibiting such flexibility. Flow of algorithm presumes PSVT is continuing. (From *Textbook of Advanced Cardiac Life Support.* Dallas, American Heart Association, 1989. Reproduced by permission.)

BRADYCARDIA

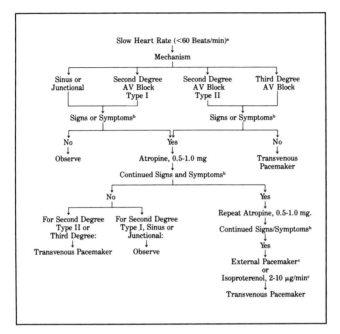

FIG 7–36.
Bradycardia. This sequence was developed to assist in teaching how to treat a broad range of patients with bradycardia. Some patients may require care not specified herein. This algorithm should not be construed to prohibit such flexibility. *AV* = atrioventricular.

[a]A solitary chest thump or cough may stimulate cardiac electrical activity and result in improved cardiac output and may be used at this point.

[b]Hypotension (blood pressure <90 mm Hg), premature ventricular contractions, altered mental status or symptoms (e.g., chest pain or dyspnea), ischemia, or infarction.

[c]Temporizing therapy. (From *Textbook of Advanced Cardiac Life Support*. Dallas, American Heart Association, 1989. Reproduced by permission.)

VENTRICULAR ECTOPY

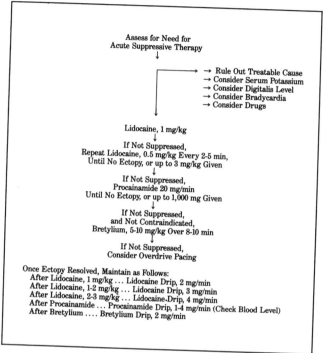

FIG 7–37.
Ventricular ectopy: acute suppressive therapy. This sequence was developed to assist in teaching how to treat a broad range of patients with ventricular ectopy. Some patients may require therapy not specified herein. This algorithm should not be construed as prohibiting such flexibility. (From *Textbook of Advanced Cardiac Life Support.* Dallas, American Heart Association, 1989. Reproduced by permission.)

DEFIBRILLATION AND SYNCHRONIZED CARDIOVERSION

TABLE 7–23.—GUIDELINE FOR DEFIBRILLATION AND SYNCHRONIZED
CARDIOVERSION

Defibrillation—Used in ventricular fibrillation and ventricular tachycardia in an un-
conscious patient with no circulation.
Synchronized cardioversion—Countershock delivered during QRS. Used to con-
vert ventricular and supraventricular tachydysrhythmias in settings where rapid
conversion is needed.
Technique
Defibrillation
  Charge paddles: 200 J for first, 300 for second, 360 for third.
  Place paddles: One to right of upper sternum, below clavicle; second to left
    of left nipple in anterior axillary line.
  Recheck rhythm on monitor.
  Clear area around patient. Make sure no one is in contact with patient or
    bed.
  Firmly press paddles against chest wall.
  Deliver countershock; simultaneously depress paddle buttons.
Synchronized cardioversion
  Sedate patient. Use diazepam 5–10 mg IV.
  Check QRS: must be upright on monitor.
  Activate synchronizer circuit.
  Charge paddle:
    Atrial fibrillation
      100 J first
      200 J second, if needed
      360 J third, if needed
    Paroxysmal atrial tachycardia
      75–100 J
    Ventricular tachycardia
      50 J, then 100 J, then 200 J, then 360 J
    Atrial flutter
      25 J
  Place paddle: as above.
  Clear area: as above.
  Press against chest wall and simultaneously depress paddle button and hold
    until countershock is delivered.
Contraindications
  Atrial fibrillation with slow ventricular response and coronary artery disease.
  Digitalis toxicity.
  Sick sinus syndrome.
  Long-standing atrial fibrillation.
  Atrial fibrillation secondary to hyperthyroidism.

CONGESTIVE HEART FAILURE

TABLE 7–24.—Congestive Heart Failure

Establish the diagnosis:

Symptoms	Signs	X-Ray
Orthopnea	Rales	Cardiomegaly
Dyspnea on exertion	S_3 gallop	Base to apex redistribution of
Fatigue	Peripheral edema	pulmonary vasculature
		Interstitial edema

Think about precipitating causes:

Alcoholism
Anemia
Arrhythmias
Emotional strain
Hypothyroidism
Hyperthyroidism
Medications: sodium retaining or
    disopyramide, propranolol

Myocardial infarction
Physical exertion, particularly in hot
    humid weather
Pregnancy
Pulmonary embolus
Sodium intake excess
Stopping medications, particularly
    cardiac stimulants and afterload
    reducers

Five goals of therapy:
1. Reduce cardiac work
       The need for hospitalization is determined by the acuteness and severity of symptoms, the precipitating cause, and an evaluation of the home care providers. Put the patient at bed rest in a relaxed atmosphere with legs and head elevated slightly.
2. Improve myocardial contractility
   a. Digitalis is the cornerstone of therapy and should be administered after: Obtaining baseline ECG to rule out AV block or dysrhythmia. ECG may define valve disease or IHSS.
      Checking renal function and potassium
   b. Other inotropic agents include:
       Dopamine, Amrinone
       Dobutamine, Milrinone
3. ACE Inhibitor (can reduce mortality of CHF)
   Captopril
   Enalapril
4. Reduce afterload
       Vasodilating agents are used for CHF not responding to digitalis and diuretics. Examples of vasodilators:
       Isosorbide dinitrate
       Sublingual nitroglycerin
       Nitroglycerin paste
       Hydralazine (arteriolar dilation)
       Prazosin (arteriolar and venous)
       Nitroprusside (arteriolar and venous)
5. Reduce excess fluid
       2–4 gm sodium chloride diet
       Diuretics

TABLE 7–25.—Digitalization

Complete familiarity with one preparation is desirable. Since digoxin is the most widely used it will be used as the model. Digitoxin is not affected as extensively by renal function and so might be used.

Digoxin
Rapid IV route for acute, severe, unstable CHF: 0.25–0.50 mg IV over 5 min, followed by 0.125–0.25 mg IV every 4–6 hr until total dose of 0.5–1.0 mg has been administered, then daily dose of 0.125–0.25 mg IV
24-hour digitalization: 0.5–0.75 mg orally followed by 0.25–.25 mg IV every 6–8 hr until total dose of 1.0–1.5 mg has been administered, then daily dose of 0.125 mg–0.375 mg
One-week digitalization: 0.125–0.25 mg PO daily

Digoxin calculations for maintenance dose estimation:
Maintenance dose $= $ (Loading dose) $\times$ (% daily loss)
Loading dose $= $ 8–10 µg/kg in CHF
$\qquad\qquad\quad = $ 13–15 µg/kg in atrial fibrillation

% Daily loss $= 14\% + \dfrac{\text{Creatinine clearance}}{5}$

Estimated creatinine clearance* $= \dfrac{(140 - \text{Age})\,(\text{Weight in kg})}{\text{Serum creatinine} \times 72} \times$ (0.85 for females)

Oral tablet is only 80% absorbed, so:

$$\text{Tablet} = \frac{\text{IV dose (or Lanoxicap)}}{0.8}$$

*Adapted from Cockroft DW, Gault MH: *Nephron* 1976; 16:31–41.

TABLE 7–26.—Estimated Digoxin Dose

SERUM CREATININE	DAILY MAINTENANCE DOSE AS % OF LOADING DOSE
100	34
75	29
60	26
50	24
30	20
15	17
10	16
5	15
0	14

Serum levels should be measured 8–12 hr after maintenance dose is given. Therapeutic level is 0.8–1.8

TABLE 7–27.—Digitalis Intoxication

SYMPTOMS	ECG CHANGES
Anorexia	PVCs
Nausea and vomiting	AV Block
Abdominal discomfort	PAT with block
Hazy or colored vision	Wenckebach second-degree
Photophobia	Complete heart block
Hallucinations	Sinus bradycardia
Drowsiness	Accelerated junctional rhythm
Disorientation	

Treatment: Discontinue digitalis; monitor cardiac rhythm and treat as needed; measure digitalis level (toxicity may occur at therapeutic levels). See poisoning chapter for charcoal treatment.

OTHER CARDIAC DISEASE

TABLE 7–28.—Bacterial Endocarditis*

Subacute—Insidious onset, usually in an abnormal heart
Acute—Fulminant, rapid, usually in normal heart
Diagnosis
  Symptoms
    Weakness
    Fatigability
    Weight loss
    Feverishness
    Night sweats
    Anorexia
    Arthralgia
  Signs
    Elevated temperature—cyclic
    Patient appears very ill
    Cardiac failure
    Petechiae—mucous membranes, retina, skin, nails
    Emboli to large arteries causing ischemia and gangrene
    New murmur—primarily diastolic
    Splenomegaly
    Arthritis
  Lab
    Leukocytosis
    ESR increased
    Positive blood cultures
    Echocardiogram—impaired valve excursion or vegetations

Continued.

TABLE 7–28.—Continued

Management
Blood cultures
Antibiotics
 Crystalline penicillin G initially 4.8–6 million units per day, with gentamicin 3–5 mg/kg/day in 3 doses (see Chapter 16)
 Adjust antimicrobial dose as indicated by blood culture sensitivities and minimum bactericidal concentration (MBC)
 Penicillin allergic, use Vancomycin alone, 0.5 gm every 6 hr
Surgery
 May be indicated when organism is resistant or prosthetic valve is infected; should be accomplished before intractable heart failure occurs

 *From Pankey GA: *Am Heart J* 1979; 98:102–118. Reproduced by permission.

TABLE 7–29.—Endocarditis Prophylaxis*[†]

	ADULTS	CHILDREN
Dental and upper respiratory procedures[‡]		
Oral[§]		
Penicillin V	2 gm 1 hr before procedure and 1 gm 6 hr later	>60 lb: adult dosage; <60 lb: half the adult dosage
Penicillin allergy		
Erythromycin	1 gm 2 hr before procedure and 500 mg 6 hr later	20 mg/kg 2 hr before procedure and 10 mg/kg 6 hr later
Parenteral[§‖]		
Ampicillin	2 gm IM or IV 30 min before procedure	50 mg/kg IM or IV 30 min before procedure
plus Gentamicin	1.5 mg/kg IM or IV 30 min before procedure	2.0 mg/kg IM or IV 30 min before procedure
Penicillin allergy		
Vancomycin	1 gm IV infused *slowly over 1 hr* beginning 1 hr before procedure	20 mg/kg IV infused *slowly over 1 hr* beginning 1 hour before procedure
Gastrointestinal and genitourinary procedures[‡]		
Oral[§]		
Amoxicillin	3 gm 1 hr before procedure and 1.5 gm 6 hr later	50 mg/kg 1 hr before procedure and 25 mg/kg 6 hr later
Parenteral[§‖]		
Ampicillin	2 gm IM or IV 30 min before procedure	50 mg/kg IM or IV 30 min before procedure
plus Gentamicin	1.5 mg/kg IM or IV 30 min before procedure	2.0 mg/kg IM or IV 30 min before procedure

Penicillin allergy		
Vancomycin	1 gm IV infused *slowly* over 1 hr beginning 1 hr before procedure	20 mg/kg IV infused *slowly* over 1 hr beginning 1 hr before procedure
plus Gentamicin	1.5 mg/kg IM or IV 30 min before procedure	2.0 mg/kg IM or IV 30 min before procedure

*From *Med Lett* 1987; 29:110. Reproduced by permission.
†For patients with valvular heart disease, prosthetic heart valves, most forms of congenital heart disease (but not uncomplicated secundum atrial septal defect), idiopathic hypertrophic subaortic stenosis, and mitral valve prolapse with regurgitation.
‡Data are limited on the risk of endocarditis with a particular procedure. For a review of the risk of bacteremia with various procedures, see Everett ED, Hirschmann JV: *Medicine (Baltimore)* 1977; 56:61, and Shorvon PJ, et al: *Gut* 1983; 24:1078. For some useful guidelines on which procedures justify prophylaxis, see Shulman ST, et al: *Circulation* 1984; 70:1123A.
§Oral regimens are more convenient and safer. Parenteral regimens are more likely to be effective; they are recommended especially for patients with prosthetic heart valves, those who have had endocarditis previously, or those taking continuous oral penicillin for rheumatic fever prophylaxis.
‖A single dose of parenteral drugs is probably adequate, because bacteremias after most dental and diagnostic procedures are of short duration. However, one or two follow-up doses may be given at 8- to 12-hr intervals in selected patients, such as hospitalized patients judged to be at higher risk.

TABLE 7–30.—OTHER CARDIAC DISEASES: MISCELLANEOUS CONDITIONS

Acute pericarditis
Signs
Pericardial friction rub: may be three-component rub
Pericardial effusion: best diagnosed with echocardiogram
Pulsus paradoxis
ECG changes: ST elevation in all leads except aV_R and only rarely in V_1.
Treatment
Watch for effusion; consider anti-inflammatory drugs

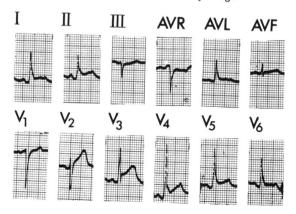

FIG 7–38.
Acute pericarditis. (From Gazes PC: *Clinical Cardiology: A Bedside Approach,* ed 2. Chicago, Year Book Medical Publishers, 1983. Reproduced by permission.)

Continued.

TABLE 7–30.—Continued

Cardiomyopathy
Either primary myocardial disease or secondary to systemic disease causing poor function of heart muscle
Three major classifications:
CONGESTIVE
Signs
Congestive heart failure, arrhythmias, cardiac chamber dilation, mitral and tricuspid valve regurgitation
Treatment
Bed rest, digitalis, diuretics, afterload and preload reduction, consider anticoagulation
RESTRICTIVE
Signs
Dependent edema, elevated jugular venous pulse, ascites, enlarged heart, enlarged liver, ECG changes
Treatment
Transvenous biopsy; treat CHF
HYPERTROPHIC (idiopathic hypertrophic subaortic stenosis)
Signs
Hypertrophy of left ventricle, murmur
Treatment
Beta-blockers; surgical excision of hypertrophy; avoid inotropic agents and limit exercise

Secondary hypertension

Causes	*Screening Test*
Coarctation	Chest PA and left lateral X-ray films
Cushing's syndrome	Plasma control after 1 mg dexamethasone suppression
Drugs	Blood and urine screens
Amphetamines, oral contraceptive, estrogens, steroid or thyroid excess	
Increased intracranial pressure	CT Scan
Pheochromocytoma	Urine metanephrine or VMA clonidine suppression test
Primary aldosteronism	Serum potassium
Conn's syndrome	Stimulated plasma renin activity
Idiopathic hyperaldosteronism	Urine potassium
Renovascular disease	Screening tests, different for each disease
Renal parenchymal disease	
Chronic pyelonephritis	
Congenital renal disease	
Diabetic nephropathy	
Glomerulonephritis	
Gout	
Interstitial nephropathy	
Obstructive uropathy	
Polycystic disease	
Renin-secreting tumors	
Vasculitis	
Renovascular hypertension	IVP Suppressed or stimulated plasma renin activity

TABLE 7–31.—RENIN AND ALDOSTERONE LEVELS IN SEVERAL DISEASE STATES*

DISEASE STATE	RENIN LEVEL	ALDOSTERONE LEVEL	CONFIRMATION OF DIAGNOSIS
Renovascular hypertension	↑ or same	↑ or same	Differential venous renin measurements Angiography
Primary aldosteronism	0	↑	Aldosterone determination Venography
Renal tumors, cysts	↑	↑	Angiographic appearance of lesion
Essential hypertension	↑ or same or ↓	↑ or same or ↓	
Low renin state	↓	↓	↓ Creatinine clearance Clinical setting
Bartter's syndrome	↑	↑	Patient normotensive Clinical setting

*Adapted from Rubinstein E, Federman D: *Scientific American Medicine.* New York, Scientific American, 1982.

PROCEDURES

TABLE 7–32.—PACEMAKER INSERTION

Indications
    Symptomatic bradydysrhythmias
    Prophylactic pacing in acute MI
        Inferior MI—Mobitz I, no pacemaker
                Mobitz II, pacemaker
        Anterior MI—Mobitz I or II, pacemaker
    Overdrive pacing of atria or ventricles in face of a tachydysrhythmia resistant to medications.
Method
    Choose either a 3F or 5F balloon-tipped catheter, a 3F or 4F semifloating catheter, or a 6F or 7F regular pacing catheter
    Choose site of insertion: subclavian, antecubital, internal jugular, or femoral vein
    Use aseptic technique
    Monitor ECG with IV in place
    Insert catheter and advance while monitoring ECG for position; a large QRS indicates right ventricular position; proper positioning is against the wall, which causes marked ST elevation.
    Secure the catheter and set the rate above the intrinsic cardiac rate or the desired rate
    Determine the threshold by decreasing the output until the capture is lost; set at 2–3 times the threshold.
    Put pacemaker in the demand mode to avoid arrhythmias due to competition with the intrinsic rate
    Obtain chest x-ray to confirm correct placement and exclude pneumothorax; catheter tip should point anteriorly on the lateral x-ray

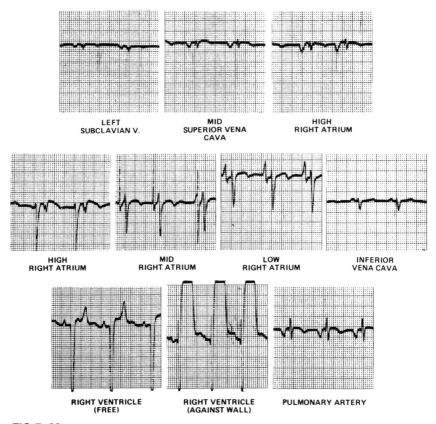

| LEFT SUBCLAVIAN V. | MID SUPERIOR VENA CAVA | HIGH RIGHT ATRIUM |

| HIGH RIGHT ATRIUM | MID RIGHT ATRIUM | LOW RIGHT ATRIUM | INFERIOR VENA CAVA |

| RIGHT VENTRICLE (FREE) | RIGHT VENTRICLE (AGAINST WALL) | PULMONARY ARTERY |

FIG 7–39.
Pacemaker location by ECG. (From Bing OHL: *N Engl J Med* 1972; 287:651. Reproduced by permission.)

TABLE 7–33.—EXERCISE STRESS TESTING

Objectives
  To diagnose ischemic heart disease
  To measure functional capacity for working, sports participation, or rehabilitation potential
Method
  Observe patient and ECG before and afterwards to see baseline
  Exercise by Masters Two Step, Treadmill or bicycle to 80%–90% of predicted maximum heart rate (see Table 7–42) or beyond if no symptoms occur
  Discontinue testing if symptoms occur
Evaluation
  To be positive the ST segment must be a flat depression of at least 1.0 mm below the baseline lasting at least 0.08 sec; if 0.5 mm is used there will be more false positives and fewer false negatives

Common causes of false positive exercise stress tests include: anemia, digitalis, hypertension, hypoxia, left bundle branch block, left ventricular hypertrophy, LGL syndrome, pectus excavatum, ST changes at rest, valvular heart disease, vasoregulatory asthenia

Many centers now do low-level exercise testing before post-MI patients are discharged to determine homegoing exercise prescriptions. See Table 7–43 for exercise prescriptions.

TABLE 7–34.—Target Heart Rate for Graded Exercise Test Based on Age and Activity*

	AGE (YR)										
GROUP	20	25	30	35	40	45	50	55	60	65	70
Untrained											
MHR[†]	197	195	193	191	189	187	184	182	180	178	176
90% MHR	177	175	173	172	170	168	166	164	162	160	158
Trained											
MHR	190	188	186	184	182	180	177	175	173	171	169
90% MHR	171	169	167	166	164	162	159	158	156	154	152

*Data from Sheffield et al: *JSC Med Assoc* 1969; 65:18.
†MHR, maximum heart rate.

TABLE 7–35.—Screening for Coronary Artery Disease*

RISK[†]	EXAMPLE	TEST
Very low <10%	Female <60 yr, male <40 yr with nonanginal chest pain Female <40 yr with atypical angina	None (Some may wish to do exercise ECG to confirm suspicion of low risk.)
Low 10%– 25%	Female 60–69 yr, male 40– 59 yr with nonanginal chest pain Female 40–49 yr, male 30– 39 yr with atypical angina	Exercise ECG
Moderate 25%– 68%	Male >60 yr with nonanginal chest pain Female >50 yr, male >40 yr with atypical angina Female <50 yr and typical angina	Stress thallium or stress MUGA
High 68%– 100%	Female >50 yr, male >30 yr with typical angina	Cardiac catheterization

*Courtesy of Mary Thoesen Coleman, M.D., Ph.D., and Donna Hosmer, M.D., Riverside Methodist Hospital, Columbus, Ohio.
†Pretest probability of coronary artery disease.

TABLE 7–36.—CARDIAC REHABILITATION AND EXERCISE*

Cardiac rehabilitation with at least educational activities should begin in the coronary care unit. When the patient has left the coronary care unit a program of progressive exercise should be begun:
Bathroom privileges
Walking in room
Progressively lengthy walks in hallway
Heart rate and blood pressure should be measured before and after exercise. Symptoms should be monitored and activity kept to a symptom-free level. In some centers a low-level exercise test is done to determine homegoing activity level. In general a patient, on discharge, should:
Walk 15 minutes per day at 80 steps per minute, 1 week after discharge.
In second week after discharge, walk same amount 2 and 3 times a day.
In third week, increase duration of walk until it reaches 1 hour twice a day,
    then increase rate to 100 steps per minute.
At 6 weeks the patient should undergo a symptom-limited exercise test. In
    general, patient is able to:
    Begin driving the car
    Resume sexual intercourse
    Enter a routine exercise program that raises the heart rate to an exercise
        target heart rate (ETHR) which is 70% of maximal oxygen uptake. For
        this exercise formula maximum heart rate (MHR) is found from Table
        7–42. The resting heart rate is the pulse: ETHR = 0.7 MHR + 0.3
        RHR. If this rate is fatiguing, 0.5 may be substituted for 0.7.
At 8–12 weeks the patient may return to work.

*Adapted from Hartley HL: *J Cardiovasc Med* January 1983.

TABLE 7–37.—Pulmonary Artery Catheterization

Indications
  Measurement of right atrial, pulmonary arterial, and pulmonary capillary wedge
    pressure.
  Measurement of cardiac output by either thermodilution or dye dilution.
  Sampling of right atrial and pulmonary arterial blood.
Technique
  Choose a 5F or 7F pulmonary artery catheter. To measure cardiac output, use
    a 7F thermodilution catheter.
  Have an IV line in place to treat arrhythmias that may arise.
  Prepare a sterile field around the chosen insertion site: antecubital venous
    cutdown, subclavian, or internal jugular vein.
  Test balloon with air and deflate.
  Insert catheter through an adequate-sized introducer.
  Inflate balloon halfway when catheter approaches central circulation. Catheter
    measurement markers will assist in knowing the approximate position of the
    catheter.
    R antecubital fossa to right atrium = 40 cm
    L antecubital fossa to right atrium = 50 cm
    Internal jugular and subclavian to right atrium = 15–20 cm
    Femoral vein to right atrium = 70 cm
  Watch the monitor for wave forms similar to those shown in Figure 7–40 to
    determine site of catheter. Vena caval pressures are low and can be in-
    creased by asking patient to cough.
  Once inside the right atrium, inflate balloon to full volume.
  Secure catheter in a position where balloon can be slowly inflated to obtain a
    wedge pressure.

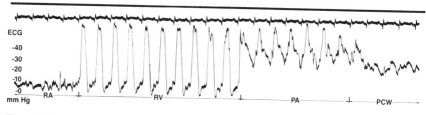

FIG 7–40.
Pressure wave forms recorded as pulmonary artery catheter is advanced through right
atrium *(RA)* and right ventricle *(RV)* into pulmonary artery *(PA)* and to wedge *(PCW)* position. (From *Textbook of Advanced Cardiac Life Support,* ed 2. Dallas; American Heart
Association, 1987. Reproduced by permission.)

TABLE 7–38.—Pericardiocentesis*

Indications
  Diagnostic fluid
  Relieve cardiac tamponade
    Causes of cardiac tamponade: trauma, infection, neoplasm, signs of cardiac
    tamponade: pulsus paradoxus, elevated central venous pressure
Methods
  Perform echocardiography to demonstrate the fluid.
  Use aseptic technique while monitoring ECG with IV line in place.
  Use atropine as premedication to avoid hypotension with puncture of pericar-
  dium.
  Attach ECG V-lead to needle. If ST changes occur the ventricle has been
  touched.
  Choose site—subxiphoid is preferred over apex and left sternal border in 5th
  intercostal space.
  Place patient in 20–30 degree supine position and infiltrate site with lidocaine.
  Insert large-bore needle 1 cm to left of xiphoid.
  Advance needle with constant aspiration at a 20–30 degree angle to frontal
  plane.
  Test aspirated fluid to see if it clots (pericardial fluid will not) or if it leaves a
  central dark red stain with peripheral clearing on a gauze pad (pericardial
  fluid will).
INTRACARDIAC INJECTIONS
  Indications
    For injection of epinephrine and calcium when IV and ET routes are unavail-
    able.
  Method
    The technique is basically the same as for pericardiocentesis except that the
    blood returned usually indicates an intracardiac position. If needle is fully
    inserted with no blood return (an 18-gauge 3½-inch needle is used), with-
    draw slowly while aspirating.
  Stop when blood returns and inject the medicines.

  *Adapted from *Textbook of Advanced Cardiac Life Support,* ed 2. Dallas, American
Heart Association, 1987.

TABLE 7-39.—PEDIATRIC HEART DEFECTS: SIGNS AND DIAGNOSTIC AIDS*

DEFECT	CYANOSIS	CHAMBER ENLARGEMENT	P₁	MURMUR	CHEST FILM	ECG	ECHOCARDIOGRAM
Valvular Pulmonic Stenosis	0	Right ventricle	Lessened intensity Wide split	Ejection murmur in pulmonic area Ejection click	Right ventricular enlargement Normal pulmonary blood flow Poststenotic dilation	Right axis deviation Right ventricular enlargement	Right ventricular-enlargement; if severe, increased a wave on the pulmonic valve
Ebstein's anomaly	20%	Quiet precordium	Single	Tricuspid insufficiency	Globular heart Clear lungs Large right atrium	Wolff-Parkinson-White syndrome (25%) Right atrial enlargement Atypical right bundle-branch block	Tricuspid valve displaced and abnormal

Continued.

TABLE 7–39.—Continued

DEFECT	CYANOSIS	CHAMBER ENLARGEMENT	P₁	MURMUR	CHEST FILM	ECG	ECHOCARDIOGRAM
Atrial septal defect (primum)	0	Right and possibly left ventricle enlargement	Wide and fixed	Flow murmur, left sternal border Mitral regurgitation murmur	Increased pulmonary blood flow Enlargement of pulmonary artery, right ventricle, and atrium Enlargement of left atrium and ventricle	Incomplete right bundle-branch block Left axis deviation	Defect in the atrioventricular valves Paradoxical septal motion
Atrial septal defect (secundum)	0	Right ventricular lift	Wide and fixed	Flow murmur, left sternal border	Increased pulmonary artery size Increased pulmonary blood flow Right ventricular and right atrial enlargement	Incomplete right bundle-branch block	Right ventricular enlargement Paradoxical septal motion

Ventricular septal defect	0	Thrill, left sternal border Left ventricle enlargement	Variable	Regurgitant murmur, left sternal border	Increased pulmonary blood flow Enlargement of right and left ventricle	Biatrial and biventricular enlargement	Increased left-atrium size Left ventricular dilation Septal defect visualized at times
Patent ductus arteriosus	0	Wide pulse pressure Left ventricle enlargement	Variable	Continuous murmur, "machinery murmur"	Increased pulmonary blood flow Left ventricular and left atrial enlargement	Left ventricular enlargement	Increased left atrium size Left ventricular dilation
Tetralogy	+	Right ventricle enlargement	Lessened intensity	Ejection murmur	Decreased pulmonary artery size Decreased pulmonary blood flow No specific chamber enlargement Boot-shaped heart	Right ventricular enlargement	Overriding of the aorta Right ventricular enlargement

*From Eich RH: *Introduction to Cardiology.* New York, Harper & Row Publishers, 1980. Reproduced by permission.

8 Pulmonary Medicine
Charles W. Smith, Jr., M.D.

NORMAL PHYSIOLOGY AND PULMONARY FUNCTION TESTS

TABLE 8–1.—PULMONARY FUNCTION TESTS

Below are short descriptions of commonly ordered pulmonary function tests. Vital capacity, inspiratory capacity, expiratory reserve volume, tidal volume, forced expiratory volume, forced mid-expiratory flow rate, and maximal breathing capacity are measured by routine spirometry. Functional residual capacity, residual volume, and total lung capacity require measurement of lung volumes by gas diffusion studies. (Normal values are listed in parentheses.)

1. *Vital capacity (VC):* The maximum volume of gas that can be exhaled from the lung following a maximal inspiration. A combination of inspiratory reserve volume, tidal volume, and expiratory reserve volume (4 L).

2. *Inspiratory capacity (IC):* The maximum amount of air that can be inspired from the expiratory position of normal breathing. A combination of tidal volume and inspiratory reserve volume (3.37 L).

3. *Expiratory reserve volume (ERV):* The maximum amount of air that can be expired from the end-expiratory position of a normal breath (.7 L).

4. *Tidal volume (TV):* The volume of inspired or expired air during each respiratory cycle (.5 L).

5. *Functional residual capacity (FRC):* The amount of air remaining in the lungs at the expiratory position of normal breathing. A combination of expiratory reserve volume and residual volume (2 L).

6. *Residual volume (RV):* The volume of gas remaining in the lungs at the end of a maximal expiration (1.3 L).

7. *Total lung capacity (TLC):* The amount of air remaining in the lungs at the end of a maximal inspiration. A combination of the four lung volumes (5.37 L).

8. *Forced expiratory volume* (1 sec and 3 sec); (FEV_1, FEV_3): The maximum amount of air that can be expired in 1 (3) sec (FEV_1 = 3.7 L).

9. *Forced mid-expiratory flow* (FEF_{25-75}): The flow rate of air measured during mid-expiration (from spirometry, during 25% and 75% of the forced vital capacity) (2.8 L).

10. *Maximal breathing capacity (MBC):* The total volume of air a patient can move with maximum effort during a given period (also known as maximal voluntary ventilation, MVV) (158 L/min).

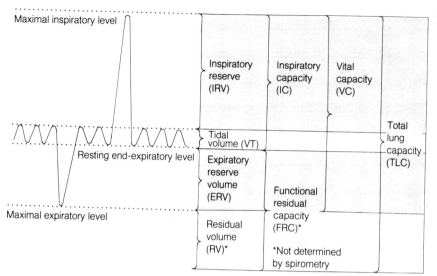

FIG 8–1.

Respiratory system. (From Netter FH, in *The Respiratory System,* vol 7, *The CIBA Collection of Medical Illustrations.* Philadelphia, CIBA-Geigy Corp, 1979, p 48. Reproduced by permission.)

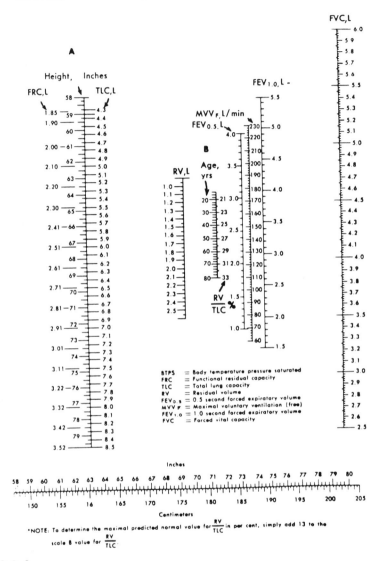

FIG 8–2.

Nomogram for predicting pulmonary function in men. The predicted FRC and TLC can be read directly from the left-hand scale *(A)* based on the patient's height. The horizontal scale at the bottom is for convenience in converting centimeters to inches. The RV/TLC % may be read directly from the age scale *(B)*. For other predicted values, lay a straight edge between the patient's height (scale A) and age (scale B). Predicted normal values can be read directly from the points where the straight edge crosses the RV, $FEV_{0.5}$, MVV, FEV_1, and FVC scales. (From Slonim NB, Hamilton LH: *Respiratory Physiology,* ed 4. St Louis, CV Mosby Co, 1981. Reproduced by permission.)

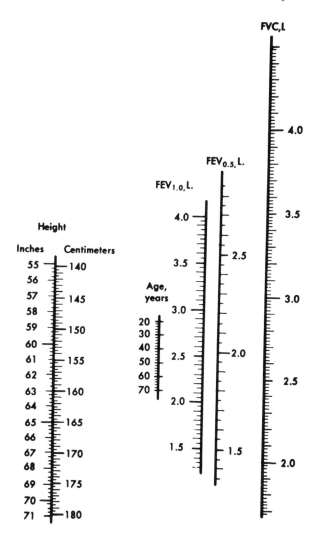

FIG 8–3.
Nomogram for predicting pulmonary function in women. To use nomogram, lay a straight edge between the patient's height as read on the height scale and her age as it appears on the age scale. Predicted normal values for *FEV₁* and *FVC* can be read directly from the points where the straight edge crosses the two right-hand axes. (From Slonim NB, Hamilton LH: *Respiratory Physiology,* ed 4. St Louis, CV Mosby Co, 1981. Reproduced by permission.)

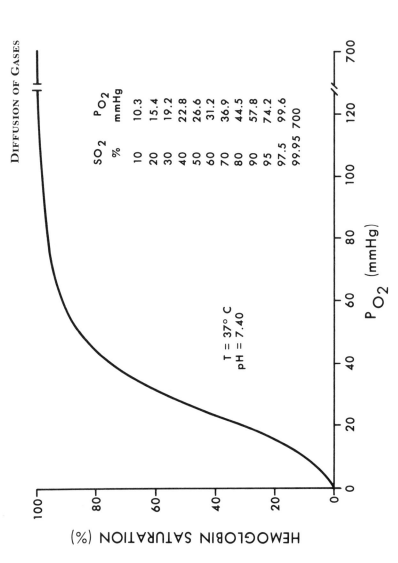

DIFFUSION OF GASES

SO₂ %	P O₂ mmHg
10	10.3
20	15.4
30	19.2
40	22.8
50	26.6
60	31.2
70	36.9
80	44.5
90	57.8
95	74.2
97.5	99.6
99.95	700

T = 37° C
pH = 7.40

FIG 8–4.
The normal oxyhemoglobin dissociation curves for man. Values for hemoglobin saturation (SO_2) at different P_{O_2} values, under standard conditions of temperature and pH, are indicated (data from Severinghaus). (From Murray JF: *The Normal Lung*. Philadelphia, WB Saunders Co, 1976, p 162. Reproduced by permission.)

RESPIRATORY INFECTIONS

TABLE 8–2.—DRUGS OF CHOICE FOR COMMON RESPIRATORY TRACT INFECTIONS*

INFECTING ORGANISM	DRUG OF CHOICE	ALTERNATE DRUG
Gram-positive organisms		
Streptococcus pyogenes (beta-strep.)	Penicillin	Erythromycin or cephalosporin
Staphylococcus aureus	Penicillinase-resistant penicillin	Cephalosporin or amoxicillin–clavulanic acid
Streptococcus pneumoniae (pneumococcus)	Penicillin	Erythromycin or cephalosporin
Gram-negative organisms		
Bacteroides:		
Oropharyngeal	Penicillin G	Clindamycin or metronidazole
Gastrointestinal	Clindamycin or metronidazole	Cefoxitin or pipericillin or imipenem

Continued.

TABLE 8–2.—Continued

INFECTING ORGANISM	DRUG OF CHOICE	ALTERNATE DRUG
Escherichia coli	Ampicillin with or without gentamicin or tobramycin	Mezlocillin or pipericillin or cephalosporin
Klebsiella pneumoniae	A cephalosporin	Gentamicin, tobramycin, or amoxicillin–clavulanic acid
Hemophilus influenzae	Ampicillin or amoxicillin	Trimethoprim-sulfamethoxazole, cefaclor, or ceftriaxone
Legionella pneumophila	Erythromycin with or without rifampin	Trimethoprim-sulfamethoxazole
Pseudomonas aeruginosa	Carbenicillin or ticarcillin plus gentamicin or tobramycin	Gentamicin with ceftazidime or ciprofloxacin
Chlamydia organisms *Chlamydia trachomatis*	Tetracycline	Sulfonamide or erythromycin
Mycoplasma organisms *Mycoplasma pneumoniae*	Erythromycin	Tetracycline

*Adapted from *Med Lett* 1988; 30:30–40.

TABLE 8–3.—GUIDELINES FOR TUBERCULOSIS CHEMOPROPHYLAXIS*

Give isoniazid 300 mg once daily for a year (children, 6–8 mg/kg) to:
1. All known recent (within the past year) tuberculin skin test converters, regardless of age.
2. All household contacts of persons with newly diagnosed active cases, regardless of skin test status.
3. Persons who have a positive tuberculin test who are under 20 years.[†]
4. Positive reactors of any age who have silicosis, severe diabetes, post-gastrectomy, healed Tb on x-ray, lung cancer, lymphoma, need for prolonged steroid treatment, and known Tb who have received inadequate treatment.

*Adapted from Des Prez R: Tuberculosis, in Cecil Textbook of Medicine, ed 16. Philadelphia, WB Saunders Co, 1982.
[†]Some authors recommend extending prophylaxis up to 35 years. Above age 35 the risk of INH hepatitis exceeds the risk of active Tb.

TABLE 8–4.—ANTITUBERCULOUS DRUGS*

DRUG	USUAL DAILY DOSE	TOXICITY
Primary drugs		
Isoniazid	5–10 mg/kg (300 mg max.)	Hepatitis, peripheral neuritis
Rifampin	10–20 mg/kg (600 mg max.)	Hepatitis
Secondary drugs		
Ethambutol	15–25 mg/kg	Optic neuritis
Para-aminosalicylic acid (PAS)	12–15 gm	Hepatotoxic, GI intolerance
Pyrazinamide	20–35 mg/kg (3 gm max.)	Hepatotoxic
Streptomycin	1 gm (IM)	Eighth cranial nerve damage, nephrotoxic
Tertiary drugs†		
Capreomycin		Eighth cranial nerve damage, nephrotoxic
Cycloserine		Convulsions, psychosis
Ethionamide		Hepatotoxic
Kanamycin		Eighth cranial nerve damage, nephrotoxic

*Adapted from Whitcomb ME: *The Lung*. St Louis, CV Mosby Co, 1982, p 327.
†Tertiary drugs are rarely used except in the treatment of drug-resistant tuberculosis.

TABLE 8–5.—CHARACTERISTICS OF PNEUMONIAS CAUSED BY PYOGENIC BACTERIA VERSUS VIRUSES, CHLAMYDIAE, RICKETTSIAE, AND MYCOPLASMAS*

CLINICAL FINDINGS	PYOGENIC BACTERIA	VIRUSES, CHLAMYDIAE, RICKETTSIAE, AND MYCOPLASMAS
Onset	Often sudden	Usually gradual
Myalgia, headache, and photophobia	Not prominent	Often prominent
Fever	>104°F (40°C)	<104°F (40°C)
Rigors	Common, often multiple	Rare, except in influenza and usually single
Toxicity	Marked	Mild to moderate
Cough	Productive—purulent, bloody sputum	Nonproductive or only scant mucoid sputum
Physical findings	Consolidation	Often minimal
Roentgenographic findings	Agree with physical examination; localized	Involvement in excess of physical findings; often multiple sites
Leukocyte count	>15,000/mm³, marked shift to the left	<15,000/mm³, possible lymphocytosis

*Adapted from Hinshaw HC, Murray JF: *Diseases of the Chest*. Philadelphia, WB Saunders Co, 1980, p 212.

TABLE 8–6.—CHARACTERISTICS OF PULMONARY MYCOSES*

	BLASTOMYCOSIS	COCCIDIOIDOMYCOSIS	HISTOPLASMOSIS
Chest roentgenogram			
Acute disease	Focal alveolar infiltrates	Focal alveolar infiltrates Pleural effusions Hilar adenopathy	Focal alveolar infiltrates Diffuse nodules Hilar adenopathy
Chronic disease	Cavities Masses	Thin-walled cavities	Cavities Parenchymal calcifications Fibrosing mediastinitis
Sites of dissemination	Skin Bone Male genital tract	Skin Bone Meninges	Liver and spleen Mucosal surfaces Adrenal glands
Diagnostic studies			
Skin test	No value	Excellent epidemiologic tool	Limited value
Serologic tests	No value	Diagnostic and prognostic value	Limited value

*Adapted from Whitcomb ME: *The Lung.* St Louis, CV Mosby Co, 1982, p 332.

ASTHMA AND COPD

Asthma results in recurrent attacks of wheezing dyspnea with coughing and sputum production. It affects 1 of 25 people. Attacks are caused by an allergic reaction in atopic patients. Nonallergic asthma (intrinsic) is caused by air pollutants, cold, humid air, exercise, respiratory tract infection, drugs, or tension.

TABLE 8–7.—CLINICAL FEATURES OF ASTHMA*

	EXTRINSIC	INTRINSIC
Family history of asthma	Usually positive	Usually negative
Etiology of attacks	Specific antigens	Infections, exercise, smoke, fumes, etc.
Skin testing	Usually positive	Usually negative
Response to hyposensitization	Favorable	Unfavorable
History of childhood eczema	Usually positive	Negative
Relationship to IgE	Yes	No
Character of attacks	Usually self-limiting	More fulminant
Natural history	Often outgrown, may become chronic	Poorer prognosis; respiratory failure not uncommon

*Adapted from Netter FH, in *The Respiratory System,* vol 7, *The CIBA Collection of Medical Illustrations.* Philadelphia, CIBA-Geigy Corp, 1979, p 120.

TABLE 8–8.—TREATMENT OF ACUTE ASTHMA*

1. Quickly assess air movement, cardiac status, and oxygenation.
2. Consider the presence of complications or other diseases such as pulmonary embolus or pulmonary edema as the cause of wheezing.
3. Begin nasal oxygen (4–6 L/min if no COPD is present).
4. Give subcutaneous epinephrine (.3 cc of 1:1000 for adults; 0.01 ml/kg for child). Repeat twice at 15-minute intervals.
5. If first or second dose of epinephrine results in minimal improvement, give nebulized terbutaline.
6. If wheezing persists, begin IV aminophylline (bolus of 6 mg/kg, which is equivalent to 5 mg of anhydrous theophylline). See following tables for maintenance infusions. Dosage must be reduced for patients with heart disease or liver disease, patients taking cimetidine or erythromycin, and the elderly.
7. Give oral or IV steroids early (they take about 12 hours to work). Dosage = 80–100 mg Methylprednisolone (or equivalent) q6h IV for adults. Dosage = 1 mg/kg q6h for children.

8. If alveolar hypoventilation occurs, intubate.
9. Avoid all tranquilizers and sedatives.
10. If wheezing doesn't totally clear after the initial treatment, admit patient to the hospital.

*Adapted from Mitchell RS: *Synopsis of Clinical Pulmonary Disease,* ed 2. St Louis, CV Mosby Co, 1978.

TABLE 8–9.—THEOPHYLLINE DOSING FOR ASTHMA*

1. For patients currently receiving theophylline (within 24 hours):
   Obtain stat serum level.
   For each 1 µg/ml desired increase in serum level, give 0.6 mg/kg of aminophylline as loading infusion over 30 minutes.
2. For patients not receiving theophylline:
   Loading dose of aminophylline is 6 mg/kg (equivalent to 5 mg/kg of anhydrous theophylline) over 30 minutes.
   Following infusion, obtain stat level.
   Begin infusion listed in Table 8–10.
   Measure level 4–6 hours after starting infusion.
   Adjust infusion.
   Obtain serum level 12–24 hours later.

*Aminophylline = theophylline/0.8.

TABLE 8–10.—INITIAL AMINOPHYLLINE MAINTENANCE INFUSIONS*†

GROUP	AGE	AMINOPHYLLINE INFUSION (MG/KG/HR)
Neonates	<24 days	1.3 mg/kg/12 hr
	>24 days	1.9 mg/kg/12 hr
Infants	6 wk to 1 yr	mg/kg/hr = (0.008) (age in weeks) + 0.21
Children	1–9 yr	1.0 mg/kg/hr
	9–12 yr	0.9 mg/kg/hr
Adolescents (cigarette or marijuana smokers)	12–16 yr	0.9 mg/kg/hr
Adolescents (nonsmokers)	12–16 yr	0.6 mg/kg/hr
Adults (healthy cigarette or marijuana smokers)	16–50 yr	0.6 mg/kg/hr
Adults (healthy nonsmokers)	16 yr	0.5 mg/kg/hr
Cardiac decompensation, cor pulmonale, or liver disease	16 yr	0.3 mg/kg/hr

*Adapted from Hendeles L, Weinberg M: *Am J Hosp Pharm* 1982; 39:249–250.
†Infusion is designed to achieve 10 µg/ml serum level. Anhydrous theophylline = aminophylline × 0.8.

TABLE 8–11.—PULMONARY FUNCTION IN PATIENTS WITH ASTHMA, CHRONIC BRONCHITIS, AND EMPHYSEMA*

TEST[†]	ASTHMA[‡]	CHRONIC SEVERE BRONCHITIS	EMPHYSEMA
Vital capacity	Decreased	Decreased	Normal or decreased
Residual volume	Increased	Increased	Increased
Total lung capacity	Normal	Normal	Increased
RV/TLC	Increased	Increased	Increased
FEV_1/FVC	Decreased	Decreased	Decreased
MMFR	Decreased	Decreased	Decreased
Single-breath O_2	Increased	Increased	Increased
Diffusing capacity	Normal or slightly increased	Normal	Decreased
Response to bronchodilators	Improvement	No change	No change
Arterial Po_2	Decreased	Decreased	Slight decrease
Arterial Pco_2	Decreased	Increased	Normal
Hematocrit	Normal	Increased	Normal

*Adapted from Hinshaw HC, Murray JF: *Diseases of the Chest.* Philadelphia, WB Saunders Co, 1980, p 94.
†Abbreviations: RV/TLC = residual volume to total lung capacity ratio; FEV_1/FVC = forced expiratory volume in 1 second to forced vital capacity ratio; MMFR = maximal midexpiratory flow rate.
‡During an attack; values should approach or be normal when properly treated.

RESPIRATORY FAILURE, ARDS, AND VENTILATORS

TABLE 8–12.—PRINCIPLES OF MANAGEMENT OF RESPIRATORY FAILURE

Respiratory failure: The sudden reduction in oxygen tension to less than 50 mm Hg.
1. If patient is apneic or nearly apneic, immediately intubate.
2. Consider narcotic as a cause and give 0.4 mg of naloxone IV, IM, or SQ (.01 mg/kg in children).
3. Measure blood gases and begin 24% oxygen.
4. Attempt to maintain Po_2 at about 50 mm Hg if patient has physical signs of COPD.
5. If pH is less than 7.20, give 44 mEq (1 ampule) sodium bicarbonate. Measure blood gases again, check electrolytes, and calculate anion gap.
6. Intubate and ventilate the patient if:
   (a) Patient cannot be adequately oxygenated without increasing CO_2 retention and acidosis.
   (b) There are respiratory depressant drugs "on board" or there is mechanical interference with chest wall function.
7. Look aggressively for the cause of the decompensation (CHF, pneumonia, pneumothorax).
8. Use bronchodilators to attempt to improve ventilation.
9. Give frequent chest physical therapy, even if patient is being mechanically ventilated.

TABLE 8–13.—Devices for Oxygen Delivery

DEVICE	FLOW (L/MIN)	RANGE (% Fi_{O_2})
Nasal cannula	1–2	23–28
	3–4	28–38
	5–6	32–45
	Advantages	*Disadvantages*
	Inexpensive	Poor humidification
	Comfortable	Drying of mucosa
	Allows eating	Uncertain Fi_{O_2}
	and exercise	Limited maximum Fi_{O_2}
Simple mask	3–4	25–30
	5–6	30–45
	7–8	40–60
	Advantages	*Disadvantages*
	Inexpensive	Bothersome
	Higher maximum Fi_{O_2}	Possible CO_2 collection
		Requires tight seal
Nonrebreathing mask	8	70–100
	Advantages	*Disadvantages*
	Useful for severely	Bothersome
	hypoxemic,	Requires tight seal
	normocapnic patients	Not tolerated for long
Rebreathing mask	8	50–60
	Advantages	*Disadvantages*
	Useful for hypoxemic,	Possible hypercapnia
	hypocapneic patients	Bothersome
		Requires tight seal
Face tent or aerosol mask	8	30–100
	Advantages	*Disadvantages*
	Versatile	Requires frequent drainage of
	High humidity	tubing and filling reservoir
	Good CO_2 washout	Contamination with gram-negative bacteria
		Noisy
Venturi mask	4	24
	4	28
	6	31
	8	35
	8	40
	Advantages	*Disadvantages*
	Comfortable, cool	More expensive
	Accurate air flow	Not tolerated for long

TABLE 8–14.—INDICATIONS FOR HOME OXYGEN THERAPY

1. Documentation of persistent Po$_2$ <55 mm Hg or
2. Presence of Po$_2$ between 55 and 59 mm Hg accompanied by one or more of the following:
   Cor pulmonale
   Evidence of pulmonary hypertension on physical exam, chest x-ray film, or ECG
   Hematocrit >55%
   Decreased mental function, improved by O$_2$ trial
   Markedly decreased exercise tolerance, improved by O$_2$ trial (requires documentation of worsening oxygenation after exercise)

TABLE 8–15.—CHECKLIST FOR PATIENTS USING A VENTILATOR*

1. Use ≥ 7.5-mm tube for adults with a high compliance cuff.
2. Keep the cuff pressure < 30 mm Hg.
3. Check the tube position with a portable chest x-ray film.
4. Keep the tidal volume at 10–13 ml/kg body weight.
5. Set the rate initially at a minute ventilation of 5–10 L (12–16 breaths/min), but adjust to keep blood gases optimal.
6. Set initial mode at assist/control.
7. Set sensitivity so that patient will trigger an inspiration at about −2 or −3 cm H$_2$O inspiratory force.
8. Select a flow rate that provides an inspiratory/expiratory flow of about 1:3 (usually about 40–60 L/min).
9. Set alarm at about 10 cm H$_2$O above pressure required to deliver the selected tidal volume, keep in continuous use, and check daily.
10. Set initial O$_2$ concentration at 100%, and adjust to keep arterial blood gases at about this level: Po$_2$ 60–90 mm Hg; pH 7.35–7.50. NOTE: Ear oximetry, when calibrated against arterial blood gases, is adequate for monitoring oxygen saturation, provided there is no need to know Paco$_2$ or pH.
11. If inadequate oxygenation persists despite 100% O$_2$, add positive end-expiratory pressure (PEEP). Start with 4 cm H$_2$O and add increments of 2–4 cm H$_2$O every 15–30 min, monitoring blood gases prior to each change. Also consider PEEP if a Pao$_2$ ≥ 50 mm Hg cannot be maintained with an inspired O$_2$ concentration of ≤ 50%.
12. Monitor vital signs frequently and look for a cause for sudden tachycardia or low blood pressure.
13. Continuously monitor cardiac rhythm.
14. Frequently monitor mentation and urine output.

*Adapted from Mitchell RL: *Synopsis of Clinical Pulmonary Disease*, ed 2. St Louis, CV Mosby Co, 1978, and Popovich J: *Postgrad Med* 1986; 79:217–227.

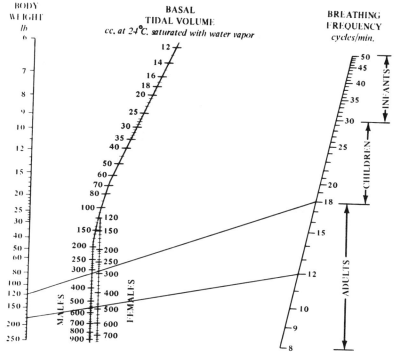

FIG 8–5.
Nomogram for predicting normal tidal volumes at different rates of breathing according to body weight. The values given represent minimum values in most clinical situations below which underventilation can be considered to have occurred. A spirometer or ventilation meter is necessary for the application of this nomogram. Correction of these values can be made in the following manner: add 10% for daily activity and eating; add 5% for each degree of fever (°F) above rectal normal, 99°; and 5% for each 2,000 feet of residence above sea level. (From Crews ER, Lapuerta L: *A Manual of Respiratory Failure.* Springfield, III, Charles C Thomas, Publisher, 1976, p 79. Reproduced by permission.)

TABLE 8–16.—Weaning Patients From Ventilators*

1. Make sure alveolar-arterial oxygen tension difference on 100% O_2 is less than 300–350 mm Hg.
2. Make sure vital capacity is 10–15 ml/kg body weight.
3. Maximum inspiratory force should be > -20 cc H_2O.
4. Ratio of dead space to tidal volume (VD/VT) should be $<.6$ for "difficult to wean" patients.
5. Place patient in a sitting position.
6. Reduce Fi_{O_2} to 25%–30%.
7. Reduce tidal volume to about 500 ml.
8. Place ventilator on assist.
9. Take patient off all respiratory depressant drugs.

Continued.

TABLE 8–16.—Continued

10. Assure that patient has FVC 2 to 3 times normal tidal volume (about 1,000 cc).
11. Try off ventilator for 15 minutes with O_2 increased by 5%–10% over baseline.
12. If Po_2 remains above 50 mm Hg and pH is above 7.25, keep off ventilator for 15 minutes of every hour. Otherwise, postpone weaning.
13. Check blood gases regularly.
14. Place back on ventilator for sleeping, first night.
15. Next day increase time off ventilator to 30 minutes per hour until morning of third day.
16. Third day allow off ventilator for 45 minutes every hour.
17. Increase time off to 1¾ hours off, 15 minutes on.
18. If tolerated, consider extubation at this point.
19. Administer IPPB treatment every 4–6 hours and continue to monitor blood gases and clinical status closely. Monitor vital signs every 5–10 minutes in first hour, then every 15–20 minutes; blood gases about every hour.
NOTE: Intermittent mandatory ventilation is an alternative weaning procedure that allows a gradual decrease in the number of ventilator-delivered breaths per minute. The criteria and monitoring are otherwise the same as for the traditional approach.

*Adapted from Berte JB: *Pulmonary Emergencies.* Philadelphia, JB Lippincott Co, 1977, p 86, and Feely TW, Hedley-Whyte J: *N Engl J Med* 1975; 292:903–905.

LUNG TUMORS AND PULMONARY NODULES

TABLE 8–17.—CONTRAINDICATIONS TO RESECTIONAL SURGERY IN PATIENTS WITH LUNG CANCER

Absolute contraindications:
1. Extrathoracic metastases.
2. Involvement of the trachea, carina, or proximal mainstem bronchus.
3. Obstruction of the superior vena cava.
4. Involvement of the recurrent laryngeal nerve.
5. Malignant effusion.
6. Positive mediastinoscopy; positive contralateral nodes.
7. Phrenic nerve, pericardial, or esophageal involvement.
8. Undifferentiated small cell (oat cell).
9. Inadequate pulmonary function to tolerate surgery.
Relative contraindications:
1. Age 70 or older.
2. Local chest wall involvement.
3. Pancoast tumor.
4. Positive mediastinoscopy; ipsilateral nodes.
5. Pleural effusion with negative cytology.

TABLE 8–18.—THE SOLITARY PULMONARY NODULE

Lesion more likely benign if:
  Previous X-ray documents no growth.
  It is totally calcified.
  It has target, "popcorn," or lamellated calcification (suggests inflammatory lesion).
  It is small (i.e., <1.5 cm).
  If it is near an interlobular fissure (characteristic of granuloma).
Lesion more likely malignant if:
  It has grown in the past year.
  It has no calcification (or only a "fleck").
  It has spicular radiations at the peripheral edge.
  It has a lobular appearance.
  It is in the center of a lobule.
  It is a large lesion.

TABLE 8–19.—INITIAL APPROACH TO EVALUATING HEMOPTYSIS

1. Determine whether sputum is blood-streaked or whether gross blood is present.
2. Look at a Gram stain.
3. Obtain a chest X-ray.
4. Apply a tuberculin test.
5. Obtain sputum cytology.
6. Further testing or referral, depending on results of above.

TABLE 8–20.—DIFFERENTIAL DIAGNOSIS OF HEMOPTYSIS*

GROSS HEMOPTYSIS	BLOOD-STREAKED SPUTUM
Tuberculosis	Upper respiratory tract infection
Bronchiectasis	Chronic bronchitis
Bronchial adenoma	Sarcoidosis
Bronchogenic carcinoma	Bronchogenic carcinoma
Aspergilloma	Tuberculosis
Necrotizing pneumonia	Pulmonary infarction
Lung abscess	Pulmonary edema
Pulmonary contusion	Mitral stenosis
Arteriovenous malformation	Idiopathic pulmonary hemosiderosis
Bleeding disorder or excessive anticoagulant therapy	
Mitral stenosis	

*Adapted from Goroll AH, May LA, Mulley AG: *Primary Care Medicine.* Philadelphia, JB Lippincott Co, 1981.

ACIDOSIS AND ALKALOSIS

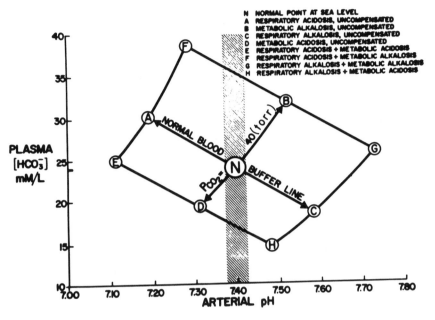

FIG 8–6.
Curve for acidosis and alkalosis. (From Slonim NB, Hamilton LH: *Respiratory Physiology,* ed 3. St Louis, CV Mosby Co, 1976, p 115. Reproduced by permission.)

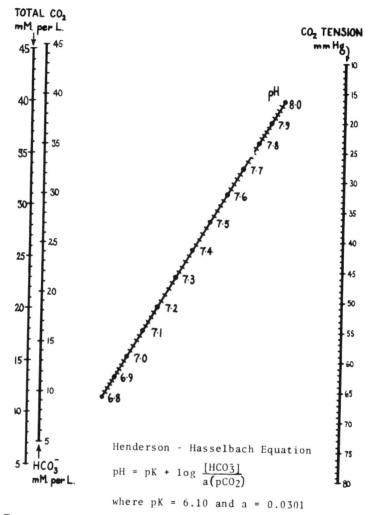

Henderson - Hasselbach Equation

$$pH = pK + \log \frac{[HCO_3^-]}{a(pCO_2)}$$

where $pK = 6.10$ and $a = 0.0301$

FIG 8–7.
Henderson-Hasselbach equation: acid-base nomogram. (From Biller JA, Yeager AM: *The Harriet Lane Handbook,* ed 9. Chicago, Year Book Medical Publishers, 1981, p 256. Reproduced by permission.)

TABLE 8–21.—ACID-BASE BALANCE

ANION GAP $= (Na^+ + K^+) - (Cl^- + HCO_3^- + Prot^-, Phos^-, Sulfate^-)$
Normally this value should not exceed 12 mmol/L. If it does, consider the following:
Renal failure
Diabetic ketoacidosis
Alcoholic ketoacidosis
Lactic acidosis
Salicylate poisoning
Ethylene glycol poisoning
Methyl alcohol poisoning
(Note: $Prot^-$, $Phos^-$, $Sulfate^-$ is estimated by a constant $= 20$ mEq/L)

*Adapted from Levinsky N: Acidosis and alkalosis, in Isselbacher K, Braunwald E, et al (eds): *Harrison's Principles of Internal Medicine,* ed 11, New York, McGraw-Hill Book Co, 1980.

TABLE 8–22.—CALCULATION OF ANION GAP*

	POSITIVE CHARGES (mEq/L)		NEGATIVE CHARGES (mEq/L)		ANION GAP
Normal	Na^+	140	Cl^-	100	
	K^+	5	HCO_3^-	25	
			Protein$^-$, phosphate$^-$, and sulfate$^-$	20	$145 - 145 = 0$ mEq/L
	Positive charges	$\overline{145}$	Negative charges	$\overline{145}$	
Organic (lactic) acidosis	Na^+	140	Cl^-	95	
	K^+	5	HCO_3^-	10	
			Protein$^-$, phosphate$^-$, and sulfate$^-$	20	$145 - 125 = 20$ mEq/L
	Positive charges	$\overline{145}$	Negative charges	$\overline{125}$	

*From Robin EG: Respiratory medicine, in Rubenstein E, Federman D (eds): *Scientific American Medicine.* New York, Scientific American Co, vol 2, chap 14, 1–10, 1984. Reproduced by permission.

INTERSTITIAL LUNG DISEASE

TABLE 8–23.—DRUGS THAT CAUSE INTERSTITIAL LUNG DISEASE*

Those indicated *in italics* are of particular clinical importance; the others are rarely encountered.

ACUTE INFILTRATIONS
With eosinophilia
Aurothioglucose (Solganal)
Chlorpropamide (Diabinese)
Disodium cromoglycate (Cromolyn)
Imipramine (Tofranil)
Isoniazid
Mephenesin carbamate
Methotrexate (Amethopterin)
Nitrofurantoin (Furadantin)
Para-aminosalicylic acid
Penicillin
Pituitary snuff
Sulfonamides
Without eosinophilia
Amitriptyline (Elavil)
Azathioprine (Imuran)
Procarbazine (Matulane)

CHRONIC INFILTRATIONS
Diffuse interstitial fibrosis
Bleomycin
Busulfan (Myleran)
Carmustine (BiCNU)
Cyclophosphamide
(Cytoxan)
Gold sodium thiomalate
(Myochrysine)
Hexamethonium
Mecamylamine (Inversine)
Melphalan (Alkeran)
Methysergide (Sansert)
Nitrofurantoin (Furadantin)
Oxygen
Pentolinium tartrate (Anso-
lysen)
Pituitary snuff
Radiation
With lupus erythematosus-like
syndrome
Digitalis
Gold salts
Griseofulvin
Hydantoin (Dilantin)
Hydralazine (Apresoline)
Isoniazid
Mephenytoin (Mesantoin)
Methyldopa (Aldomet)
Methylthiouracil
Oral contraceptives
Penicillin
Phenylbutazone (Butazoli-
din)
Procainamide (Pronestyl)
Propylthiouracil
Reserpine
Streptomycin
Sulfonamides
Tetracyclines
Thiazides

*From Hinshaw HC, Murray JF: *Diseases of the Chest.* Philadelphia, WB Saunders Co, 1980, p 573. Reproduced by permission.

TABLE 8–24.—Chest X-Ray Changes in Chronic Intrinsic Lung Disease*

CHANGE	USUAL CAUSE
Reduced lung volumes	Decreased pulmonary compliance
Reticular pattern	Interstitial granuloma, cell infiltrate, or fibrosis
Nodular pattern	Intra-alveolar or interstitial abnormalities
Reticulonodular pattern	Intra-alveolar or interstitial abnormalities
Ground-glass appearance with or without air bronchogram	Intra-alveolar accumulation of non-air-bearing material
Miliary pattern	Filling of pulmonary acinus with fluid or other non-air-bearing material
Kerley's A, B, and C lines	Thickened interlobular septa
Honeycombing	Advanced interstitial fibrosis
Dilated central pulmonary artery branches with attenuated peripheral branches	Pulmonary hypertension
Pleural alterations	Pleural effusion, fibrosis, or calcification
Increased right ventricular size	Cor pulmonale

*From Robin EG: Respiratory medicine, in Rubenstein E, Federman D (eds): *Scientific American Medicine.* New York, vol 2, chap 14, V–14, 1984. Reproduced by permission.

CHEST FILMS

TABLE 8–25.—Short Guide to Reading Chest Films

1. Check exposure technique for lightness or darkness.
2. Verify left and right by looking at stomach bubble and heart shape.
3. Check for rotation: does the thoracic spine shadow align in the center of the sternum between the clavicles?
4. Make sure film is taken in full inspiration (10 posterior or 6 anterior ribs should be visible).
5. Is the film a portable, anteroposterior, or posteroanterior film? (The heart size cannot be accurately judged from an AP film.)
6. Check the soft tissues for foreign bodies or subcutaneous emphysema.
7. Check all visible bones and joints for osteoporosis, old fractures, metastatic lesions, rib notching, or presence of cervical ribs.
8. Look at diaphragm for tenting, free air, and position.
9. Check hilar and mediastinal areas for:
    Size and shape of aorta
    Presence of hilar nodes
    Prominence of hilar blood vessels
    Elevation of vessels (left normally slightly higher)

Continued.

TABLE 8–25.—Continued

10. Look at heart for size, shape, calcified valves, and enlarged atria.
11. Check costophrenic angles for fluid or pleural scarring.
12. Check pulmonary parenchyma for infiltrates, increased interstitial markings, masses, absence of normal margins, air bronchograms, or increased vascularity, and "silhouette" signs.
13. Look at lateral film for:
    Confirmation and position of questionable masses or infiltrates
    Size of retrosternal air space
    Anteroposterior chest diameter
    Vertebral bodies for bony lesions or overlying infiltrates
    Posterior costophrenic angle for small effusion

PLEURAL EFFUSIONS

TABLE 8–26.—PLEURAL FLUID TRANSUDATES AND EXUDATES*

CHARACTER OF PLEURAL EFFUSION	RELATED DISORDERS
Transudate	
Protein less than 2.5 gm/dl	Cardiac, renal or hepatic failure
Clear, yellow; specific gravity	Myxedema (protein content increased)
less than 1.016	Severe anemia
Fluid/serum protein	Nephrotic state
ratio < 0.5	Hypoproteinemic states
Fluid/serum LDH	Pancreatic disease
ratio < 0.6	Liver disease (cirrhosis)
Fluid LDH < 2/3 upper limit	Meig's tumor
of nl for serum LDH	Superior vena cava obstruction
Exudate	
Protein greater than 3 gm/dl	Bacterial infections
Cloudy; specific gravity	Viral infections
greater than 1.016	Tuberculosis
At least one of the	Thoracic neoplasms
following:	Rheumatic fever
Fluid/serum protein	Septicemia
ratio > 0.5	Postmyocardial infarction
Fluid/serum LDH	Infectious mononucleosis
ratio > 0.6	Pulmonary infarct
Fluid LDH > 2/3 upper	Rheumatoid arthritis
limit of nl for serum	SLE (lupus)
LDH	

Increased eosinophils

Hydatid cyst
Loeffler syndrome
Tropical eosinophilia
Polyarteritis nodosa
Hodgkin's disease
Carcinoma
Pulmonary infarct

Decreased pleural glucose

SLE
TBC (tuberculosis)

(as low as 6 mg/dl)   R.A. (rheumatoid arthritis)

*Adapted from Berte JB: *Pulmonary Emergencies.* New York, JB Lippincott Co, 1977, p 149 and Sahn SA: *Hosp Med* 1988; 24(8):77–87.

COMMON PULMONARY DIAGNOSTIC PROCEDURES

TABLE 8–27.—Thoracentesis*

Materials:
  Antiseptic solution and swabs
  Sterile field
  Small and large syringes
  25-gauge needle and 1% Xylocaine
  15- to 18-gauge needle
  Three-way stopcock
  Sterile specimen containers
Procedure:
  1. Determine puncture site by x-ray and percussion.
  2. Entry site should be directly above the rib (nerve and vessels are under the rib surface).
  3. Raise a skin wheal and inject 1–2 cc along the rib periosteum.
  4. Inject 3–5 cc near the pleural surface.
  5. Use a large syringe and needle with three-way stopcock and draw off fluid as needed. An intracath or angiocath can be used to minimize risk of lung puncture.
  6. When attempting to draw all the fluid off, stop when aspiration begins to block further drainage (the pleura is being drawn into the end of the needle at this point).
  7. Send fluid for all needed studies. Routinely these should include cell count and differential, protein, glucose, LDH, routine culture, Gram stain, and specific gravity. If indicated, include cytology, AFB, and fungal cultures.
  8. A post-tap chest x-ray film should be obtained to rule out traumatic pneumothorax.

*Adapted from Fishman NH: *Thoracic Drainage: A Manual of Procedures.* Chicago, Year Book Medical Publishers, 1983, pp 27–32.

TABLE 8–28.—Pʟᴀᴄᴇᴍᴇɴᴛ ᴏꜰ Cʜᴇsᴛ Tᴜʙᴇ*

Materials:
Applicators for antiseptic
Antiseptic (Iodophor)
Sterile gloves
Lidocaine, 1% without epinephrine
Syringes, 10 ml and 30 ml
Needles: ½-inch, 25-gauge; 1½-inch, 22-gauge
Scalpel with No. 11 and 15 blades
Suture, 2–0 silk or synthetic with cutting skin needle
Hemostats, one sharp pointed "mosquito," one Kelly or Mayo clamp
Scissors, preferably pointed
Connectors, two "five-in-one" double-tapered
Test tubes for laboratory specimens
Dressings, four 4 × 4 inches
Chest tubes (usually kept separately): 12 F Trocarcath; 20 or 36 F multifenestrated vinyl tube
Suction/underwater seal apparatus, e.g., Pleurevac (kept separately)
Tubing, to connect apparatus to vacuum source
Procedure (see corresponding letters in Figure 8–8):
1. Prepare patient in the appropriate area.
2. Anesthetize skin, periosteum, and pleura as for thoracentesis procedure. Insert needle and aspirate to confirm presence of air or fluid *(A)*.
3. Make a 1–1½-inch transverse incision just above the rib in the appropriate interspace. The incision should be carried through the dermis *(B)*.
4. Work a closed Kelly clamp through the subcutaneous tissue, intercostal muscles, and into the pleural space. Turn the clamp with a "screw-like" motion but maintain control of the clamp. Entering the pleura may require additional pressure and will probably be accompanied by a sudden "popping" into the space *(C)*.
5. Enlarge the opening in the chest wall and pleura by spreading the clamp in several different planes.
6. Insert a 12 F trocar along same path. After tube is through pleura, withdraw stylet a few mm *(D)*.
7. Insert the tube into the opening and advance the tube until it is suitably placed within the pleural space, withdrawing stylet as you go. Clamp tube to avoid entry of air into the chest *(E)*.
8. Attach the tubing to the bottle with an underwater seal.
9. Secure the chest tube to the chest wall with a skin suture *(inset)*.
10. Further secure and protect the tube by taping.

*Adapted from Fishman NH: *Thoracic Drainage: A Manual of Procedures.* Chicago, Year Book Medical Publishers, 1983, pp 32–37.

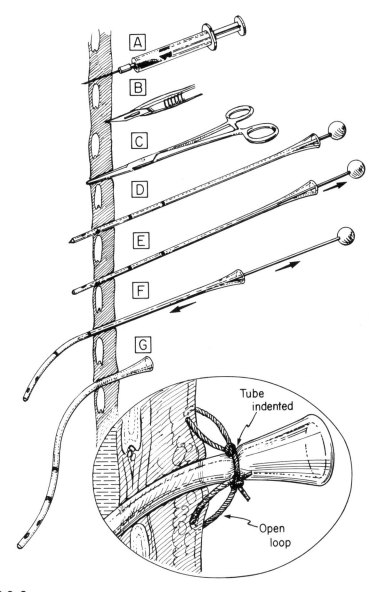

FIG 8–8.
Technique of chest tube placement. (From Fishman NH: *Thoracic Drainage: A Manual of Procedures*. Chicago, Year Book Medical Publishers, 1983, p 34. Reproduced by permission.)

TABLE 8–29.—MAKING AND INTERPRETING GRAM STAINS

Materials:
  Gram's iodine
  Crystal violet
  Acetone or 95% ethyl alcohol
  Safranin
Procedure
  1. Spread sputum in thin layer over slide. Use another slide to obtain good uniformity. Do not use cotton swab.
  2. Fix slide with match, burner, or by placing in incubator for 3–5 minutes.
  3. Flood slide with crystal violet for 15–30 seconds and rinse with tap water.
  4. Flood slide with Gram's iodine for 15–30 seconds and rinse with tap water.
  5. Decolorize with acetone or alcohol by rinsing just until the blue color disappears.
  6. Counterstain for 15 seconds with safranin.
  7. Dry by leaving in open air, placing in incubator, or by carefully blotting with soft, absorbent paper.
Tips on interpretation:
  1. Obtain the sputum yourself if you feel it important to have accurate information.
  2. Check for the presence of epithelial cells and, if large numbers are present, obtain another specimen. The one you have isn't sputum, it's saliva.
  3. If there are five or more polymorphonuclear cells per high power field, it is probably an infectious or inflammatory process.
  4. There will almost always be various kinds of bugs on the slide. Look for the predominant organism.
  5. Look especially for intracellular organisms. They are a certain indicator of the infecting process.
  6. Even if the slide isn't technically ideal, look for an interpretable area, e.g., not overdecolorized, few or no epithelial cells, numerous polys, etc.

TABLE 8–30.—Arterial Puncture

Materials:
10-cc glass syringe
Heparin 1:1,000 dilution
22- to 25-gauge needle
Rubber stopper or other occlusive device for needle
Ice

Procedure

1. Line the glass syringe with heparin by aspirating 1 cc and pumping the plunger twice and squirting out all but what remains in the hub and the needle.
2. Palpate the pulse with two or three fingers to "map" the course of the vessel.
3. Prepare the area with an alcohol swab.
4. Insert the needle at about 90 degrees (45 degrees for radial samples).
5. A short, quick, downward motion will be more likely to enter the artery. The depth of insertion depends on the site of the puncture (2 cm for brachial and 3–4 cm for femoral punctures).
6. Allow the arterial pressure to fill the syringe to about 3 cc volume.
7. If first insertion not successful, gently and slowly withdraw needle, since artery may have been overshot on the way in.
8. If still unsuccessful, repalpate pulse, redirect needle, and reinsert.
9. Do not aspirate except as a last resort. If aspiration is necessary to get the specimen, it is much more likely to contain venous blood.
10. Place pressure over the puncture with a dry gauze pad for at least 5 minutes.
11. Occlude needle and transport specimen to lab in ice.

9 Gastroenterology
Charles W. Smith, Jr., M.D.

REFLUX ESOPHAGITIS

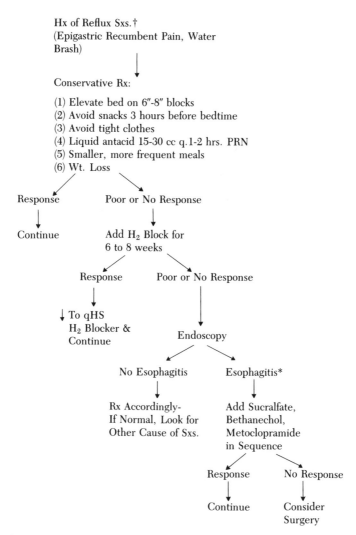

FIG 9–1.
Evaluation and treatment of reflux esophagitis. *If findings are equivocal, consider Bernstein test. †If symptoms are not typical, consider barium swallow to exclude peptic ulcer disease, cancer, etc. (Adapted from Crump WJ: *Primary Care Clinics in Office Practice* 1988; 15(1):13–30.)

PEPTIC ULCER DISEASE

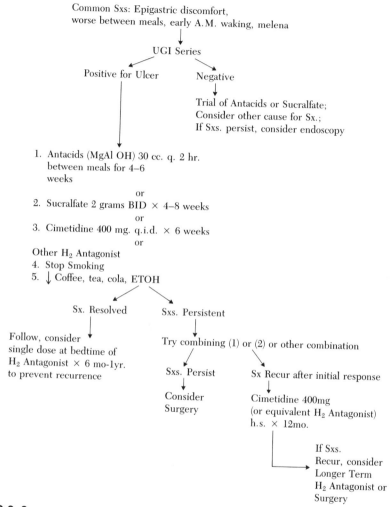

FIG 9–2.
Evaluation and treatment of peptic ulcer disease.

TABLE 9–1.—DIFFERENTIAL FEATURES OF PEPTIC ULCER*

TYPE OF LESION	INCIDENCE	PATHOPHYSIOLOGY	CLINICAL FEATURES	COURSE
Duodenal ulcer	M:F ratio, 3:1 Peak incidence, 5th–6th decades Prevalence, 10–12%	Normal to increased parietal cell mass Normal to increased gastric acid secretion Normal to mildly elevated circulating gastrin levels Excessive gastrin response to meals, excessive parietal cell sensitivity Genetic factors: familial tendency, frequent blood group O, nonsecretor Positive associations: chronic obstructive lung disease, hepatic cirrhosis, pancreatic insufficiency, hyperparathyroidism Located in duodenal bulb, pyloric channel, postbulbar area	Pain: rhythmic, periodic, chronic Pain-food-relief-pain pattern	Remissions and exacerbations for 10–25 years after onset. "Once an ulcer, always an ulcer"; seasonal trend (spring and fall)

Gastric ulcer	M:F ratio, 3–4:1 Peak incidence, 6th–7th decades Duodenal ulcer: gastric ulcer, 4:1	Normal to decreased parietal cell mass Normal to decreased gastric acid secretion (not achlorhydria) Normal to elevated circulating gastrin level Presence of gastritis Abnormal gastric mucosal barrier Abnormal pyloric function, bile reflux Ulcerogenic drugs	Pain-food-relief-pain pattern, or food-pain pattern Weight loss, anorexia	Remissions and exacerbations less than in duodenal ulcer: high recurrence rate: no seasonal trend
Gastric erosions or stress ulcer	No sex difference Related to severe stress, sepsis, burns, trauma, head injuries	Head injuries; marked gastric acid hypersecretion Others: gastric mucosal ischemia, acid back-diffusion, acute gastritis	Bleeding frequent in recognized cases; may be severe, persistent (actual frequency unknown)	Half of those who bleed require surgery

*From Greenberger NJ: Gastrointestinal Disorders, ed 2. Chicago, Year Book Medical Publishers, 1981, p 72. Reproduced by permission.

TABLE 9–2.—Sources of Gastrointestinal Tract Bleeding[*]

CATEGORY	UPPER GI TRACT	LOWER GI TRACT
Inflammatory	Peptic ulcer[†] Esophagitis[†] Gastritis[†] Stress ulcer Pancreatitis	Ulcerative colitis[†] Crohn's disease[†] Diverticulitis Enterocolitis; tuberculosis bacterial, toxic, radiation
Mechanical	Hiatal hernia Mallory-Weiss syndrome[†] Hematobilia	Diverticulosis[†] Anal fissure[†]
Vascular	Esophageal or gastric varices[†] Mesenteric vascular occlusion Aortoduodenal fistula Malformations: hemangioma, Osler- Weber-Rendu syndrome, blue nevus bleb	Hemorrhoids[†] Mesenteric vascular occlusion Aortointestinal fistula Aortic aneurysm Malformations: hemangioma, Osler-Weber-Rendu syndrome, blue nevus bleb, angiodysplasia
Neoplastic	Carcinoma Polyps; single, multiple, Peutz-Jeghers syndrome Leiomyoma Carcinoid Leukemia Sarcoma Metastatic (e.g., melanoma)	Carcinoma[†] Polyps[†]; adenomatous and villous, familial polyposis, Peutz-Jeghers syndrome Leiomyoma Carcinoid Leukemia Sarcoma Metastatic (e.g., melanoma)
Systemic	Blood dyscrasias and clotting abnormalities Collagen diseases Uremia	Blood dyscrasias and clotting abnormalities Collagen diseases Uremia
Anomalies	Gastric and duodenal diverticula	Meckel's diverticulum

[*]Adapted from Greenberger NJ, Norton J: *Gastrointestinal Disorders,* ed 2. Chicago, Year Book Medical Publishers, 1981.
[†]Most common disorders.

UPPER AND LOWER GI BLEEDING

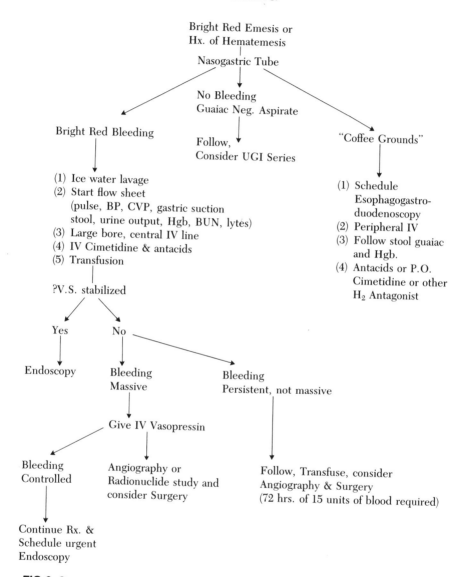

FIG 9–3.

Evaluation and treatment of upper gastrointestinal tract bleeding.

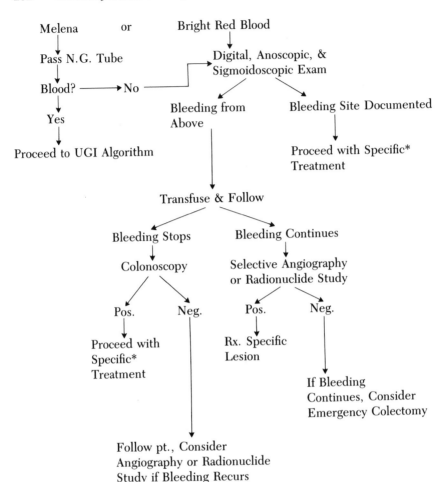

Melena   or   Bright Red Blood

Pass N.G. Tube → Digital, Anoscopic, & Sigmoidoscopic Exam

Blood? → No

Yes → Bleeding from Above   Bleeding Site Documented

Proceed to UGI Algorithm   Proceed with Specific* Treatment

Transfuse & Follow

Bleeding Stops   Bleeding Continues

Colonoscopy   Selective Angiography or Radionuclide Study

Pos.   Neg.   Pos.   Neg.

Proceed with Specific* Treatment   Rx. Specific Lesion

If Bleeding Continues, Consider Emergency Colectomy

Follow pt., Consider Angiography or Radionuclide Study if Bleeding Recurs

*Diverticular Disease——→Vasopressin or Surgery
Angiodysplasia——→Same or Electrocautery
Polyp——→Biopsy and Electrocautery
Tumor——→Definitive Surgery

FIG 9–4.
Management of lower gastrointestinal tract bleeding. (Adapted from Bope ET: *Primary Care* 1988; 15:93–97.)

ABDOMINAL PAIN

TABLE 9–3.—Evaluation of Acute Abdominal Pain

TEST	METHOD	INTERPRETATION	SIGNIFICANCE
Rebound tenderness	Gentle, deep pressure over abdomen, quick release	Severe pain on release = pos. test	Localized or generalized peritonitis
Guarding (rigidity)	Careful gentle pressure on abdominal wall	Pt. resists palpation; may be voluntary or involuntary	May be pos. in some normal pts.; consider nervous state of pt.; "board-like" indicates perforated viscus
Hyperesthesia	Lightly stroke abdominal wall with point of a pin at slight angle	Stroke feels sharper in pos. area	Pos. along dermatome affected or in distribution of affected peripheral nerve
Iliopsoas sign	Place pt. on side opposite pain; extend and hyperextend thigh	Causes pain or pt. resists maneuver due to psoas spasm	Caused by direct or indirect psoas (retroperitoneal) irritation
Obturator sign (thigh rotation test)	Flex knee and thigh on affected side; rotate lower leg medially and thigh laterally	Pos. test causes lower quadrant pain	Pos. when focus in contact with obturator internus (e.g., perforated appendix)

DIARRHEA AND MALABSORPTION

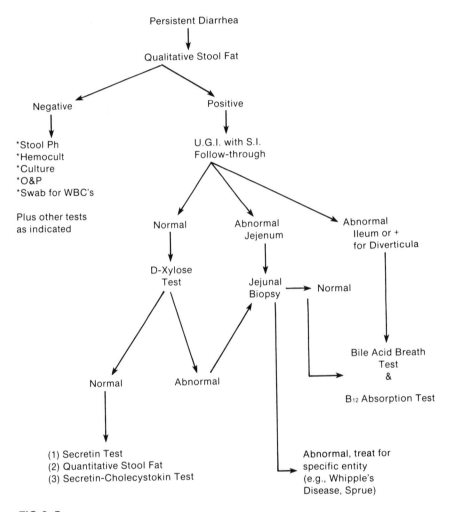

FIG 9–5.
Evaluation of chronic diarrhea.

TABLE 9–4.—TESTS FOR MALABSORPTION*

TEST	NORMAL VALUES	MALABSORPTION (NONTROPICAL SPRUE)	MALDIGESTION (PANCREATIC INSUFFICIENCY)	COMMENT
Quantitative determination of stool fat	<6 gm/24 hr; >95% coefficient of fat absorption	>6 gm/24 hr	>6 gm/24 hr	Best test for establishing presence of steatorrhea
D-Xylose absorption (25 gm oral dose)	5-hr urinary excretion >4.5 gm; peak blood level >30 mg/dl	↓	Normal	A good screening test for carbohydrate absorption
Small intestinal x-rays		Malabsorption pattern	Normal or minimal malabsorption pattern; occasionally pancreatic calcification	Moulage sign and other abnormalities may be present in several disorders
Small intestinal mucosal biopsy		Abnormal	Normal	A specific diagnosis can be established in a small number of disorders
Schilling test for vitamin B12 absorption	>8% urinary excretion in 48 hr	Frequently ↓	Frequently ↓	Useful in determining whether vitamin B12 malabsorption is due to gastric or small intestinal disorders
Secretin test	Volume >1.8 (ml/kg)/hr Bicarbonate concentration >80 mEq/L	Normal	Abnormal	
Serum calcium	9–11 mg/dl	Frequently ↓	Usually normal	

Continued.

TABLE 9-4.—Continued

TEST	NORMAL VALUES	MALABSORPTION (NONTROPICAL SPRUE)	MALDIGESTION (PANCREATIC INSUFFICIENCY)	COMMENT
Serum albumin	3.5–5.5 gm/dl	Frequently ↓	Usually normal	Decreased levels of both serum albumin and globulins should raise the question of protein-losing enteropathy
Serum cholesterol	150–250 mg/dl	↓	Frequently ↓	Usually decreased in disorders associated with significant steatorrhea
Serum iron	80–150 µg/dl	Frequently ↓	Normal	Low values may reflect decreased body iron stores
Serum carotenes	>100 IU/dl	↓	Usually ↓	Fairly satisfactory screening tests for malabsorption
Serum vitamin A	>100 IU/dl	↓		
Prothrombin time	70%–100%; 12–15 sec	Frequently ↑	Frequently ↑	
Urine 5-hydroxyindoleacetic acid (5-HIAA)	2–9 mg/24 hr	↑	Normal	Slightly increased level (12–16 mg/24 hr) characteristically found in nontropical sprue
Breath H_2 (after 50 gm lactose)	Minimal breath H_2	May be ↑	Normal	Secondary to lactase deficiency

Duodenal fluid analysis:				
Conjugated bile salts	>2 mmoles/ml	Normal	Normal	May be decreased with bacterial overgrowth, ileal resection, or ileal inflammatory disease
Unconjugated bile salts	Not present	Normal	Normal	Increased with bacterial overgrowth
Micellar lipid	$>50\%$ ingested lipid in micellar phase	Normal or decreased	Decreased	Decreased with a deficiency of conjugated bile salts or pancreatic lipase
Bacteria (culture)	$<10^3$ organisms/ml	Normal	Normal	$>10^5$ organisms/ml indicates bacterial overgrowth
Glycocholic acid metabolism (oral glycine-1-[^{14}C]glycocholate)	$<1\%$ of dose excreted as $^{14}CO_2$ in 4 hr	Normal	Normal	Increased $^{14}CO_2$ excretion with bacterial overgrowth or bile acid malabsorption (due to ileal resection or inflammatory disease)
	$<4\%$ of dose excreted in stools	Normal	Normal	Increased fecal excretion of ^{14}C in bile acid malabsorption
[^{14}C]Triolein absorption (breath test)	$>3.5\%$ of dose as breath $^{14}CO_2$ per hour	Decreased	Decreased	Correlates well with chemical stool fat; recently introduced test

*Adapted from MacDonald WC, Rubin CE: Gastric tumors, gastritis, and other gastric diseases, in Braunwald E (ed): Harrison's Principles of Internal Medicine, ed 11. New York, McGraw-Hill Book Co, 1987, p 64.

INFLAMMATORY BOWEL DISEASE

TABLE 9–5.—DIAGNOSIS OF ACUTE COLITIS/PROCTITIS*

DIAGNOSIS	SIGMOID APPEARANCE	BARIUM ENEMA	RECTAL BIOPSY
Ulcerative colitis	Diffuse erythema and ulceration (no normal mucosa)	Pseudopolyposis; loss of haustra; involvement from rectum proximally	Goblet cell depletion, pseudopolyps
Crohn's disease	Diffuse erythema and ulceration (some normal mucosa)	"Skip" lesions (thickening and luminal narrowing with areas of normal bowel between)	Crypt abscesses, epithelioid granulomas
Salmonella, Shigella, or Campylobacter	Same as ulcerative colitis	Usually normal	Crypt abscesses
Amebiasis	Diffuse inflammation, ulceration	Usually normal	Trophozoite in ulcer base
Antibiotic-associated colitis	Multiple, discrete yellow plaques	Usually normal	Fibrinous pseudomembrane over inflammation
Gonorrheal proctitis	Erythema and ulceration, limited to rectum	Normal	Intracellular diplococci
Lymphogranuloma venereum	Same as gonorrhea	Normal	Nonspecific inflammation

*Adapted from Lewis JH, et al: Postgrad Med 1981; 70:145–162.

TABLE 9–6.—CLINICAL DISTINCTIONS BETWEEN CROHN'S DISEASE
AND ULCERATIVE COLITIS*

FEATURE	CROHN'S DISEASE	ULCERATIVE COLITIS
In the intestine:		
Rectal bleeding	Uncommon	Very common
Sigmoidoscopic findings	Normal or spotty lesions	Diffusely abnormal
Spontaneous fistulas	Common	Never occurs
Perianal disease	Common	Uncommon
Abdominal pain	Very common	Uncommon
Abdominal mass	Common	Only with cancers
Strictures	Common	Rare, suspect cancer
Distribution	Discontinuous, entire GI tract	Continuous, colon and rectum
Shortening due to incidence of cancer	Fibrosis increased	Muscle thickening greatly increased
Extraintestinal manifestations:		
Arthritis	Occurs	Occurs
Dermatitis	Occurs	Occurs
Episcleritis and uveitis	Occurs	Occurs
Hydronephrosis	Occurs	Occurs
Liver disease	Occurs	Occurs
Metabolic manifestations:		
Amyloidosis	Incidence increased	Rare
Anemia	Common	Common
Fever	Occurs	Occurs
Gallstones	Incidence increased	Incidence normal
Growth retardation	Occurs	Occurs
Kidney stones	Occurs	Occurs

*From Sessions T Jr: *Viewpoints Dig Dis* Sept 7, 1975. Reproduced by permission.

MALIGNANCIES

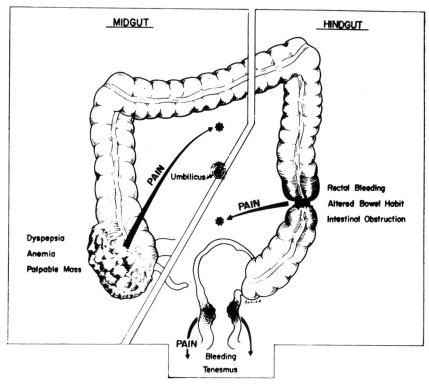

FIG 9–6.
Symptoms of carcinoma of the colon. (From Cohn I, Nance FC: Intermediate or precancerous lesions and malignant lesions, in Sabiston DC [ed]: *Textbook of Surgery,* ed 12. Philadelphia, WB Saunders Co, 1981, p 1098. Reproduced by permission.)

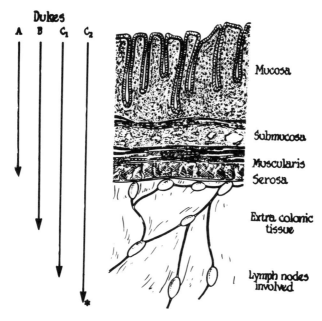

FIG 9–7.
Duke's classification of colon cancer. Grade *A*: cancer confined to the colon, without serosal invasion. Grade *B*: cancer through the colon but without lymph node involvement. *C1*: cancer affecting lymph nodes, no other tissue involvement. *C2*: cancer affecting lymph nodes, plus other tissue invasion. (From Cohn I, Nance FC: Intermediate or precancerous lesions and malignant lesions, in Sabiston DC [ed]: *Textbook of Surgery*, ed 12. Philadelphia, WB Saunders Co, 1981, p 1092. Reproduced by permission.)

TABLE 9-7.—Approach for Detecting Colonic Neoplasms*

SCREENING TEST	ASYMPTOMATIC	HIGH RISK	POSTSPLENECTOMY	POST RESECTION FOR CARCINOMA
Fecal occult blood	Annually	Annually (except in ulcerative colitis)	Annually	Annually plus annual CEA
Proctosigmoidoscopy	Annually for 2 yr after age 50, then every 5 yr	Annually	Every 2–3 yr when necessary to supplement colonoscopy	Annually
Air contrast barium enema (ACBE)	Only for positive findings	ACBE; frequency depends on underlying risk factors	ACBE every 2–3 yr	ACBE annually for 2 yr then every 2–3 yr
Colonoscopy	Only for positive findings	May be required annually in certain diseases (e.g., ulcerative colitis after 10 yr)	Every 2–3 yr	Every 2–3 yr

*Adapted from Stouffer JQ: Polypoid tumors of the colon, in Sleisenger MH, Fordtran JS (eds): *Gastrointestinal Disease*, ed 2. Philadelphia, WB Saunders Co, 1981, p 1780.

TABLE 9–8.—CHANGING DISTRIBUTION OF COLON CANCER*

PERIOD	NO. OF CASES	RIGHT (%)	LEFT (%)	RECTUM (%)
1950–54	453	19.6	28.0	52.0
1955–59	520	21.5	33.3	45.2
1960–64	513	24.8	35.5	39.8
1965–69	382	30.4	43.2	26.5

*From Cohn I, Nance FC: Intermediate or precancerous lesions and malignant lesions, in Sabiston DC (ed): *Textbook of Surgery,* ed 12. Philadelphia, WB Saunders Co, 1981, p 1089. Reproduced by permission. Data are from Charity Hospital, New Orleans.

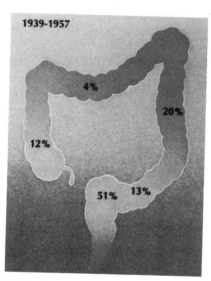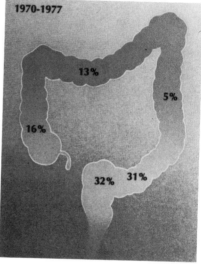

FIG 9–8.
Changing site distribution of colorectal cancer. *Left,* 1939–1957 figures. *Right,* 1970–1977 figures. (From Hocutt JE: *Am Fam Physician* 1982; 26(5):133. Reproduced by permission.)

TABLE 9–9.—Diagnosis of Pancreatic Cancer*

PROCEDURE	HEAD	BODY	TAIL
Ultrasound	+ +	+ +	+ +
Pancreatic function tests	+ +	+ +	+ +
Duodenal aspirate cytology	+	+	+
CT scan	+ + +	+ + +	+ + +
ERCP	+ + +	+ + +	+ + +
Percutaneous cholangiography	+ + +	+	0
Angiography	+ + +	+ + +	+ + +
Percutaneous biopsy with CT	+ + + +	+ + + +	+ + + +
UGI	+	+	+

+ = Occasionally helpful
+ + = Useful as initial screen
+ + + = Frequently helpful (>50% sensitive)
+ + + + = Often diagnostic

*Adapted from Greenberger NJ, Toskes PP, Isselbocher KJ: Diseases of the pancreas, in Petersdorf RG (ed): *Harrison's Principles of Internal Medicine,* ed 10. New York, McGraw-Hill Book Co, 1981, p 1846.

HEPATITIS

TABLE 9–10.—Epidemiologic and Clinical Features of Viral Hepatitis*

	HEPATITIS VIRUS		
FEATURE	A	B	Non-A, Non-B
Oral transmission	+	+	+
Parenteral transmission	–	+	+
Chronic infection	–	+	+
Fulminant hepatitis	Rare	+	+
% of seropositive adults in U.S.	25%–50%	10%	Unknown
% of sporadic hepatitis	40%	40%	20%
% of posttransfusion hepatitis	0%	20%	80%

*From Branch WT: Diseases of the liver, in Branch WT (ed): *Office Practice of Medicine.* Philadelphia, WB Saunders Co, 1982, p 679. Reproduced by permission.

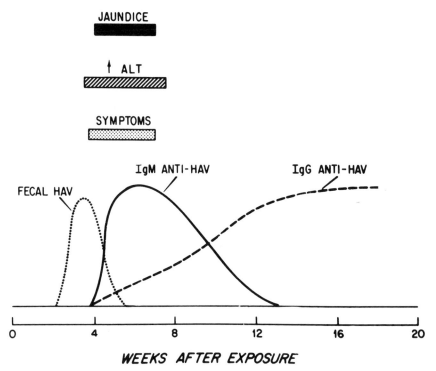

FIG 9–9.
Clinical and virologic events during acute type A hepatitis. (From Dienstag JL, Wands JR, Koff RS: Acute hepatitis, in Petersdorf RG [ed]: *Harrison's Principles of Internal Medicine,* ed 10. New York, McGraw-Hill Book Co, 1981, p 1792. Reproduced by permission.)

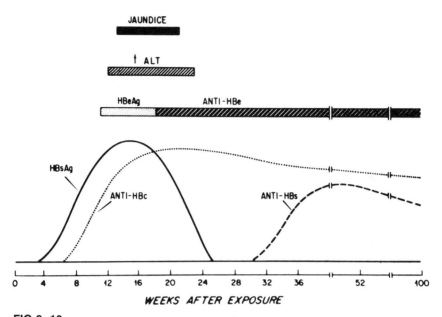

FIG 9–10.
Clinical and virologic events during a typical self-limiting episode of acute viral hepatitis type B. (From Dienstag JL, Wands JR, Koff RS: Acute hepatitis, in Petersdorf RG [ed]: *Harrison's Principles of Internal Medicine,* ed 10. New York, McGraw-Hill Book Co, 1981, p 1793. Reproduced by permission.)

TABLE 9–11.—γ-GLOBULIN PROPHYLAXIS IN VIRAL HEPATITIS*

TYPE OF HEPATITIS	TYPE OF EXPOSURE	RECOMMENDATIONS
Hepatitis A	Sexual or family contacts	Immune serum globulin 0.02 ml/kg/M body weight
	Travelers to Asia, Africa, South America, Pacific Islands, rural Mexico, Central America	Same as above
	School or office contacts	Not recommended
Hepatitis B	Sexual or family contacts	Hepatitis B immune globulin, 3–5 ml; repeat in 1 mo. + hepatitis B vaccination
	Needle stick from surface antigen-positive donor[†]	Same as above
	Dialysis unit personnel and others at high risk[†]	Hepatitis B immunization (Heptavax-B), IM, 20 μg, 0, 30, and 180 days
Non-A, non-B	Sexual or family contacts	Same as for hepatitis A
	Needle stick from surface antigen-negative donor	3.5 ml regular γ-globulin; repeat in 1 mo.

*From Branch WT: Diseases of the liver, in Branch WT (ed): *Office Practice of Medicine,* ed 2. Philadelphia, WB Saunders Co, 1987, p 472. Reproduced by permission.
[†]Individuals should be tested for HB_s antibody prior to receiving HBIG. Those with naturally acquired HB_sAb do not require passive immunization with HBIG.

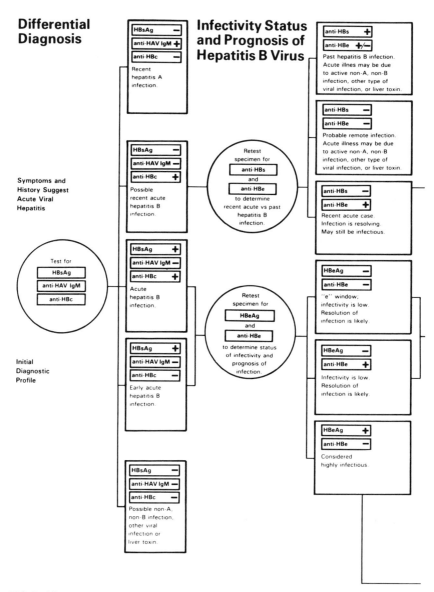

FIG 9–11.
Laboratory evaluation of acute hepatitis. *HBsAg* = hepatitis B surface antigen; *anti-HAV IgM* = hepatitis A antibody; *anti-HBc* = hepatitis B "core" antigen; *anti-HBs* = hepatitis B surface antibody; *anti-HBe* = hepatitis B "E" antibody; *HBeAg* = hepatitis B "E" antigen. (Adapted from *Perspectives on Viral Hepatitis.* New York, Biomedical Information Corp.)

Clinical Result:
Chronicity
or Resolution

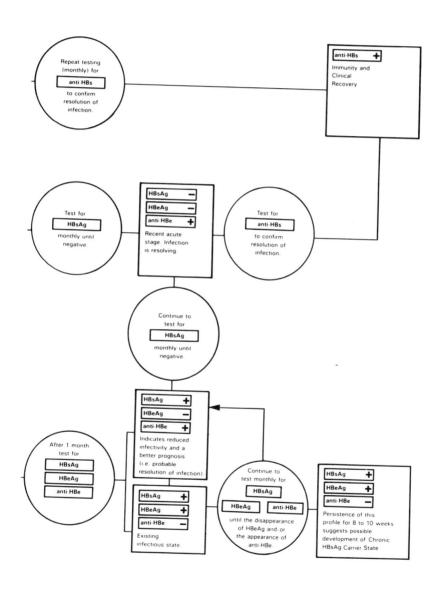

Repeat testing (monthly) for **anti-HBs** to confirm resolution of infection.

anti-HBs **+** Immunity and Clinical Recovery

Test for **HBsAg** monthly until negative.

HBsAg **−**
HBeAg **−**
anti-HBe **+**
Recent acute stage. Infection is resolving.

Test for **anti-HBs** to confirm resolution of infection.

Continue to test for **HBsAg** monthly until negative.

HBsAg **+**
HBeAg **−**
anti-HBe **+**
Indicates reduced infectivity and a better prognosis (i.e. probable resolution of infection).

After 1 month test for **HBsAg** **HBeAg** **anti-HBe**

HBsAg **+**
HBeAg **+**
anti-HBe **−**
Existing infectious state.

Continue to test monthly for **HBsAg** **HBeAg** **anti-HBe** until the disappearance of HBeAg and/or the appearance of anti-HBe.

HBsAg **+**
HBeAg **+**
anti-HBe **−**
Persistence of this profile for 8 to 10 weeks suggests possible development of Chronic HBsAg Carrier State

PROCEDURES

TABLE 9–12.—PROCEDURES IN THE GASTROINTESTINAL TRACT*

Rigid sigmoidoscopy
1. In general, should be performed without preparation to preserve mucosal character.
2. Position patient in knee-chest, lateral (Sim's) position, or on sigmoidoscopy table.
3. Fully explain procedure to patient prior to beginning.
4. Perform external anal and digital rectal exam.
5. Hold sigmoidoscope in right hand with obturator firmly in place.
6. Lubricate scope with K-Y jelly and insert into the rectum. Scope should be deflected slightly posteriorly after passing through the anorectal ring.
7. Withdraw the obturator.
8. Advance slowly with the lumen in view at all times.
9. The rectosigmoid junction occurs at 12–15 cm and appears to be a cul-de-sac because of a sharp forward, left bend.
10. Place gentle anterior pressure on the tip of the scope to enter the sigmoid.
11. If possible, insert the scope its full length.
12. Observe the lumen circumferentially on removal of the scope. Pay special attention on entering the rectum because of increased lumen size. Note the areas above the rectal valves (of Houston).

Flexible sigmoidoscopy
1. The patient should administer 2 Fleet's enemas on the morning of the procedure. If patient has chronic constipation, preparation of the bowel requires 3 bisacodyl (Dulcolax) tablets the afternoon prior to the test in addition to the enemas on the morning of the procedure.
2. Place patient in left lateral decubitus position.
3. Perform digital exam and anoscopy first.
4. Hold shaft of instrument in right hand and control head of endoscope with left hand.
5. Apply water-soluble lubricant to endoscope shaft.
6. Guide scope into rectum with finger.
7. Advance scope, always with lumen in view.
8. Insufflate air periodically to distend collapsed bowel.
9. Aspirate liquid with suction control as needed.
10. Extra care is required to negotiate the angle at the rectosigmoid junction.
11. If colonic spasm occurs, pull back 3–4 cm and reinsert.
12. Examine mucosa on withdrawal of scope.
13. Biopsy suspicious lesions on withdrawal.

Diagnostic paracentesis
1. Turn patient on left side for 5 min.
2. After the bladder has been emptied, insert 19-gauge short beveled spinal needle halfway between umbilicus and pubis at the left lateral edge of rectus sheath.
3. Do *not* use local anesthesia (pain signals entering peritoneum).
4. Apply gentle suction with 15–20 cc syringe.
5. If no fluid is obtained, repeat on right side.

Alternate method
1. Use intracath.
2. Insert in lower abdominal midline, 1 inch below umbilicus.
3. Pass catheter, withdraw needle; apply gentle suction.
4. If no fluid is obtained, infuse 500 cc of sterile saline over 10–15 min.
5. Aspirate and check fluid for pH, bile, amylase, WBCs, RBCs, cytology, and cultures, as indicated.

String test (for localization of chronic GI blood loss)
This procedure is indicated to evaluate guaiac-positive stools when barium studies and colonoscopy are negative.
1. Pass weighted umbilical tape with radiopaque markers (available from Advanced Laboratory Associates, New Brunswick, N.J.) orally. It will advance by peristalsis through the small bowel over 2–3 hr.
2. Document the position of the tape with abdominal x-ray.
3. Inject 20 ml of fluorescein IV over 2–3 min.
4. Withdraw tape and examine under fluorescent light and with guaiac reagent.
5. Correlate presence of blood with position on x-ray.

Bedside test for gastric outlet obstruction (saline load test)
1. Empty stomach and irrigate with normal saline until clear through a No. 30 Ewald tube.
2. Insert soft nasogastric tube to 65 cm.
3. Infuse 750 cc of normal saline over 3–5 minutes.
4. Aspirate after 30 minutes: aspirate with patient in supine, upright, and both right and left decubitus positions.
5. A residual of 400 cc or more indicates probable obstruction; 300–400 cc is suggestive.
6. Repeat daily to assess results of medical therapy; if positive after 72 hours of suction, surgery will usually be required.

Insertion of nasogastric tube
1. Measure from the xiphoid to either ear lobe. This is the distance the tube should be passed.
2. The tube should be placed in ice or refrigerated prior to insertion to facilitate passage through the pharynx.
3. Insert gently through the nose to the posterior pharynx.
4. Ask the patient to swallow, or have patient drink sips of water. Tube should be passed synchronous with swallowing.
5. Aspiration of gastric contents and/or auscultation of borborygmi with air insertion confirms proper placement in the stomach.
6. Tube should be carefully taped to the nose, avoiding excessive pressure of the tube on the nares.

Routine stool examination
Observe for odor, color, consistency, mucus, blood, concretions, adult parasites, pus, and fat (a putty-like appearance).

Qualitative stool examination for fat (Sudan stain)
1. Emulsify a small portion of stool with normal saline.
2. Add 1 drop of glacial acetic acid.
3. Add 1 drop of Sudan III or IV stain.

Continued.

TABLE 9–12.—Continued

4. Place a drop on a slide, cover with a cover slip, and examine for fat droplets.
5. Neutral fat appears as deep orange or red drops.

Ova and parasites
1. Obtain a fresh, preferably warm stool specimen.
2. Emulsify a 1–2 mm portion of fecal material with normal saline using an applicator stick.
3. Emulsify a second specimen as above, but add 2–3 drops of Gram's iodine.
4. Make two thin wet preparations and cover each with a cover slip.
5. Look for trophozoites in the saline prep.
6. Look for cysts in the iodine solution (will stain light brown).

White blood cells in stool
1. Emulsify stool in normal saline as above.
2. Add one drop of methylene blue.
3. Place a drop on a slide and cover with a cover slip.
4. Observe under high dry. White cell nuclei will stain blue. More than 5 WBCs per high-power field suggests inflammation.

*Flexible sigmoidoscopy procedure adapted from Quan M, Rodney WM, Johnson RA: *Postgrad Med* 1982; 72:151–156, and Rodney WM, Felmar E: *Your Patient and Cancer* February 1984. Diagnostic paracentesis procedure adapted from Baker RJ: Differential diagnosis of abdominal pain, in Condon RE, Nyhus LM (eds): *Manual of Surgical Therapeutics*, ed 2. Boston, Little, Brown & Co, 1972, p 286. String test and bedside test for gastric outlet obstruction adapted from Boedeker EC: Gastrointestinal disease, in Boedeker EC, Dauber JH (eds): *Manual of Medical Therapeutics*, ed 21. Boston, Little, Brown & Co, 1974, p 256.

TABLE 9–13.—GALLBLADDER DISEASE

Indications for cholecystectomy
Recurrent biliary colic
Acute cholecystitis
The presence of multiple small stones that were symptomatic but are now quiescent
NOTE: Most authors agree that asymptomatic gallstones do not need medical or surgical intervention.

Indications for gallstone dissolution therapy
Patients with chronic or recurrent dyspeptic symptoms compatible with gallbladder disease, *plus*
a radiologically "functional" gallbladder, *plus*
the presence of radiolucent, small stones, *plus*
relative contraindications to elective surgery or a patient who doesn't wish to have surgery.

Guidelines for initiation of chenodiol therapy
1. Begin at 250 mg b.i.d. for 2 weeks. Divide dose between morning and evening meals.
2. Increase the dose gradually to about 15 mg/kg/day in 2 divided doses or until symptoms such as diarrhea and flatulence become unacceptable.
3. Monitor liver hepatocellular enzymes periodically (about once per month) for the first 12 months of therapy.

4. Perform gallbladder ultrasound at 6- to 9-month intervals to monitor dissolution rate.
5. If reduction in stone size is not obvious by 16 months, therapy should be discontinued.

NOTE: Only about 15%–30% of patients have experienced complete dissolution over 2 years of therapy.

TABLE 9–14.—ANORECTAL DISORDERS

Hemorrhoids
Thrombosed external hemorrhoids
Pain is prominent and bleeding is infrequent.
Examination reveals a bluish perianal mass just below the mucocutaneous junction.
Treatment consists of sitz baths and stool softeners.
Pain usually disappears within 1 week, the mass within 2 weeks.
Residual skin tags are common and do not indicate chronic hemorrhoidal disease.
If acutely painful, overlying skin may be anesthetized with 1% lidocaine, incised, and the clot removed with resultant immediate pain relief.
Internal hemorrhoids
Symptoms usually limited to bright red bleeding, almost always *painless.*
Large hemorrhoids may prolapse out of the rectum at bowel movement.
Digital exam is often negative; diagnosis requires anoscope with a good light source.
Even if hemorrhoids are present on exam, other sources of bleeding such as colon cancer must be excluded.
Small, minimally symptomatic lesions may be treated with observation and a high-fiber diet.
Larger lesions may be treated with sclerotherapy with injection of 5% phenol solution in oil into the submucosal area. (Care must be exercised not to inject into the vein!)
Very large, prolapsing lesions are best treated by rubber band ligature technique.
Anal fissure
Characterized by pain associated with a hard bowel movement with minor bleeding on the toilet tissue.
Patients usually mistake them for hemorrhoids.
Mucosal tears are demonstrable, usually at 6 or 12 o'clock, by everting the buttocks. Will often be missed unless specifically sought.
Treat with sitz baths, stool softeners, high-fiber diet, and hydrocortisone suppositories.
Chronic, recalcitrant cases may require sphincterotomy and/or fissurectomy.
Pruritis ani
Causes are multiple and poorly understood but include poor perianal hygiene, trauma from scratching or excessive cleaning or wiping, excessive moisture, yeast infections, hypersensitivity reactions to local or systemic agents, dietary irritants such as jalapeno peppers, or personality or psychological factors.

Continued.

TABLE 9–14.—Continued

Once started, a vicious cycle occurs and is hard to break.
Treatment approaches should include:
1. Correct all predisposing anatomic conditions (e.g., hemorrhoids)
2. Direct attention to meticulous perianal hygiene; use water, not soap. If sitz bath is unavailable, use premoistened towelettes.
3. Avoid scratching at all cost; use oral Vistaril, Phenergan, or Benadryl as antipruritic, if necessary.
4. Keep the area dry with loose clothing; consider tucking gauze into the buttocks; cornstarch or other drying powder may help.
5. Medications should be minimized; topical steroids are contraindicated except for a short, initial course; avoid local anesthetic such as benzocaine, which is highly sensitizing. Yeast infections are often secondary and should be treated with nystatin or miconazole cream.
6. Efforts should be directed toward complete normalization of stool patterns. Overly soft stool may be as irritating as constipated stool.
7. Consider the importance of psychological factors.

---

10 Nephrology/Urology
Charles E. Driscoll, M.D.

URINE COLLECTION, ANALYSIS, AND RENAL FUNCTION

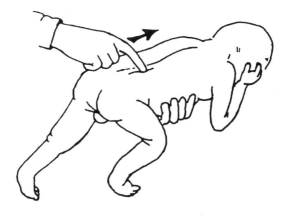

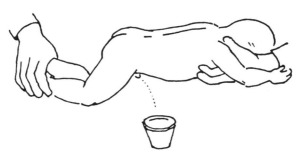

FIG 10–1.
Collection of urine from children may be done noninvasively in the male by stimulating the Perez reflex. Holding the infant in ventral suspension, stroke along the midline cephalad. As the infant's back is arched, position the infant over a sterile collection cup. (From Kuhlberg A: *Top Emerg Med* 1983; 5:50. Reproduced by permission.)

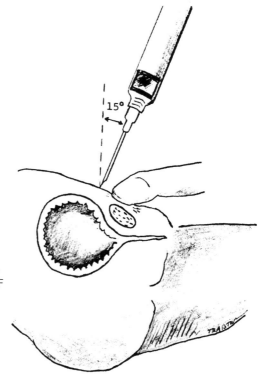

FIG 10–2.
For collecting urine from female infants, use a lubricated 5 or 8 F pediatric polyethylene feeding tube or perform suprapubic bladder aspiration. (From Kuhlberg A: *Top Emerg Med* 1983; 5:49. Reproduced by permission.)

TABLE 10–1.—SUPRAPUBIC BLADDER ASPIRATION

1. Give liquids prior to procedure to ensure a full bladder.
2. Place child supine in a frog leg position with assistant providing gentle restraint.
3. Cleanse suprapubic area above symphysis with povidine-iodine solution.
4. With sterile gloved finger, palpate symphysis; usually at or just above crease in fat.
5. Use 10-cc syringe with 1½-inch 22-gauge needle.
6. Insert above symphysis in midline, applying negative pressure while advancing needle until urine appears in syringe.
7. Urination can be prevented during procedure by applying digital pressure to urethral opening.

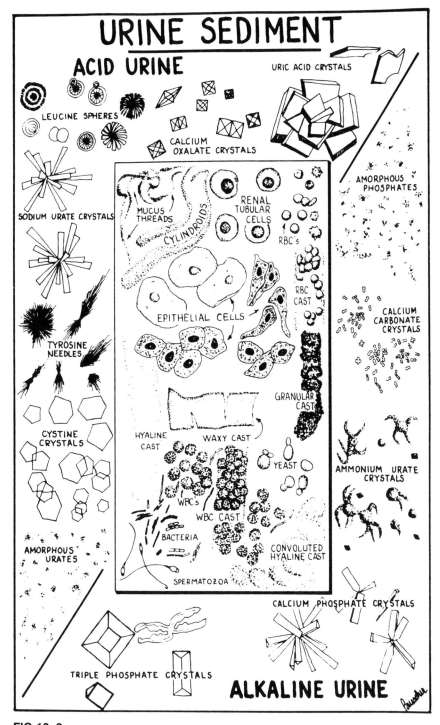

FIG 10–3.
Microscopic appearance of urine sediment. (From Biller JA, Yeager AM [eds]: *The Harriet Lane Handbook,* ed 10. Chicago, Year Book Medical Publishers, 1984, Reproduced by permission.)

TABLE 10–2.—Substances in Urine That May Change Urine Color*

SUBSTANCE	COLORS PRODUCED IN URINE
Acetanilid	Yellow to red
Acetophenetidin (metabolite)	Yellow (dark brown to wine color)
Alcohol	Lightens color
Aloin	Red-brown to yellow-pink (alkaline urine), yellow-brown (acid urine)
Aminopyrine	Red-brown
Aminosalicylic acid (para-aminosalicylic acid)	Discoloration (no distinctive color)
Amitriptyline	Blue-green
Anisindione	Orange (alkaline urine), pink to red-brown
Anthraquinone laxatives	Reddish (alkaline urine)
Antipyrine	Yellow to red-brown
Azuresin	Blue or green
Beets	Red
Benzene	Red-brown
Biliverdin	Yellow-green
Carbon tetrachloride	Red-brown
Carrots	Yellow
Cascara	Yellow-brown (acid urine), yellow-pink (alkaline urine), darkens to brown to black on standing
Chloroquine	Rust-yellow to brown
Chlorzoxazone	Orange to purple-red
Cinchophen	Red-brown
Creosote	Dark green
Cresol	Dark color on standing
Danthron	Pink to red
Deferoxamine mesylate	Reddish
Dihydroxyanthraquinone	Pink to orange (alkaline urine)
Dinitrophenol	Red-brown
Diphenylhydantoin (see phenytoin)	
Dithiazanine hydrochloride	Blue
Doan's kidney pills	Greenish blue
Doxorubicin	Red-brown
Emodin (in cascara)	Pink to red to red-brown (alkaline urine)
Ethoxazene	Orange to red
Ferrous salts	Black
Fluorescein (intravenous)	Yellow-orange
Furazolidone (metabolite)	Brownish or rust-yellow
Ibuprofen	Red or pink
Indanediones	Orange (alkaline urine)
Indomethacin	Green (biliverdinemia)
Iron sorbitex	Dark to black on standing
Lead	Red-brown

Levodopa	Dark red-brown
Melanin	Black-brown
Mercury	Red-brown
Methocarbamol	Dark brown, black or green on standing
Methyldopa	Dark (red to black) on standing
Methylene blue	Greenish yellow to blue
Metronidazole	Dark brown in acidic urine
Naphthol	Dark color on standing
Nitrobenzene	Dark color on standing
Nitrofurantoin and derivatives	Brown or rust-yellow
Oxamniquine	Red-orange
Pamaquine naphthoate	Rust-yellow or brown
Phenacetin (see acetophenetidin)	
Phenazopyridine	Orange-red to red-brown (HNO_3 turns orange to pink)
Phenindione	Reddish brown to pink, orange in alkaline urine
Phenolphthalein	Pink to red to magenta (alkaline urine), yellow-brown (acid urine)
Phenolsulfonphthalein	Red (alkaline urine)
Phenols	Dark green to brownish black (darkens on standing)
Phenothiazines	Pink to red-brown
Phensuximide	Pink to red to red-brown
Phenyl salicylate	Dark green
Phenytoin	Pink to red to reddish brown
Picric acid	Yellow to red-brown
Porphyrins	Burgundy red, darkens on standing
Primaquine phosphate	Rust-yellow to brown
Pyocyanin	Blue-green
Pyrogallol	Brown to black (darkens on standing)
Quinacrine hydrochloride	Yellow (deep yellow on acidification)
Quinine and derivatives	Brown to black
Resorcinol	Dark green to greenish-blue, darkens on standing
Rhubarb	Yellow-brown (acid urine), yellow-pink (alkaline urine), darkens to brown to black on standing
Riboflavin	Yellow
Rifampin	Red to orange
Salicylazosulfapyridine	Orange-yellow (alkaline urine)
Salol	Dark color on standing
Santonin	Bright yellow (NaOH changes to pink or scarlet)
Senna	Yellow-brown (acid urine), yellow-pink (alkaline urine), darkens on standing

Continued.

TABLE 10–2.—Continued

SUBSTANCE	COLORS PRODUCED IN URINE
Sulfonamides	Rust-yellow or brown
Sulfonethylmethane	Red
Sulfonmethane	Red-brown
Tetralin	Greenish blue
(tetrahydronaphthalene)	
Thiazosulfone	Pink to red
Thymol	Greenish blue
TNT (trinitrotoluene)	Red-brown
Tolonium (Blutene)	Blue-Green
Triamterene	Bluish color (pale blue fluorescence)
Warfarin sodium	Orange

*Adapted from Kulberg A: *Top Emerg Med* 1983; 5: 52–53, and Raymond JR, Yarger WE: *South Med J* 1988; 81:837–841.

RENAL FUNCTION

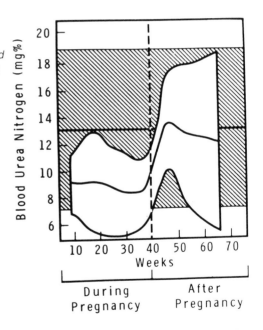

FIG 10–4.
Genitourinary system during pregnancy and after delivery. *Solid area* depicts range of *BUN* during normal pregnancy and after delivery. *Hatched area* depicts range in nonpregnant women. (From Harris JP, et al: *Am Fam Physician* 1978; 18:97–102. Reproduced by permission.)

TABLE 10-3.—CREATININE CLEARANCE ESTIMATES*†

Cockroft-Gault equation:

$$CrCl = \frac{(140 - Age) \times Weight\ (kg)}{72 \times S_{cr}}$$ Multiply by 0.85 for females.

Weight: Lean weight in kg
CrCl: Creatinine clearance
S_{cr}: Serum creatinine

NOTE: A 75-year-old woman (60 kg/lean) who has a "normal" serum creatinine value of 1.0 may not have "normal" renal function:

$$\frac{(140 - 75) \times 60\ kg}{72(1.0)} \times 0.85 = 46\ cc/min$$

*Adapted from Cockroft DW, Gault MH: *Nephron* 1976; 16:31–41.
†In young healthy persons with stable renal function. May be less accurate in the elderly.

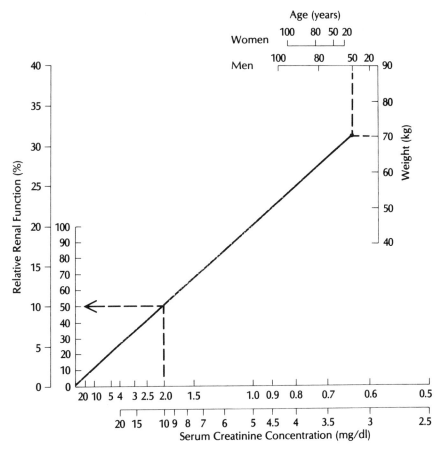

FIG 10–5.
Estimating relative renal function. Nomogram graphically depicts patient's relative renal function from the serum creatinine concentration. To prepare, a line is drawn from the point of intersection of individual's sex, age, and weight to the origin; the percent of renal function remaining for a given serum creatinine value is read on the ordinate, using the outer scales for serum creatinine values above 2.5 mg/dl. For example, renal function is 50% of normal in a 50-year-old man weighing 70 kg, with a serum creatinine of 2 mg/dl. (From Anderson R: *Hosp Pract* 1983; 18:155. Reproduced by permission. Adapted from Bjornsson TD: *Clin. Pharmacokinet* 1979; 4:200.)

CYSTOMETRICS

A Capacity : Normal
Proprioception (sense of fullness and desire to void at
normal volume) : Intact
Exteroception (normal voiding
sensation) : Intact
Motor Function : Voluntary
control of normal voiding
contraction
Post-Void Residual : Negligible
or increased in patients with
true outlet obstruction (e.g. BPH)

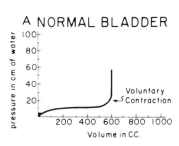

A NORMAL BLADDER

B Capacity : Reduced
Proprioception : Present or absent
Exteroception : Present or absent
Motor Function : absent voluntary
control
Post-Void Residual : Variable

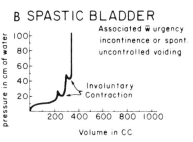

B SPASTIC BLADDER

C Capacity : Increased except when
catheter has been indwelling
Proprioception : Diminished or
absent
Exteroception : Present or absent
Motor Function : Cannot initiate
bladder contraction
Post-Void Residual : Large

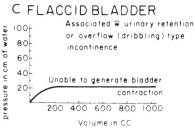

C FLACCID BLADDER

FIG 10–6.
Typical cystometrograms. Patients with pattern *A* may be expected to benefit from prostatectomy. Patients with pattern *B* deserve a more thorough urodynamic workup before
surgery is considered. Although these patients have symptoms that mimic prostatic obstruction, they usually are not obstructed, and surgery may aggravate the problem. Patients with pattern *C* may benefit from surgery. Although the neurogenically induced flaccid bladder is not relieved by prostatectomy, the procedure reduces the resistance to
emptying and thereby may improve function. (From Branch WT Jr: *Office Practice of Medicine.* Philadelphia, WB Saunders Co, 1982, p 516. Reproduced by permission.)

TABLE 10–4.—SIMPLE OFFICE TESTING OF LOWER URINARY TRACT FUNCTION

TEST	PROCEDURE	INTERPRETATION
1. Stress test	With full bladder, cough 3 times in standing position with filter paper at urethra.	Urine leakage indicates stress incontinence.
2. Normal voiding volume	Patient asked to empty bladder into measuring "hat."	Small volumes may indicate obstruction; check for straining, hesitancy.
3. Residual urine	Pass sterile 14 F catheter into bladder after voiding.	Obstruction is indicated by difficult passage; $\geq$ 100 ml urine indicates obstruction or contractility problem.
4. Bladder filling	Fill bladder with sterile water through 14 F catheter attached to 50-cc catheter tip syringe without piston. Pinch catheter while filling 50-cc measure to ensure accurate volumes.	Note volume at first urge to void; note involuntary contractions and volume of urine lost. Severe urgency or urine involuntarily lost at $\leq$300 cc suggests urge incontinence.

*Adapted from Ouslander JG, Leach GE, Staskin DR: *J Am Geriatr Soc* 1989; 37:706–714.

CATHETER CARE

TABLE 10–5.—CATHETER CARE

Insert with careful aseptic technique, use 16–18 F size with 5-cc balloon.
Secure catheter to leg to minimize urethral trauma.
Cleanse perineum twice daily with Hibiclens® antiseptic soap.
Keep system closed; open only at bag.
Irrigate only *after* infection is established (use 0.25% acetic acid solution).
Obtain specimens for culture by sterile needle aspiration from distal catheter (after cleansing with antiseptic soap and sterile water).
Always place collection bag below bladder.
Topical antibiotic ointment should be applied to meatus once daily.
Change catheter only if obstructed or malfunctioning.
Separate bacteriuric from nonbacteriuric patients.
Discontinue use as soon as possible.
Symptomatic (temp < 102° F and normotensive) beyond 24 hr, give broad-spectrum antibiotics. If serious (temp > 102° F and hypotensive), obtain urine and blood cultures, hospitalize, prescribe parenteral antibiotics.

ACID BASE BALANCE

TABLE 10–6.—THE GOLDEN RULES OF ACID-BASE BALANCE

1. A change in Pa_{CO_2}, either up or down, of 10 mm Hg is associated with an increase or decrease of pH by 0.08 unit (as Pa_{CO_2} increases pH falls).
2. A pH change of 0.15 is the result of a base change of 10 m Eq/L.
3. Total body bicarbonate deficit equals =

$$\text{Base deficit (mEq/L)} \times \frac{[\text{Pt. weight (kg.)}]}{4}$$

Use 100% correction for acute conditions (CPR) and 50% correction for sub-acute/chronic conditions.

Example: 70-kg man in cardiac arrest with Pa_{CO_2} of 52 mm Hg and pH of 7.17: Since Pa_{CO_2} is increased by 12 mm Hg, respiratory acidosis is present. Calculating pH from change in Pa_{CO_2} gives an expected pH of 7.30. There is an unexplained pH difference of 0.13 (7.30 − 7.17), which is attributed to metabolic acidosis.

Calculation of base deficit by rule 2 $\left(\dfrac{0.15}{10}\right) \times \left(\dfrac{0.13}{X}\right)$

Bicarbonate deficit = $9 \times \dfrac{70}{4} = 157$ mEq.

The patient requires increased ventilation for respiratory acidosis and 157 mEq of sodium bicarbonate for metabolic acidosis.

INFECTIONS

TABLE 10–7.—WORKUP AND TREATMENT OF URINARY TRACT INFECTIONS IN CHILDREN*

Causes	*Workup*
30%–50% have anomalies. All boys and girls < 6 yr and girls > 6 yr with ≥ 2 UTIs should be worked up as soon as urine becomes sterile. Vesicoureteral reflux should be considered a medical (antibiotic suppression) problem; 20%–30% resolve per 2-yr period; overall long-term disappearance rate is 80%. Obstruction is a surgical problem.	Renal sonogram and voiding cystogram; *isotope cystogram* is more sensitive for vesicoureteral reflux in girls; *contrast cystograms* are better to evaluate the urethra in boys ^{99m}Tc-DTPA renal scan for diagnosing obstruction ^{99m}Tc-DMSA if reflux is detected to look for renal scarring or interstitial pyelonephritis

Continued.

TABLE 10–7.—Continued

NOTE: Radionuclide scanning is now preferred over IV urogram for children.
Treatment for acute UTIs

Infants	Amoxicillin	5–7 days of 20 mg/kg/day given in 3 doses
Child > 3 mo	Trimethoprim-sulfamethoxazole	5–7 days of 8 mg of TMP and 40 mg of SMX/kg/day in 2 doses
Child with high fever, vomiting, sepsis, known vesicoureteral reflux	Parenteral antibiotics	Ampicillin + aminoglycoside until afebrile for 48 hr; then oral antibiotic specific to culture (for 4–6 wk)

*Adapted from O'Brien WM, Gibbons MD: *Am Fam Physician* 1988; 38(1)101–112.

TABLE 10–8.—SELECTING PATIENTS FOR SINGLE-DOSE THERAPY OF ACUTE CYSTITIS

Selection
Patient is reliable female who will return for follow-up.
None of the following conditions is present:
Pregnancy, diabetes, renal disease, anatomic urinary anomaly, allergy to drug, upper urinary tract infection (fever > 100.4°F, flank pain, shaking chills, costovertebral angle tenderness)
Treatment
Amoxicillin, 3 gm PO or
TMP-SMX, 2 or 3 double-strength tablets PO
Follow-up
Culture 14 days after treatment.

TABLE 10–9.—OVERVIEW OF OUTPATIENT ANTIMICROBIAL THERAPY FOR LOWER URINARY TRACT INFECTIONS IN ADULTS*

INDICATION	ANTIMICROBIAL AGENT (ORAL ADMINISTRATION)	DOSE	INTERVAL	DURATION (DAYS)
Lower urinary tract infection	Trimethoprim-sulfamethoxazole, double-strength tablet†	2 tablets	Single dose	—
		1 tablet	Every 12 hr	3
		1 tablet	Every 12 hr	7–10
	Amoxicillin, 250- or 500-mg capsule	6 500-mg capsules	Single dose	—
		1 250-mg capsule	Every 8 hr	7–10
	Sulfisoxazole, 500-mg tablet	4 tablets	Single dose	—
		2 tablets	Every 6 hr	7–10
	Trimethoprim, 100-mg tablet	1 tablet	Every 12 hr	7–10
	Nitrofurantoin macrocrystals (Macrodantin), 100-mg capsule	1 capsule	Every 6 hr	7–10
	Norfloxacin, 400-mg tablet	1 tablet	Every 12 hr	7–10
"Acute urethral syndrome" Initial therapy	Trimethoprim-sulfamethoxazole, double-strength tablet†	2 tablets	Single dose	—
	Amoxicillin, 500-mg capsule	6 capsules	Single dose	—

Continued.

TABLE 10-9.—Continued

INDICATION	ANTIMICROBIAL AGENT (ORAL ADMINISTRATION)	DOSE	INTERVAL	DURATION (DAYS)
After failure	Doxycycline, 100-mg capsule	1 capsule	Every 12 hr	10
Long-term prophylaxis against recurrent bacteriuria				
First-choice agents	Trimethoprim-sulfamethoxazole, single-strength tablet‡	½ tablet	Every evening	≥6 mo
	Macrodantin, 50-mg capsule	1 capsule	Every evening	≥6 mo
	Trimethoprim, 100-mg tablet	½ tablet	Every evening	≥6 mo
Alternatives	Cephalexin, 250-mg capsule	1 capsule	Every evening	≥6 mo
	Methenamine mandelate, 1-gm tablet	1 tablet	Every 6 hr	≥6 mo
	Methenamine hippurate, 1-gm tablet	1 tablet	Every 12 hr	≥6 mo

*From Wilhelm MP, Edson RS: *Mayo Clin Proc* 1987; 62:1025–1031. Reproduced by permission.
†Each double-strength tablet consists of 160 mg of trimethoprim and 800 mg of sulfamethoxazole.
‡Each single-strength table consists of 80 mg of trimethoprim and 400 mg of sulfamethoxazole.

SEXUALLY TRANSMITTED DISEASES (STDs)

TABLE 10–10.—TREATMENT OF SEXUALLY TRANSMITTED DISEASES*

TYPE/CONDITION	RECOMMENDED REGIMEN	ALTERNATIVE
Gonorrhea		
Urethral, cervical, rectal	Ceftriaxone 250 mg IM once *plus* doxycycline 100 mg PO b.i.d. × 7d	Spectinomycin 2 gm IM once *plus* erythromycin 500 mg PO QID × 7d
Pharyngeal	Ceftriaxone 250 mg IM once *plus* erythromycin 500 mg PO q.i.d. × 7d	Spectinomycin 2 gm IM once *plus* erythromycin 500 mg PO q.i.d. × 7d
Disseminated	Ceftriaxone 1 gm IM or IV q24h until symptoms resolve	Spectinomycin 2 gm IM q12 h
Ophthalmic (adult)	Ceftriaxone 1 gm IM once	Spectinomycin 2 gm IM once *plus* erythromycin 500 mg PO QID × 7d
Meningitis	Ceftriaxone 1–2 gm IV q12h × 10–14d	Spectinomycin 2 gm IM q12h × 10–14d
Endocarditis	Ceftriaxone 1–2 gm IV q12h × 4 wk	
Infants	Ceftriaxone 25–50 mg/kg/ day, give IV or IM once	
Children	If ≥ 45 kg, use adult regimen; if < 45 kg, ceftriaxone 125 mg IM once; and if ≥ 8 yr, add doxycycline 100 mg PO b.i.d. × 7d.	
Syphilis		
Early	Benzathine penicillin G, 2.4 million units IM once	Doxycycline 100 mg PO b.i.d. × 2 wk *or* ceftriaxone 125 mg IM daily × 10d *or* erythromycin 500 mg PO q.i.d. × 2 wk if compliance assured.
Late latent (> 1 yr)	Benzathine penicillin G 2.4 million units 1 time/wk for 3 doses (total 7.2 million units)	Doxycycline 100 mg PO b.i.d. × 4 wk
Neurosyphilis	Aqueous crystalline penicillin G 2–4 million units IV q4h × 10–14d (total 12–24 million units per day)	Desensitize PCN allergic pts.
Congenital	Aqueous crystalline penicillin G 50,000 units/kg IV q8– 12 h × 10–14d (total 100,000–150,000 units)	

Continued.

TABLE 10–10.—Continued*

TYPE/CONDITION	RECOMMENDED REGIMEN	ALTERNATIVE
Chancroid	Erythromycin 500 mg PO q.i.d. × 7d *or* ceftriaxone 250 mg IM once	Trimethoprim-sulfamethoxazole 160/800 mg PO b.i.d. × 7d
Lymphogranuloma venereum	Doxycycline 100 mg PO b.i.d. × 21d	Erythromycin 500 mg PO q.i.d. × 21d
Genital herpes simplex		
First clinical episode	Acyclovir 200 mg PO 5×/d for 7–10d	
Severe disease	Acyclovir 5 mg/kg IV q8h for 5–7d	
Herpes proctitis	Acyclovir 400 mg PO 5×/d for 5d	
Recurrent	Acyclovir 200 mg PO 5×/d for 5d	
Daily suppressive	Acyclovir 200 mg PO 2–5×/d *or* 400 mg PO 2×/d	
Genital warts	Cryotherapy with liquid nitrogen or cryoprobe	10%–25% podophyllin *or* 80%–90% trichloracetic acid (TCA) *or* electrodesiccation
Chlamydial infections		
Urethral, endocervical or rectal	Doxycycline 100 mg PO b.i.d. × 7d *or* tetracycline 500 mg PO q.i.d. × 7d	Erythromycin 500 mg PO q.i.d. × 7d
Pregnant	Erythromycin 500 mg PO q.i.d. × 7d	Erythromycin 250 mg PO q.i.d. × 14d
Epididymitis	Ceftriaxone 250 mg IM once *plus* doxycycline 100 mg PO b.i.d. × 10d	
Pelvic inflammatory disease Outpatients (no concern for fertility)	Ceftriaxone 250 mg IM once *or* Cefoxitin 2 gm IM *plus* Probenecid 1 gm PO *plus* doxycycline 100 mg PO b.i.d. for 10–14d	If patient cannot tolerate doxycycline, use erythromycin 500 mg PO q.i.d. for 10–14d.
Inpatients	Cefoxitin 2 gm IV q6h *plus* doxycycline 100 mg PO b.i.d. until 48 hr after clinical improvement, then continue doxycycline dose for 10–14d	Clindamycin 900 mg IV q8h *plus* gentamycin 2 mg/kg loading dose (IM or IV) followed by 1.5 mg/kg q8h; 48 hr after clinical improvement, continue clindamycin 450 mg PO 5×/d for 10–14d *or* switch to doxycycline 100 mg PO b.i.d. for 10–14d.

Vaginal
trichomoniasis

Nonpregnant	Metronidazole 2 gm PO in 1 dose *or* 500 mg PO b.i.d. × 7d	
Pregnant	Avoid metronidazole in 1st trimester only.	
Vaginal candidiasis	Miconazole nitrate 200 mg vaginal suppository qhs × 3d *or* clotrimazole 200-mg vaginal tablet qhs × 3d *or* terconazole 80 mg suppository *or* 0.4% cream vaginally qhs × 3d	Alternatively, use agent of choice for 7d.
Bacterial vaginosis	Metronidazole 500 mg PO b.i.d. × 7d	Clindamycin 300 mg PO b.i.d. × 7d
Hepatitis B	Postexposure, hepatitis B immune globulin (HBIG) 0.06 ml/kg IM once *plus* immediately begin hepatitis B vaccine series	
Cytomegalovirus	No therapy exists.	

*Adapted from Centers for Disease Control: *MMWR* 1989; 38(S-8).

TABLE 10–11.—Androscopy: Detection of Occult
Papillomavirus Infection*

HPV types 16 and 18 are clearly associated with precancers and invasive cancers of the lower female genital tract. Since HPV is an STD, male partners of these women should be examined for subclinical infection that may be present in up to 80% of cases.

Indications
  Men who have sexual partners with known HPV infection
  Men who have had sex with prostitutes or ≥ 20 sexual partners
  Men who have (or who have had) penile warts
  Men who have bowenoid papillosis

Technique for detection
  An initial colposcopic examination should be made prior to staining to identify any lesions. The supine patient may be placed in stirrups in the lithotomy position, and if uncircumcised, foreskin should be withdrawn and held back by the patient for exam of the glans. Examine glans, shaft and scrotal skin, perineal body, and perianal tissues.
  Soak gauze 4 × 4's in a 5% acetic acid solution and allow to remain in contact with the skin that needs to be examined for approximately 5 minutes. More dilute solutions (e.g., 3%) is less effective on the keratinized squamous epithelium; however, 3% acetic acid may be more comfortable for mucosal surfaces such as the glans of the uncircumcised male.
  Carefully repeat the colposcope examination looking for acetowhite lesions.

Continued.

TABLE 10–11.—Continued

Biopsy of acetowhite lesions may be performed using local anesthetic with 0.1 to 0.2 cc of 1% lidocaine inserted sublesionally. The lesion may be shaved with a scalpel blade and removed with conventional colposcopic biopsy forceps, or a skin biopsy may be taken using punch biopsy technique. Accomplish hemostasis with topical styptic.

Biopsy specimens may be submitted in formalin for histological exam.

Aftercare

When biopsy report returns indicating HPV infection, lesions identified by their acetowhite change may be treated with topical application of 75% trichloroacetic acid, cryotherapy, or carbon dioxide laser fulguration. Recurrence rates may be as high as 10%–50%.

*Adapted from Driscoll CE: *Patient Care* 1990 (in press).

TABLE 10–12.—HIV Infection

Acute retroviral syndrome
 3 days–3 wk after exposure
 Mononucleosis-like syndrome
 Fever, skin rash, myalgias, arthralgias, lymphadenopathy, malaise, sore throat, headache, photophobia, GI symptoms
 (Neuologic symptoms, weight loss, elevated SGOT level in some patients)
Chronic HIV infection
 PGL (persistent generalized lymphadenopathy) = nodes ≥ 1 cm at ≥ 2 extrainguinal sites persisting > 3 mo.
 Patients with clinical disease may also have fever, fatigue, diarrhea, weight loss (10% of ideal), night sweats.
 Declining T-lymphocyte count
 Oral hairy leukoplakia
 Herpes infections
 Enlarged liver and spleen
 Chronic vaginitis
 Dermatologic disorders
History questions
 Prior blood transfusions
 IV drug use
 Sex with men, women, or both
 Number of sexual partners
 Known HIV+ sex partner or partner of high risk
 Oral, anal, or vaginal sex
 Exchanged money or drugs for sex, sex with prostitute
Pretest Counseling
 Informed consent obtained
  Benefits
   Reduce risky behavior
   Diminish anxiety
   Reduce further transmission
   Conception counseling
   Immunomodulation therapy

Risks
    Psychological trauma
    Social ostracism and discrimination
    Insurance problems
    Preoccupation and exaggeration of symptoms
Ask why patient wants test.
Give estimate of how likely they are to be positive.
Ask how they will feel and what they will do if positive.
Explain limits of HIV antibody test; false positives/negatives.
Educate regarding safe sex.
Testing
HIV antibodies develope within 3 mo. of infection for most patients but can remain seronegative for up to 36 mo.
Lab abnormalities supporting need for HIV testing
    Low serum cholesterol level, lymphopenia, anemia, thrombocytopenia; high ESR, low LDH, low serum globulin levels, or positive VDRL result
Two-step testing
    ELISA: enzyme-linked immunosorbent assay
      Repeat if positive and if positive second time, then do next step
    WESTERN BLOT TEST (WBT): identification of specific antibody bands

	Negative	False Positive	True Positive	False Negative
ELISA	−	+/+ or −	+/+	− Within 3 mo. of exposure
WBT	Not run	−	+	Not run

Post-test Counseling
Done in person, never over the phone.
Educate concerning prognosis, medical and social resources, how to prevent transmission of infection, sexual contact notification, danger signals of infection.
Evaluate and manage emotional response.
Refer to support group.

INTERSTITIAL CYSTITIS

TABLE 10–13.—Interstitial Cystitis

Underdiagnosed and difficult to treat condition of the bladder.
Urinalysis results are usually normal; 10% of patients may have $\geq$ 5 RBCs/HPF; urine culture is sterile despite occasional pyuria.
Patients must have all 3 of the following criteria:
1. Irritative voiding symptoms: urgency, frequency, suprapubic or pelvic pain relieved by voiding, dyspareunia.
2. Absence of other urologic disease: normal x-ray and cystometric studies.
3. Cystoscopic evidence: focal ulceration, edema, perineural-perivascular infiltrates, increased Mast cells in detrussor muscle biopsy specimens.
Treatments vary from medical, surgical, to laser therapy with less than optimal success.

CALCULI

TABLE 10–14.—Urinary Calculi

Urinary calculi are manifested by pain over the T12–L1 dermatomes, hematuria (10%–15% gross), and dysuria. Fever, urinary retention, and vomiting may be present. Urinary calculi composition:

Type	Incidence	X-ray
Calcium oxalate or phosphate	75% of stones	Opaque
Calcium phosphate with magnesium ammonia phosphate	15% of stones	Opaque
Uric acid	7% of stones	Lucent
Cystine	2% of stones	Opaque
Other types	1% of stones	? Opaque

Diagnosis

Family history, diet history (high calcium, vitamin D, drugs).
Complete physical exam to rule out malignancy and chronic disease.
Urinalysis and C&S.
Serum BUN and creatinine, creatinine clearance rates.
Serum electrolytes, calcium, phosphorus, uric acid, glucose, alkaline phosphatase and total protein; serum parathormone if calcium elevated.
24-hour urine for uric acid, cystine, and oxylate.
IVP with delayed films; retrograde pyelogram if obstruction.

Management

Increase urine volumes to dilute urinary crystalloids.
Vigorously treat any infection, consider prophylaxis.
Rule out hyperparathyroidism.
Stones caused by renal tubular acidosis: treat with alkalinization (citrate mixture of sodium bicarbonate).
Thiazide diuretics to reduce urinary calcium.
Orthophosphates decrease urinary calcium and improve solubilizing effect.
Low oxalate diet and pyridoxine to treat hyperoxaluria.
Magnesium oxide (200 mg t.i.d.) plus pyridoxine (25 mg/day) for treatment of calcium oxalate stones.
Methylene blue (65 mg t.i.d.) for recurrent calcium stones.
Alkalinization of urine to pH 7.0 to prevent uric acid stone formation.
Add allopurinol if serum uric acid is elevated.
Alkalinization of urine to pH of 7.8 or more, high fluid intake, low calcium diet for cystine stones. (Low methionine diet raises cystine.)
Add D-penicillamine and pyridoxine for large amounts of urinary cystine.
Single stone, young and healthy, normal lab and IVP: increase fluid volumes only.

TABLE 10–15.—WORKUP OF HYPERCALCIURIA AND NEPHROLITHIASIS*

| | PRIMARY HYPERPARA-THYROIDISM | ABSORPTIVE HYPERCALCIURIAS | | HYPOPHOSPHATEMIC HYPERCALCIURIA | RENAL HYPERCALCIURIA | HYPEROXALURIA OF ENTERIC CAUSE | HYPERURICOSURIC CALCIUM OXALATE NEPHROLITHIASIS |
		TYPE I	TYPE II				
Serum calcium	E	N	N	N	N	L/N	N
Serum phosphorus	L/N	N	N	L	N	L/N	N
Urinary calcium	E/N	E	E	E/N	E	L	N
Serum PTH†	E	L/N	L/N	L/N	E	E/N	N
Urinary cyclic AMP	E	L/N	L/N	L/N	E	E/N	N
Urinary uric acid	E/N	E/N	E/N	E/N	E/N	L	E
Urinary oxalate	E/N	E/N	E/N	E/N	E/N	E	N
Urinary citrate	N	L/N	L/N	L/N	L/N	L	L/N
Bone density‡	L/N	N	N	N	L/N	L	N
Fractional calcium absorption§	E/N	E	E/N	E/N	E/N	L	N

*E = elevated; N = normal; L = low.
†PTH = parathyroid hormone.
‡Bone density—in distal 1/3 of radius by photon absorptiometry.
§Fractional calcium absorbtion—fecal recovery of radioactivity after oral ingestion of 100 mg radioactive calcium.

TABLE 10–16.—EXTRACORPOREAL SHOCK-WAVE LITHOTRIPSY (ESWL)*

Successful clearance in 3 mo. (50%–90%); kidney stone prognosis better than ureteral.
Contraindications to ESWL:
  Obstruction distal to stone
  Coagulopathy, bleeding dyscrasia
  Pregnancy
  Marked obesity (> 300 lb)
Postprocedure problems; monitor for occurrence
  Ureteral obstruction, 4%
  Hemorrhage (usually inconsequential but up to ⅓ require transfusion), 20%–30%
  Hypertension, 10% up to 1 yr
  Cardiac dysrhythmias, 1%

*Adapted from Atala A, Steinbock GS: *Am J Surg* 1989; 157:350–358.

HEMATURIA AND PROTEINURIA

TABLE 10–17.—DIFFERENTIAL DIAGNOSIS OF ASYMPTOMATIC HEMATURIA

AGE GROUP	DIAGNOSTIC POSSIBILITIES	CHARACTERISTICS
Neonates and toddlers	Nephroblastoma, renal vein thrombosis, polycystic kidney disease, obstructive uropathy, medullary sponge kidney, occult trauma, abuse	Usually manifested by gross hematuria, invariably serious in nature; aggressive workup indicated
Children aged 5–15 yr	Glomerulonephritis, sickle cell disease or trait, acute hemorrhagic cystitis, trauma	Usually benign disorders with a good prognosis; workup needs to exclude reduced renal function
Young adults (after puberty to age 40)	Honeymoon cystitis, urinary schistosomiasis, exercise-induced, associated with pregnancy, urinary calculi, inflammatory bladder conditions, bladder tumor, essential hematuria, urethritis	Rarely due to a life-threatening or surgical lesion; evaluation can usually stop after IVP and cystoscopy
Adults 40 and older	Renal or bladder neoplasm, urinary calculi, analgesic nephropathy, prostatic disease	Suspect neoplastic disorder until proved otherwise; complete workup indicated

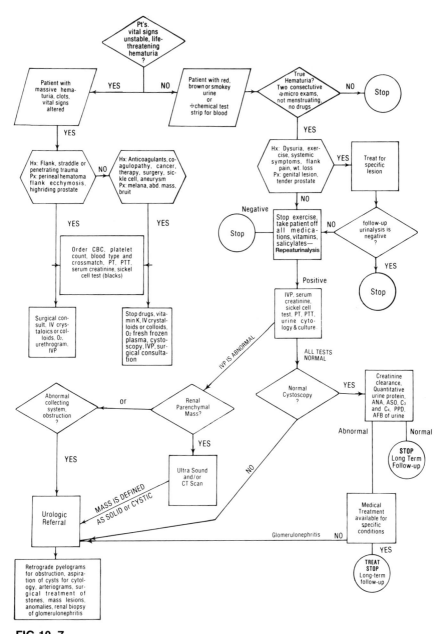

FIG 10–7.
Primary care of hematuria. (Adapted from Driscoll CE: *Emerg Decisions* 1985; 1[4]:35–40.)

TABLE 10–18.—Determining the Significance of Proteinuria

True proteinuria
When urinalysis dipstick test is positive for protein you may perform sulfosalicylic acid (Exton's) test:
1. Collect fresh, concentrated urine by clean catch method.
2. Add 8 drops of 20% sulfosalicylic acid to 2 ml of urine.
Exton's test also detects nonalbumin proteins. Protein concentration is directly proportional to white turbidity.
  + dipstick/ − Exton's → false positive dipstick
  + dipstick/ + + Exton's → suspect nonalbumin protein
  + dipstick/ + Exton's → confirms presence of protein

Orthostatic proteinuria:
Caused by upright body posture; prognosis probably benign. Instruct patient to:
Void at 7:00 A.M. and discard urine.
Collect all urine 7:00 A.M. to 9:00 P.M. in container #1.
Assume recumbent position from 9:00 P.M. until 7:00 A.M.
Void 11:00 P.M. urine into container #1.
All urines 11:00 P.M. to and including 7:00 A.M. voiding collected in container #2.
Determine urinary protein and creatinine for both containers.

Orthostatic proteinuria: total 24-hour protein greater than 150 mg with less than 75 mg excreted over 8 hours in recumbent position.

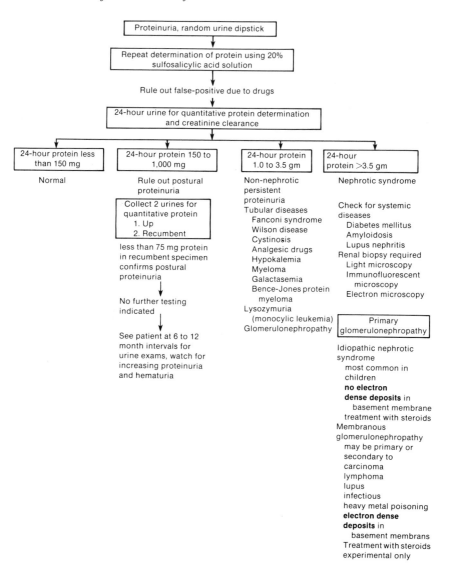

FIG 10–8.

Evaluation for asymptomatic proteinuria. (From Weber H Jr: *Contin Ed Fam Physician* 1978; 8:18–25. Reproduced by permission.)

PROSTATE DISEASE

TABLE 10–19.—PROSTATIC DISEASES

CONDITION	SYMPTOMS	EXAM	LAB STUDIES	TREATMENT
Benign hypertrophy	Nocturia, hesitancy, urge incontinence, dribbling, decreased urine flow, obstruction	Smooth, symmetrical enlargement	>150 cc postvoid residual, urinalysis, IVP, cystoscopy, urine flow studies	TURP, balloon dilatation, prazosin 1–2 mg PO b.i.d.
Acute bacterial prostatitis	Sudden onset of fever, chills, malaise, arthralgia, frequency, dysuria, pain in perineum	Tender and warm prostate, boggy enlargement (examine gingerly)	Urine culture, blood culture, avoid catheterization	IV antibiotics, analgesics, stool softeners, NSAIDs
Prostatic abscess	Acute bacterial prostatitis with spiking fevers and rectal pain, chills	Firm, tender, or fluctuant mass	Elevated blood glucose level, persistent leukocytosis despite antibiotics	Surgical drainage and antibiotics

Continued.

TABLE 10–19.—Continued

CONDITION	SYMPTOMS	EXAM	LAB STUDIES	TREATMENT
Chronic bacterial prostatitis	Recurrent UTIs, irritative voiding symptoms, no systemic signs	Prostatic calculi, boggy enlargement	Persistent bacteria in prostatic fluid, hematospermia, split-voided urinalysis	4–6 wk of antibiotic therapy, surgery if calculi
Nonbacterial prostatitis	Frequency, urgency, dysuria, testicular or penile pain; no systemic signs and no recurrent UTIs	Prostate may be normal on exam	$\geq$ 10 WBCs/HPF in prostatic secretions, no bacteria, lipid-laden prostatic macrophages, cystoscopy to rule out interstitial cystitis	Oxybutynin 5 mg PO t.i.d. or propantheline 15 mg PO t.i.d. or diazepam 2 mg PO t.i.d.
Prostatodynia	Painful prostate, symptoms similar to chronic bacterial or nonbacterial prostatitis, history of sexual or marital difficulties	Normal prostate on exam, pelvic muscle tension	Prostatic secretions without WBCs	Prazosin 1 mg PO b.i.d. or baclofen 5–10 mg PO t.i.d., warm sitz baths, psychosocial support

TABLE 10–20.—PROSTATITIS

Acute inflammation increases vascular permeability and antibiotics may gain easier access; chronic prostatic infection is "protected" from most antibiotics, which fail to diffuse into prostatic fluid.

Best antibiotics to use will:
  Be lipid soluble
  Have ionization potential (pKa) $\geq$ 8.6
  Have gram-negative spectrum at pH of 6.6
  Have low degree of protein binding

Type	Organisms	Drug	Duration
Acute infection	Gram-neg. coliforms, enterococci	Aminoglycoside or ampicillin	7–10 days
Chronic infection	Gram-neg. coliforms, *Chlamydia*	Trimethoprim-sulfamethoxazole or doxycycline or erythromycin	2–3 mo.

TABLE 10–21.—SCROTAL PROBLEMS

	CLINICAL DIFFERENTIATION	DIAGNOSTIC STUDIES	TREATMENT
Epididymo-orchitis	Gradual onset (hours–days), worsening incrementally; late adolescence to young adults	Nuclear scan with technetium reveals increased blood flow; normal Doppler study; >10 WBCs/HPF in prostatic secretions	Bed rest, heat or cold to scrotum, NSAID, doxycycline
Trauma	Painful trauma, gross swelling with ecchymosis	Urethrography; ultrasonography	Exploratory surgery
Torsion	Sudden onset, extreme pain; nausea, vomiting; young boys to early teens	Thicker ipsilateral spermatic cord; unequal Doppler flow; testicle higher in scrotum; no blood flow by nuclear scan	Surgery within 6 hr
Hydrocele	Rule out hernia; irreducible painless mass, occurs in all age groups; may communicate intraabdominally.	No bowel sounds on auscultation; transilluminates	May be sclerosed with tetracycline or surgically removed

Condition	Clinical Features	Diagnosis	Treatment
Varicocele	"Bag of worms" or "spaghetti" of spermatic cord usually on left; be suspicious of serious problem if acute onset on right side	IVP or CT scan of retroperitoneal space if acute onset	Surgically remove if painful or infertility a problem
Spermatocele	Painless lump in spermatic cord	Transillumination shows fluorescence	Surgical removal if large or cosmetically undesirable
Testicular cancer	Painless firm enlarging mass; often ignored for months	Ultrasonography; exploratory surgery	Biopsy of mass; removal and lymph node dissection
Cryptorchidism	Nonexistant testicle, asymptomatic	Chromosome studies if bilateral	Surgical exploration

TABLE 10–22.—Assessment and Treatment of Penile Curvature*

Presentation: Congenital or acquired curvature noted during a spontaneous erection. May be associated with urethral stricture. In Peyronie's disease, patient palpates mass in shaft of penis.

Congenital	Acquired
With epispadias or hypospadias	Stricture of urethra
Chordee without hypospadias	Penile trauma
Penile torsion	Peyronie's disease

Clinical evaluation: History, physical exam and special studies are needed

History	Physical	Studies
Onset	Palpable plaque	At-home polaroid pictures of
Degree of curvature	Other penile	curvature with erection
Pain	abnormalities	X-ray or ultrasound of plaque
Erectile failure		Evaluation for erectile failure
Sexual difficulties		(NPT, Rigiscan)
		Corporacavernosogram

Treatment: Treatment may be necessary if curvature severe, problem has been stable over time and it interferes with intercourse.

Nonsurgical (for Peyronie's disease)	Surgical
None has been documented to be successful but may serve to show concern for patient's problem; the condition tends to abate somewhat over time; vitamin E, aminobenzoate potassium.	Urethral repair
	Release of inelastic integument
	Nesbit plication of corpora
	Excision of plaque with skin graft if not impotent
	Impotent patients may have excision and prosthesis.

*Adapted from Gregory JG, Purcell MH: Med Aspects Hum Sexuality 1989; 23:64–70.

TABLE 10–23.—Emergency Management of Priapism

Since impotence is a known complication of priapism, this possibility should be explained to the patient early on; informed consent for an emergency procedure is obtained.

Aspiration

Thoroughly cleanse penis with povidine-iodine to prep the skin.

Wearing sterile gloves, drape off surrounding area to create a sterile field.

Locate the 3 o'clock or 9 o'clock position on the shaft of the penis, approximately 1 inch proximal to the corona. Avoid the dorsal neurovascular bundle and the ventral urethral areas. Inject 0.5–1.0 cc of lidocaine to anesthetize skin over the aspiration site. Only one side of the penis needs to be aspirated due to the cross-flow of circulation.

Insert a 19-gauge butterfly needle into the corpora through the anesthetized skin and aspirate blood into a sterile 20-cc syringe. If blood gases on sludged penile blood are desired, use a 5-cc glass heparinized syringe to do the first aspiration, then change to the 20-cc syringe. If the condition has persisted for >36 hr and/or pH is <7.25, Po_2 <30 and Pco_2 is >60 mm Hg, a significant ischemic condition exists, and the patient should be referred for surgical shunt procedure.

Continue aspiration until all possible blood is obtained and the penis loses its rigidity. Squeezing, or "milking," of blood from the penis may help in removing blood.

When aspiration is no longer productive, move to the irrigation stage of the procedure.

Irrigation

Add 1 ml of epinephrine 1:1,000 to a 1-L bag of sterile saline. Attach an IV administration set, run some fluid through the tubing, and fill a clean sterile 20-cc syringe from it.

Slowly inject epinephrine/saline solution into cavernosa and aspirate back into syringe and discard.

Repeat the step above until satisfactory detumescence has occurred and blood returned from the penis is bright red instead of dark and viscous. Then withdraw the butterfly needle from the penis and cover the aspiration site with sterile dressing. If no satisfactory results are obtained after 200 cc of irrigation, abandon the procedure and plan for surgical shunting.

Hospitalize the patient for 24 hours of observation to ensure that priapism does not recur. Success should be anticipated in $\geq$ 75% of the cases regardless of etiology.

*Adapted from Driscoll CE: *Patient Care* 1990; 24(10):117–118.

POLYCYSTIC KIDNEY DISEASE

TABLE 10–24.—POLYCYSTIC KIDNEY DISEASE (PCKD)*

EXPECTED FINDINGS	% OF CASES[†]
Proteinuria	75
Palpable kidneys	66
Abdominal pain	66
Pyuria	50
Hematuria	50
Hypertension	50
Liver cysts	33
Renal insufficiency	33
Intracranial aneurysm[‡]	16
Stones	10

Incidence: 1 in 500 at autopsy; typically a middle-aged patient with abdominal pain and hematuria.

Infection is the most common complication.

Hypertension and azotemia associated with eclampsia of pregnancy.

Diagnose by ultrasound (or by IVP or renal scanning).

Aggressively treat hypertension to minimize risk of intracerebral hemorrhage; avoid manipulations of lower urinary tract.

*Adapted from Chester AC, Harris JP, Schreiner GE: *Am Fam Physician* 1977; 16:94.
[†]Based on a number of large series.
[‡]Responsible for 15% of deaths in patients with PCKD.

SEXUAL PROBLEMS

TABLE 10–25.—DIFFERENTIATION OF PSYCHOGENIC AND ORGANIC
ERECTILE DYSFUNCTION[*†]

FEATURE	PSYCHOGENIC	ORGANIC
History		
Onset	Usually abrupt with temporal relationship to specific stress	Usually gradual
Course	Selective, intermittent, episodic	Persistent, progressive
Severity	Variable, erection may occur with masturbation or with alternate partners; nocturnal or morning erections generally present	Unable to achieve erection in any setting; nocturnal erections absent or markedly reduced
Physical		
Nocturnal penile tumescence (NPT)	Normal	Absent or decreased in number, duration, or rigidity
Penile blood pressure	Penile index 0.90; systolic pressure no more than 20 mm Hg below brachial systolic	Penile index 0.60; systolic pressure 30 mm Hg below brachial systolic
Bulbocavernosus reflex latency	Normal (33.5–35 m/sec)	Prolonged (>40 m/sec)
Lab		
Serum-free testosterone	Normal	Low
Leutinizing hormone (if low testosterone)	Normal	Low (pituitary), high (testicular)
Serum prolactin	Normal	Elevated

*Adapted from Vliet LW, Meyer JK: *Johns Hopkins Med J* 1982; 151:246.
†Erectile dysfunction is defined as erectile failure in 25% or more of attempts at intromission.

TABLE 10–26.—Possible Causes of Organic Erectile Dysfunction*

Inflammatory	Urethritis, prostatitis, seminal vesiculitis, cystitis, gonorrhea, tuberculosis, elephantiasis, mumps
Mechanical	Congenital deformities, Peyronie's disease, morbid obesity, hydrocele, spermatocele, varicocele, phimosis, priapism, urethral stricture
Postoperative	Perineal prostatic biopsy, perineal prostatectomy, abdominal aortic aneurysmectomy, aortofemoral bypass, retroperitoneal lymphadenectomy, sympathectomy (lumbar, dorsal, pelvic), cystectomy, abdominoperineal resection, external spincterotomy
Occlusive-vascular	Atherosclerosis, arteritis, thrombosis, embolism, aneurism, Leriche syndrome
Traumatic	Penectomy, urethral rupture, pelvic fracture
Endurance-related	Myocardial failure, angina pectoris, related insufficiency, anemia, leukemia, systemic illness, renal or hepatic failure, sickle cell disease
Neurologic	Myasthenia gravis, multiple sclerosis, parkinsonism, amyotrophic lateral sclerosis, stroke, cerebral tumors, temporal lobe, infections, head trauma, spinal cord trauma, spinal cord compression, tabes dorsalis, temporal lobe epilepsy, spina bifida, syringomyelia, subacute combined degeneration of the cord, peripheral neuropathy, cerebral palsy, electroconvulsive treatment (occasionally)
Chemical	Multiple pharmacologic agents affect sexual function, notably antihypertensives, anticholinergics, antidepressants, sedatives, and narcotics
Endocrine	Acromegaly, chromophobe adenoma, craniopharyngioma, pituitary ablation, hyperprolactinemia, Addison's or Cushing's syndrome, hyperthyroidism, hypothyroidism, castration, postinflammatory fibrosis; exogenous estrogens; Klinefelter or male Turner syndromes, feminizing interstitial cell tumor, diabetes, Fröhlich syndrome

*Adapted from Vliet LW, Meyer JK: *Johns Hopkins Med J* 1982; 151:246.

TABLE 10–27.—Anabolic-Androgenic Steroid Side Effects*

RATE OF OCCURRENCE (%)	CONDITION
Rare	Cholestatic jaundice, peliosis hepatitis, hepatic carcinoma, infection or nerve trauma from injections, tendon pain
1–2	Intolerance reaction consisting of anorexia, burning tongue, nausea and vomiting, abdominal pressure, diarrhea
5–10	Increase in liver enzymes
20–30	↓ HDL, ↑ LDL, voice deepening, alopecia, acne, aggressiveness, gynecomastia
> 60	Testicular atrophy, altered libido, virilization

*Adapted from Frankle MA: *J Musculoskeletal Med* November 1989; pp 69–88.

HYPERTENSION

TABLE 10–28.—Differentiation of Renovascular
and Essential Hypertension*

PARAMETER	RENOVASCULAR	ESSENTIAL
Age at onset (yr)	<30 or >50	30–50
Family history of high BP	46% of pts.	71% of pts.
Abdominal bruits	46%	9%
Urinary casts	20%	9%
Grade 3 or 4 eye ground changes	15%	7%
More prone to malignant, accelerated, severe hypertension	Positive	Positive
Response to usual drugs	Poor	Good
Prone to adverse drug effects	Negative	Negative

*Adapted from Ram CVS: *Diagnosis* 1983; 5:41.

RENAL FAILURE

TABLE 10–29.—RENAL FAILURE

Acute renal failure
    Diagnosis can be made if urine volume falls below 400 ml/24 hr, elevated serum BUN and creatinine. BUN rises 10–20 mg/day; creatinine rises 0.5–1.0 mg/day. Mortality is about 50%.

Types of Renal Failure

Characteristic	Prerenal	Renal	Postrenal
Causes	Volume depletion, reduced cardiac output, vascular obstruction	Glomerular or tubular lesions	Bladder or ureteral obstruction
Urine osmolality (mOsm/kg H_2O)	>500	<350	Usually <350
Urine to serum osmolar ratio	>1.2	<1.1	<1.1
Urine sodium (mEq/L)	<20	>40	Variable
Urine to serum urea ratio	>8	<3	<3
Urine to serum creatinine ratio	>40	<20	<20

Causes of renal azotemia
    Glomerular
        Glomerulonephritis, lupus, allergic angiitis, polyarteritis nodosa, Wegener's granulomatosis, streptococcal disease.
    Tubular
        Ischemic hypotension, contrast materials, antibiotics, heavy metals, methoxyflurane anesthesia, ethylene glycol, methanol, carbon tetrachloride, rhabdomyolysis, septic abortion, eclampsia, uric acid, sulfonamide, hypercalcemia, Bence Jones protein.

TABLE 10–30.—CLINICAL MANAGEMENT OF RENAL FAILURE

CONDITION	OBSERVATION	MANAGEMENT
Hyperkalemia	Serum K^+, ECGs	Kayexalate (oral or enema) 50 gm in 200 ml of 20% sorbitol, repeat q4h and/or dialysis
Acidosis	Serum pH, serum bicarbonate	Oral bicarbonate solutions if serum bicarbonate <15 mEq/L; guard against hypernatremia; dialysis
Protein/calorie malnutrition	Daily weights	Consider hyperalimentation; restrict Na^+, K^+, H_2O
Hypermagnesemia	Serum Mg	Avoid laxatives and antacids, dialysis
Hypocalcemia	Serum Ca^{++}	Accompanied by rise in phosphorus, if Ca^{++} < 7.5 administer replacement with 2 gm/day; restrict dietary phosphate, bind phosphorus in gut with aluminum carbonate or hydroxide antacids
Fluid overload	Observe for loss of thirst response, serum sodium, urine specific gravity	At least 2 L of fluid daily, free water access; if dilutional hyponatremia occurs, restrict fluids

Indications for dialysis:
  Volume expansion with life-threatening CHF
  Severe uncontrollable hypernatremia and/or hyperkalemia and/or acidosis
  When serum calcium × serum phosphate (mmd) product is ≥ 6
  Poisoning with salicylates, ethanol, methanol, short-acting barbiturates
  Chronic renal failure with acute temporary decline
  Terminal renal failure awaiting transplantation

TABLE 10–31.—Drug-Related Renal Syndromes*

RENAL SYNDROME	MECHANISM	CAUSATIVE AGENTS[†]
Acute renal failure (acute tubular necrosis)	Direct tubular injury	Aminoglycosides; radiocontrast agents; cisplatin; amphotericin B; cephaloridine; heavy metals
Acute renal failure (prerenal)	Decreased renal perfusion	NSAIDs; converting enzyme inhibitors; radiocontrast agents; cyclosporine
Acute renal failure (interstitial nephritis)	Immunologic, inflammatory	Penicillins; sulfonamides; cephalosporins; dilantin; allopurinol; NSAIDs; diuretics
Acute renal failure (obstruction)	Intratubular obstruction; retroperitoneal fibrosis	Methotrexate; acyclovir; radiocontrast agents; methysergide
Chronic renal failure	Chronic tubulointerstitial nephritis	Analgesics; lead; nitrosoureas; lithium; cyclosporine
Nephrotic syndrome	Primary glomerulopathy	Gold; penicillamine; captopril; NSAIDs; heroin
Hyperkalemia	Altered renal and extrarenal potassium homeostasis	β-Blockers; NSAIDs; captopril; thiazides; spironolactone; triamterine; calcium-channel blockers; cyclosporine
Hyponatremia	Decreased free-water excretion	NSAIDs; chlorpropamide; thiazides; clofibrate; vincristine; lithium; demeclocycline;
Nephrogenic diabetes insipidus	—	—

*From Cooper K, Bennett WM: *Arch Intern Med* 1987; 147:1213–1218. Reproduced by permission.
†NSAIDs indicates nonsteroidal anti-inflammatory drugs.

TABLE 10–32.—Characteristic Features of Renal Masses on Various Imaging Methods*

	IV UROGRAPHY	ULTRASOUND	CT	ANGIOGRAPHY
Benign masses				
Cyst	Sharp demarcation from surrounding renal parenchyma; pencil-thin wall	Thin, smooth wall; lack of internal echoes with through-transmission	Smooth, sharply marginated nonenhancing homogeneous lesion	Nonspecific avascular mass (this method rarely necessary)
Angiomyolipoma	Nonspecific renal mass	Increased echogenicity similar to that of renal sinus fat	Fat within tumor	
Adenoma (oncocytoma)	Nonspecific well-demarcated mass	Homogeneous well-encapsulated mass	Homogeneous mass with attenuation value similar to that of normal renal tissue; central fibrous scar	Quite vascular with sharp, smooth-rimmed homogeneous appearance ("spoke wheel" cortical pattern)

Malignant masses

Renal cell carcinoma[†]	Possible calcification, irregularity in renal contour, distortion of collecting system	Isoechoic mass with inhomogeneity caused by hemorrhage and necrosis	Solid mass that may be necrotic or have cystic components and variable contrast enhancement	Often hypervascular and neovascular
Metastasis	Often appears normal; if abnormal, solid contour-deforming mass is compressing collecting system	Possible multiple homogeneous hypoechoic masses that do not display through-transmission	Enhanced after administration of contrast medium but less than surrounding normal parenchyma	Hypovascular infiltrating mass with truncation and encasement of segmental renal arteries
Transitional cell carcinoma	Lucent filling defects with irregular surface	Low-echogenic mass in renal pelvis surrounded by normal, highly echogenic renal sinus	Flat or rounded solid intrapelvic mass outlined by contrast medium in renal pelvis	Mass that is hypovascular or avascular

Continued.

TABLE 10–32.—Continued

	IV UROGRAPHY	ULTRASOUND	CT	ANGIOGRAPHY
Pseudoneoplasms				
Xanthogranulomatous pyelonephritis	Nonspecific renal mass	Kidney appears enlarged with echogenic foci and acoustic shadowing if stone is present	Renal parenchyma is replaced by nonenhancing xanthogranulomatous deposit	
Hydronephrosis	Obstructed kidney may be enlarged with delayed nephrogram; visualization of collecting system delayed	Parenchyma is thin; loss of normal cortical medullary junction	Kidneys enlarged; renal parenchyma thinned	
Abscess	Focal enlargement of kidney	Mature abscess: anechoic mass with irregular margins; septations and floating debris may be present Chronic abscess: thick rim	Air-fluid level, fascial thickening, perirenal spread of infection	Chronic abscess: similar to renal neoplasm with stretched vessels and surrounding hyperemia
Hematoma	Mass distorts kidney	Localized fluid collections; focal low-attenuation mass with dispersed internal echoes	Nonenhancing mass	Distal renal branch or capsular artery may show site of active bleeding

*From Graham TE, Rockey KE: *Postgrad Med* 1990; 87:111–126. Reproduced by permission.
†Magnetic resonance imaging may also be used and shows intravascular tumor thrombus, perirenal adenopathy, and tumor extension.

11 *Neurology*

Charles W. Smith, Jr., M.D.

NEUROANATOMY AND NEUROLOGICAL EXAM

TABLE 11–1.—Pathologic Reflexes*†

REFLEX	STIMULUS	RESPONSE
Babinski	Stroke outer edge of side of foot	Extension great toe, flexion small toes, spreading small toes
Chaddock	Stroke lateral aspect of dorsum of foot and external malleolus	Extension great toe
Oppenheim	Firm stroke, medial tibia	Extension great toe
Rossolimo	Tap balls of toes	Plantar flexion of toes
Mendel-Bechterew	Tap dorsum of foot on outer surface	Plantar flexion of toes
Palm-chin (palmomental)	Stroke thenar eminence	Elevation of corner of mouth, contraction of chin
Thumb-adductor	Stroke hypothenar area	Adduction and flexion, thumb
Hoffman's sign	Snap nail of middle finger	Flexion of thumb and fingers
Gordon's sign	Compression of pisiform bone	Extension of flexed fingers
Chaddock's sign	Pressure of palmaris longus tendon	Flexion of wrist; extension of fingers

*Adapted from Mancall EL: *Essentials of the Neurologic Examination,* ed 2. Philadelphia, FA Davis Co, 1981, pp. 94–95.
†All pathologic reflexes listed in the table are indicative of pyramidal tract disease.

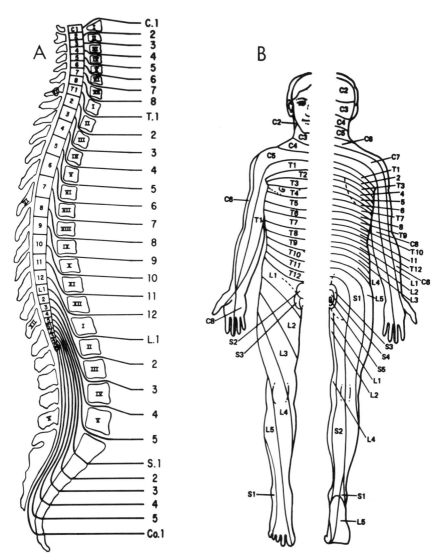

FIG 11–1.
Neuroanatomy. **A,** relationship of spinal nerves to the vertebral column. **B,** dermatome chart. (**A** from Van Allen MW, Rodnitzky RL: *Pictorial Manual of Neurologic Tests,* ed 2. Chicago, Year Book Medical Publishers, 1981, p 80. Redrawn from Favill J: Outline of the Spinal Nerves. Springfield, Ill, Charles C Thomas, Publisher, 1946. **B** from Chaplin JP, Demers A: *Primer of Neurology and Neurophysiology.* New York, John Wiley & Sons, 1978, p 57. Reproduced by permission.)

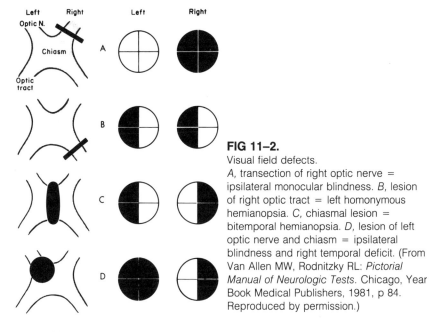

FIG 11–2.
Visual field defects.
A, transection of right optic nerve = ipsilateral monocular blindness. *B,* lesion of right optic tract = left homonymous hemianopsia. *C,* chiasmal lesion = bitemporal hemianopsia. *D,* lesion of left optic nerve and chiasm = ipsilateral blindness and right temporal deficit. (From Van Allen MW, Rodnitzky RL: *Pictorial Manual of Neurologic Tests.* Chicago, Year Book Medical Publishers, 1981, p 84. Reproduced by permission.)

TABLE 11–2.—EFFECTS OF AUTONOMIC STIMULATION ON SELECTED BODY ORGANS*

ORGAN	SYMPATHETIC EFFECTS	PARASYMPATHETIC EFFECTS
Eye		
Pupil	Dilation	Contraction
Ciliary process	None	Excitation
Gastrointestinal glands	Inhibition or no effect	Copious serous or watery secretion and enzymes
Salivary gland	Thick, viscous secretion	Serous or water secretion
Sweat glands	Copious secretion	None
Heart	Increase in rate and force of contraction	Decrease in rate and force of contraction
Lungs	Constricts blood vessels, dilates bronchi	Constricts bronchi
Gastrointestinal	Inhibits peristalsis, stimulates sphincters	Stimulates peristalsis, inhibits sphincters
Liver	Release of glucose	None
Genitalia	Ejaculation, orgasm	Erection, lubrication
Blood vessels	Constricts abdominal muscles, constricts or dilates other smooth muscles depending on receptors in tissue	None
Bladder	Uncertain	Stimulates smooth muscle for emptying, contracts detrusor, relaxes internal sphincter

*Adapted from Chaplin JP, Demers A: *Primer of Neurology and Neurophysiology.* New York, John Wiley & Sons, 1978, p 97.

TABLE 11–3.—Reflex Interpretation Chart*

REFLEX	ELICITED BY	RESPONSE	SEGMENTAL LEVEL
Corneal	Touch cornea with cotton wisp	Contraction, orbicularis oculi	Pons
Pharyngeal	Touch posterior wall of pharynx	Contraction of pharynx	Medulla
Palatal	Touch soft palate	Elevation of palate	Medulla
Scapular	Stroke interscapular skin	Contraction of scapular muscles	C5 to T2
Epigastric	Stroke skin from nipples to epigastrium	Epigastrium "dimples" toward stroke	T7 to T9
Abdominal	Stroke skin along and under costal margins and inguinal ligaments	Contraction of abdominal muscles in quadrant stimulated	T8 to T12
Cremasteric	Stroke medial surface of upper thigh	Elevation of testicle, same side	L1 to L2
Gluteal	Stroke skin of buttock	Contraction of glutei	L4 to L5
Bulbocavernous	Pinch dorsum of glans	Contraction of bulbous urethra	S3 to S4
Anal	Prick perianal skin	Contraction of rectal sphincter	S5
Jaw Jerk	Tap mandible, mouth open	Jaw closes	Pons
Triceps	Tap triceps tendon	Elbow extends	C7 to T1
Biceps	Tap biceps tendon	Elbow flexes	C5 to C6
Radial	Tap styloid process of radius	Supinator longus contracts	C5 to C6
Knee	Tap patellar tendon	Knee extends	L3 to L4
Ankle	Tap achilles tendon	Ankle extends	S1 to S3

*Adapted from Mancall EL: *Alper's and Mancall's Essentials of the Neurologic Examination,* ed 2. Philadelphia, FA Davis Co, 1981, pp 23, 25.

TABLE 11–4.—LUMBOSACRAL DISK SYNDROMES*

NERVE ROOT	DISK	PAIN	SENSORY LOSS	STRAIGHT LEG RAISING	ANKLE JERK	KNEE JERK	MOTOR SIGNS
L3	L2–L3	Back, buttock, anterior thigh and knee region	Knee region	Usually –	+	+	Quadriceps weakness
L4	L3–L4	Back, buttocks, posterior thigh, inner calf region	Inner aspect of lower leg	Usually – may be +	+	–	Quadriceps weakness
L5	L4–L5	Back, buttocks, lateral calf, dorsum of foot and big toe	Dorsum of foot and big toe	+ +	+	+	Weakness of anterior tibialis, big toe extensor, gluteus medius
S1	L5– S1	Back, buttocks, posterior calf, outer sole of foot and heel	Heel or lateral foot and toes	+ + +	–	+	Weakness of gastrocnemius, hamstring, toe flexors

*Adapted from Rakel RE: Textbook of Family Practice, ed 3. Philadelphia, WB Saunders Co, 1984.

TABLE 11–5.—COMMON PERIPHERAL NERVE LESIONS*

NERVE	MANIFESTATION
Median (at wrist)	Weakness and atrophy thumb and thenar eminence; sensory loss palm and first 3 digits, palmar surface; paresthesia and pain lateral hand, first 3 digits
Ulnar (at elbow)	Drooping 4th and 5th digits (hand of benediction); atrophy of hypothenar eminence; sensory loss of medial palm and 5th digit
Radial	Wrist drop; sensory loss dorsal hand and thumb (variable)
Femoral	Loss of knee jerk; weakness of knee extension and hip flexion
Peroneal	Foot drop
Sciatic	Pain lateral thigh; absent ankle jerk

*Adapted from Van Allen MW, Rodnitzky RL: *Pictorial Manual of Neurologic Tests.* Chicago, Year Book Medical Publishers, 1981, pp 130–133; and McKhann GM: Neurology, in Baughman KL, Green BM (eds): *Clinical Diagnostic Manual for the House Officer.* Baltimore, Williams & Wilkins Co, 1981.

TABLE 11–6.—CLINICAL USE OF EVOKED POTENTIALS*

TYPE	CLINICAL USE
Pattern shift	Abnormal in lesions of visual pathway anterior to optic chiasm (e.g., optic neuritis); helpful in diagnosis of hysteria
Brain stem auditory EPs	Useful in evaluating site of neurosensory hearing loss (e.g., acoustic neuroma)
Short latency somatosensory EPs	Evaluates integrity of plexi and dorsal roots; helpful in evaluation of radiculopathies; evaluation of extent of cord injuries; evaluation of MS

Evoked potentials are an electrical manifestation of brain response to an external stimulus.
May help distinguish abnormal sensory function when history is equivocal or presence of disease is questionable.
Can define anatomical distribution of a disease process.
Technically difficult to perform.

*Adapted from Chiappa KH, Robber AH: *N Engl J Med* 1982; 306:1140–1150.

NEUROLOGIC TESTS AND PROCEDURES

TABLE 11–7.—CEREBROSPINAL FLUID STUDIES IN MULTIPLE SCLEROSIS*

TEST	INCIDENCE OF POSITIVE FINDINGS	ABNORMAL VALUE	CAUSES OF FALSE POSITIVE RESULTS
γ-Globulins	60%–75%	>12% of protein	Neurosyphilis Guillain-Barré syndrome Systemic gammopathy
IgG index	80%–90%	>0.66	Viral encephalitis Neurosyphilis Subacute sclerosing panencephalitis (SSPE)
Oligoclonal bands	85%–95%	>2 bands	Guillain-Barré syndrome Chronic meningitis Optic neuritis
Myelin basic protein	70%–90%	Positive	Central pontine myelinolysis CNS lupus erythematosus Leukoencephalopathies Intrathecal chemotherapy Cranial irradiation Progressive multifocal leukoencephalopathy Encephalitis Anoxia Stroke

*From Schwankhaus JD: *Am Fam Physician* 1984; 29:234. Reproduced by permission.

TABLE 11–8.—TECHNIQUE OF LUMBAR PUNCTURE

1. Place patient on side on a firm mattress or padded exam table.
2. Flex patient with thighs on abdomen and neck moderately flexed.
3. Palpate L4 spinous process at level of iliac crest. Needle should be inserted into interspace either above (L3–4) or below (L4–5) this landmark.
4. Clean skin if necessary with soap and water.
5. Swab an area from the puncture site with an 8- to 10-inch radius with merthiolate, iodine, or povidone solution.
6. Drape sterile towels over area, leaving an opening at the puncture site.
7. Use sterile gloves and inject 1–2 cc of local anesthetic (e.g., 1% Xylocaine) about 2 cm into the interspace.
8. Use 20-gauge spinal needle with stylet, in the midline, angulated 5–15 degrees cephalad; advance slowly.
9. If needle meets bone withdraw partially and redirect needle.
10. Withdraw stylet every 2–3 mm to see if CSF appears; usually a slight "click" will be felt on entering the subdural space.
11. When this occurs, advance the needle 2–3 mm more and withdraw the stylet.
12. Determine opening pressure with manometer.
13. Withdraw 1 cc in each of four tubes and send first tube for cultures and Gram stain, second for WBC and RBC, third for glucose and protein, and fourth for other indicated studies (e.g., viral titers or cultures, India ink prep, fungal cultures, VDRL, rickettsial titers, or cytologies).
14. Use same procedure for infant, except use a 22-gauge, 1½-inch spinal needle; have assistant hold patient in sitting position, obtain approximately 0.5 cc/tube.
15. If tap is bloody, centrifuge 1–2 cc. If supernatant is clear, the tap is probably traumatic; if xanthochromic, blood was probably present before the tap.

TABLE 11–9.—ELECTROENCEPHALOGRAPHY*

EEG TECHNIQUES	USEFULNESS
Resting EEG	Clinical evaluation of any CNS disorder
Hyperventilation 3 min	Alkalosis and vasoconstriction may activate seizure focus
Photic stimulation (1–20/sec strobe light)	May activate certain abnormal discharges
Sleep EEG	Activates some EEG abnormalities, especially temporal lobe seizures
Nasopharyngeal leads	May show lesion in temporal lobe or deep frontoparietal area

About 12%–18% of normal persons have nonspecific EEG abnormalities.
Localized EEG activity is always significant.
Focal abnormalities do not distinguish brain pathology.
Some 20%–40% of patients with seizures have normal EEGs.

*Adapted from Adams RD, Victor M: *Principles of Neurology,* ed 2. New York, Mc-Graw-Hill Book Co, 1981, p 22.

TABLE 11–10.—PATTERNS OF EEG ABNORMALITIES*

EEG ABNORMALITY	DIAGNOSTIC CONSIDERATIONS
Focal delta wave activity	Tumor, abscess, subdural hematoma, intracranial bleed, cerebral infarct
Diffuse slow wave activity	Infratentorial tumor, cerebral edema, CNS hypoxia, meningitis, encephalitis, metabolic or toxic encephalopathy
Focal or generalized spike and wave activity	Petit mal epilepsy
Focal or generalized spike and slow wave complexes	Focal or generalized motor seizure disorder
No activity (flat line)	Brain death

*Adapted from Department of Neurology, Physiology, and Biophysics of the Mayo Clinic: *Clinical Examinations in Neurology,* ed 4. Philadelphia, WB Saunders Co, 1976, pp 284–295.

TABLE 11–11.—EMG in Neurologic Diagnosis*

NEUROLOGIC DEFICIT	CLINICAL EXAMPLE	EMG FINDINGS	DIAGNOSTIC USEFULNESS
Normal	Hysteria/malingering	Irregular firing rhythm of action potentials	+ + + +
Upper motor neuron lesions	Stroke	Diminished rate of action potential firing with contractions	0 to +
Myelopathy	Amyotrophic lateral sclerosis	Increased polyphasic potentials High amplitude and duration of action potentials	+ + +
Mononeuropathy	Carpal tunnel syndrome	Normal action potentials; diminished nerve conduction	+ + + to + + + +
Polyneuropathy	Diabetes	Same as mononeuropathy but in multiple sites	+ + + +
Neuromuscular transmission defects	Myasthenia gravis	Increased polyphasic potentials; low amplitude and duration of potentials; progressive decline of action potentials	+ + + to + + + +
Myopathies	Polymyositis	Increased polyphasic potentials; decreased amplitude and duration of action potentials	+ + to + + +

*Adapted from Departments of Neurology, Physiology, and Biophysics of the Mayo Clinic: *Clinical Examinations in Neurology*, ed 4. Philadelphia, WB Saunders Co, 1976, pp 299–316.

Key:
0   Not useful
+   Rarely useful
+ +   Occasionally useful
+ + + Usually helpful
+ + + + Always helpful

SEIZURE DISORDERS

TABLE 11–12.—CLASSIFICATION OF EPILEPSIES*

Primary Generalized Epilepsies
　Absence
　　Classic absence of childhood with diffuse 3-Hz spike-and-wave complexes
　　Absence of juvenile myoclonic epilepsy: staring, with diffuse 3-Hz to 6-Hz multispike-and-wave complexes during adolescence
　　Juvenile absence with diffuse 8-Hz to 12-Hz rhythms
　　Myoclonic absence with diffuse 3-Hz to 6-Hz multispike-and-wave complexes
　　Myoclonus absence: staring, fragmentary myoclonus, automatisms, and diffuse 12-Hz rhythms
　Myoclonic
　　Myoclonic seizures of early childhood, with 3-Hz to 6-Hz multispike-and-wave complexes without mental retardation (Doose syndrome)
　　Juvenile myoclonic seizures of Janz or benign myoclonic seizures of adolescence and late childhood, with diffuse 4-Hz to 6-Hz multispike-and-wave complexes
　Clonic-tonic-clonic (grand mal)
　Tonic-clonic (grand mal)
Partial epilepsies
　Simple partial
　Complex partial
　　Simple partial at onset followed by impairment of consciousness and automatisms
　　Impairment of consciousness at onset
　　　Motionless stare and impaired consciousness followed by automatisms (temporal lobe epilepsy)
　　　Complex motor automatisms at start of impaired consciousness (frontal lobe, somatosensory, or occipital lobe epilepsy)
　　　Drop attack with impaired consciousness and automatisms (temporal lobe syncope)
Secondary generalized epilepsies
　Simple partial evolving to tonic-clonic (secondary tonic-clonic)
　Infantile spasms (propulsive petit mal, infantile myoclonic encephalopathy with dysarrhythmia or West syndrome)
　Myoclonic astatic or atonic epilepsies (epileptic drop attacks of Lennox-Gastaut in children with mental retardation)
　Progressive myoclonic epilepsies in adolescents and adults with dementia (myoclonic epilepsies of Lafora, Lundborg, Hartung, Hunt, or Kuf)

*Adapted from Delgado-Escueta AV, Treiman DM, Walsh GO: *N Engl J Med* 1983; 308:1509.

TABLE 11–13.—COMMON DRUG REGIMENS FOR
GENERALIZED GRAND MAL CONVULSIONS AND FOCAL EPILEPSY*

CHOICE[†]	DRUGS
1	Phenytoin (Dilantin)
2	Phenobarbital (Luminal)
3	Phenytoin plus phenobarbital
4	Phenytoin plus primidone (Mysoline)
5	Carbamazepine (Tegretol)
6	Phenytoin plus carbamazepine
7	Phenobarbital plus carbamazepine
8	Primidone plus carbamazepine
9	Phenytoin plus phenobarbital plus carbamazepine
10	Phenytoin plus primidone plus carbamazepine

*From Samuels MA: *Manual of Neurologic Therapeutics.* Boston, Little, Brown & Co, 1982, p 97. Reproduced by permission.
†Choices 1 and 2 may be reversed if specifically indicated (such as in children and adolescents). Choices should be used in order of listing if currently used medication is not effective in controlling seizure activity after several weeks, assuming the patient is taking medication properly.

TABLE 11–14.—COMMON ANTIEPILEPTIC DRUGS*

| GENERIC NAME | TRADE NAME | USUAL DAILY DOSAGE | | PRINCIPAL THERAPEUTIC INDICATIONS | SERUM HALF-LIFE (hr) | EFFECTIVE BLOOD LEVEL (mg/ml) |
		Children	Adults, mg			
Phenobarbital	Luminal	4–15 mg/kg (8 mg/kg infants)	60–300	Tonic-clonic seizures; simple and complex partial seizures; absence	96 ± 12	15–30
Phenytoin	Dilantin	4–7 mg/kg	300–400	Tonic-clonic seizures; simple and complex partial seizures	24 ± 12	10–20
Carbamazepine	Tegretol	20–30 mg/kg	400–1,200	Tonic-clonic seizures; complex partial seizures	12 ± 3	4–12
Primidone	Mysoline	10–25 mg/kg	750–1,500	Tonic-clonic seizures; simple and complex partial seizures	12 ± 6	6–12
Ethosuximide	Zarontin	20–30 mg/kg	750–1,500	Absence	30 ± 6	40–100
Methsuximide	Celontin	10–20 mg/kg	500–1,000	Absence	30 ± 6	40–100
Diazepam	Valium	0.15–0.25 mg/kg (IV)	10–150	Status epilepticus	30 ± 6	40–100
ACTH		40–60 units/day		Infantile spasms		
Valproic acid	Depakene Depakote	15–60 mg/kg	1,000–3,000	Absence; simple and complex partial seizures	8 ± 2	25–100
Clonazepam	Klonopin	0.01–0.2 mg/kg	1.5–20	Absence; myoclonus	18–50	0.01–0.07

*From Adams RD, Victor M: *Principles of Neurology*, ed 2. New York, McGraw-Hill Book Co, 1981, p 227. Reproduced by permission.

TABLE 11–15.—MANAGEMENT OF STATUS EPILEPTICUS*

Definition: Continuous seizures lasting 30 minutes or more where (1) multiple tonic-clonic attacks occur without return of consciousness, (2) there is a continuous, prolonged "absence" or "twilight" state, or (3) consciousness is preserved, but with continuous partial motor seizures (epilepsia partialis continuans).

Time from starting Rx.	Procedure
Immediate	1. Assess cardiovascular status. 2. Insert oral airway. 3. Start O_2 and IV line. 4. Draw blood for anticonvulsant levels, glucose, BUN, electrolytes, and CBC. 5. Draw blood for arterial blood gas measurements. 6. Obtain ECG.
5 minutes	1. Give 100 mg of thiamine IV. 2. Give 50 cc of 50% glucose.
10 minutes	1. Give IV Valium ($\leq$2 mg/min) until seizures stop, up to 20 mg. 2. Start phenytoin ($\leq$50 mg/min) to a dose of 18 mg/kg.
30–40 minutes	If still seizing: 1. Give phenobarbital IV ($\leq$100 mg/min) up to 20 mg/kg, or 2. Give Valium IV (100 mg in 500 ml D5W) at 40 cc/hr.
50–60 minutes	1. If still seizing, place patient under general anesthesia with halothane and neuromuscular junction blockade, or 2. Start 4% paraldehyde in normal saline IV (give as fast as needed to stop seizures), or 3. Give 50–100 mg of lidocaine as IV push, followed by 50–100 mg of lidocaine in 250 cc D5W at 1–2 mg/min.
80 minutes	1. If above medications are ineffective after 20 minutes, general anesthesia with neuromuscular blockade must be given.

*Adapted from Delgado-Escueta AV, Wasterlain C, Treiman DM, et al: *N Engl J Med* 1982; 306:1339.

STUPOR AND COMA

TABLE 11–16.—Various Methods of Giving Phenytoin*

THERAPEUTIC RANGE† REACHED (AFTER INITIAL DOSE)	RATE OF ADMINISTRATION	ROUTE	COMMENT
20 min	1,000 mg at 50 mg/min in adults (10–15 mg/ kg at 25 mg/min in children)	IV	Always with pulse, BP, and respiration monitored; given by syringe; not mixed in bottle
4–6 hr	1,000 mg stat in adults; then 300 mg/ day (about 15 mg/kg stat in children; then 5 mg/kg/day)	PO	Local gastric upset is common; give with meals or milk
24–30 hr	300 mg every 8 hr for three doses; then 300 mg/day in adults (5 mg/kg every 8 hr for three doses; then 5 mg/kg in children)	PO	Mild ataxia is common initially
5–15 days	300 mg/day in adults (5 mg/kg day in children)	PO	No unusual side effects

*From Samuels MA: *Manual of Neurologic Therapeutics*. Boston, Little, Brown & Co, 1982, p 94. Reproduced by permission.
†The therapeutic range is 5–20 µg/ml of serum.

TABLE 11–17.—Harvard Criteria for Brain Death*

Unresponsive: No vocal or motor response to intensely painful stimuli.
Apneic: Room air breathing for 10 minutes; normal arterial CO_2 tension; turn off ventilator and observe; apnea for at least 3 minutes meets criteria.
Areflexic: Pupils fixed and dilated; corneal and doll's eyes reflexes absent; no response to cold water calorics; flaccid extremities; no spontaneous blinking; no deep tendon reflexes.
EEG: Flat EEG; repeated in 24 hours; patient must not be hypothermic or on barbiturates

*Adapted from Black P: *N Engl J Med* 1978; 299:7.

TABLE 11–18.—STAGES OF ROSTROCAUDAL DETERIORATION WITH CENTRAL HERNIATION*

LEVEL	CONSCIOUSNESS	PUPILS	EYE MOVEMENTS	OCULOVESTIBULAR RESPONSES	RESPIRATORY PATTERN	MOTOR FUNCTION
Diencephalic	Somnolence, stupor, or coma	Small, slightly reactive	Roving and conjugate	Abnormal calorics; doll's eyes response brisk	Sighing or Cheyne-Stokes	Generalized hypertonicity, bilateral pyramidal tract signs or decorticate posturing
Midbrain—upper pontine	Coma	Mid-size, fixed	Disconjugate	Difficult to elicit	Central neurogenic hyperventilation	Bilateral decerebrate posturing
Lower pontine—upper medullary	Coma	Mid-size, fixed	Absent	Absent	Tachypnea	Generalized flaccidity; bilateral extensor plantars, minimal flexion withdrawal
Medullary (terminal)	Coma	Dilated, fixed	Absent	Absent	Ataxic, gasping or apnea	Flaccidity

*Adapted from Mancall EL: *Alper's and Mancall's Essentials of the Neurologic Examination*, ed 2. Philadelphia, FA Davis Co, 1981, p 37.

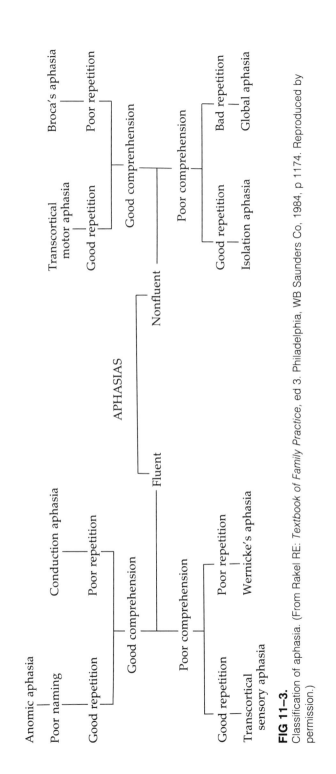

FIG 11-3.
Classification of aphasia. (From Rakel RE: *Textbook of Family Practice*, ed 3. Philadelphia, WB Saunders Co, 1984, p 1174. Reproduced by permission.)

TABLE 11–19.—COMPARISON OF MAJOR FORMS OF APHASIA*

FORM	EXPRESSION	VERBAL COMPREHENSION	REPETITION	NAMING	READING COMPREHENSION	WRITING	LESION
Expressive (Broca's)	Nonfluent	Rel. intact	Impaired	Impaired	Variable	Impaired	Posterior-inferior frontal (Broca's area)
Receptive (Wernicke's)	Fluent	Impaired	Impaired	Impaired	Impaired	Impaired	Posterior-superior temporal (Wernicke's area)
Global	Nonfluent	Impaired	Impaired	Impaired	Impaired	Impaired	Frontotemporal
Conduction	Fluent	Rel. intact	Impaired	Impaired	Variable	Impaired	Arcuate fasciculus; supramarginal gyrus
Nominal	Fluent	Rel. intact	Intact	Impaired	Variable	Variable	Angular gyrus; posterior-superior temporal
Transcortical motor	Nonfluent	Rel. intact	Intact	Impaired	Variable	Impaired	Anterior perisylvian
Transcortical sensory	Fluent	Impaired	Intact	Impaired	Impaired	Impaired	Posterior perisylvian

*From Mancall EL: Alper's and Mancall's Essentials of the Neurologic Examination, ed 2. Philadelphia, FA Davis Co, 1981, p 113. Reproduced by permission.

TUMORS

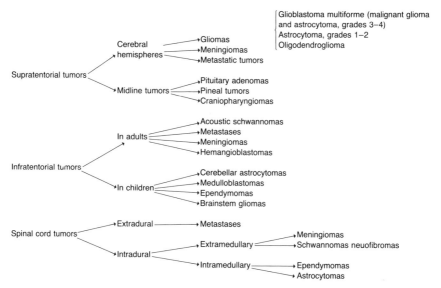

FIG 11–4.
Most frequent CNS tumors and their sites of predilection. (Adapted from Samuels MA: *Manual of Neurologic Therapeutics*. Boston, Little, Brown & Co, 1982, p 216.)

PARKINSON'S DISEASE

TABLE 11–20.—DRUGS COMMONLY USED FOR PARKINSON'S DISEASE*

DRUG	AVAILABILITY	FREQUENCY OF ADMINISTRATION	COMMENTS
Amantadine HCl (Symmetrel)	100-mg capsules	b.i.d. (reduce with renal impairment)	Excreted unchanged in urine; initial effect reached 48 hr after administration; half-life, 2–4 hr; adjunct to main therapy; initial dose 100 mg daily
Benztropine mesylate (Cogentin)	0.5, 1.0, and 2.0 mg tablets; injectable, 1 mg/ml	b.i.d.	Initial effect of PO dose requires 24 hr; if given parenterally, effect takes only minutes; cumulative action; initial dose 0.5 mg b.i.d.; half-life, 12–24 hr
L-dopa (Dopar, Larodopa)	100, 250, and 500 mg capsules and tablets	q.i.d. or more often	Half-life < 2 hr; cumulative action; start with 250 mg t.i.d. after meals
L-dopa with carbidopa (Sinemet)	10/100, 25/100, and 25/250 mg tablets	t.i.d.	Supplements of carbidopa or L-dopa may be needed
Trihexyphenidyl HCl (Artane)	2.0 and 5.0 mg tablets; 0.4 mg/ml elixir; 5 mg sustained-release capsules	t.i.d. for tablets and elixir; q.d. or b.i.d. for sustained-release capsules	Initial effect requires 24 hr; half-life 6–12 hr; cumulative action; start with 1 mg t.i.d.
Bromocriptine (Parlodel)	2.5 and 5 mg capsules	1.25 mg b.i.d., increase by 2.5 mg in 2 wk	May use adjunctively with L-dopa or Sinemet

*From Samuels MA: *Manual of Neurologic Therapeutics.* Boston, Little, Brown & Co, 1982, pp 336–337. Reproduced by permission.

12 *Psychiatry*

Edward T. Bope, M.D.

MOOD DISORDERS

These disorders represent a disturbance of mood with a manic or depressive syndrome. Mood is a prolonged emotion and is usually depression or elation (sad or happy). In the *DSM-III* these were called the affective disorders, but the *DSM-III-R* regroups them as mood disorders. The mood disorders are subdivided into bipolar disorders and depressive disorders. To qualify as a bipolar disorder, there must have been one or more manic or hypomanic episodes.

Bipolar Disorders

Bipolar Disorder (296.60)

The incidence is 0.45% to 1.25%, and it occurs at higher rates in first-degree relatives with the disorder. This disorder must have one or more of both manic and major depressive episodes. The cycle may be short or long, and either the manic or the depressive episode may be the predominant component for an individual.

Cyclothymia (301.13)

This disorder must have occurred for 2 years for adults or 1 year for children and involves numerous hypomanic episodes (essentially like manic episodes except do not interfere with function) as well as recurrent periods of depressed mood (not severe or prolonged enough to be diagnosed as major depression). There is a prevalence of 0.45% to 3.55%.

Depressive Disorders

This is a very common disorder affecting the mood. There cannot be an organic factor as the etiology, nor is it a normal reaction to bereavement. Delusions or hallucinations may occur but not in the absence of mood symptoms. Naturally, there must be a depressive episode in which there is either or both a depressed mood and a loss of interest or pleasure in daily activities. If both are present, then there must be at least three of the following findings (four if only one is present): increase or decrease in weight, increase or decrease in sleep, psychomotor agitation or retardation, fatigue, feelings of worthlessness or guilt, cognitive changes, and recurrent thoughts of death.

Major Depression (296.2)

The essentials of the diagnosis are a major depressive episode as described earlier without a history of a manic episode. Fifty percent of people who have major depression will have another episode. The range of incidence for females is 9% to 26% and for males is 5% to 12%. The disorder is 1.5 to 3 times more common in first-degree relatives.

Dysthymia (Depressive Neurosis) (300.4)

Individuals with the disorder have never had a manic episode. Symptoms of depressed mood have existed for 2 years (1 year for children) without evidence of a major depressive episode as defined before. While feeling depressed these individuals must have at least two of the following symptoms: increased or decreased appetite, increase or decrease in sleep, fatigue, low self-esteem, poor concentration or difficulty making decisions, and feeling of hopelessness.

Treatment of Mood Disorders

Bipolar Disorders

Psychotherapy is generally helpful in conjunction with medication but may be impossible in presenting episodes. Safety for the individual must be ensured since they could harm themselves in either the manic or depressive phase. Lithium carbonate is the most often used drug, but other modalities and medications are common.

Depressive Disorders

Assessing the risk of suicide is of immediate importance. When necessary or in doubt, force hospitalization. Rely on your judgment, not the patient's. Psychotherapy is certainly important, and drug therapy may be needed. Medication is generally selected, taking into account the side effect profile (some of which may be desirable). Table 16–8 lists these medications.

ANXIETY DISORDERS

TABLE 12–1.—Anxiety Disorders

ICDA-9 CODE	DSM-III CLASSIFICATION	DEFINITION: EXCESSIVE, IRRATIONAL WORRY PLUS
300.22	Agoraphobia without panic disorder	Fear of being in a place where escape might be embarrassing.
300.21	Panic disorder without agoraphobia	Fear of having a panic attack
300.01	Panic disorder with agoraphobia	Fear of having a panic attack in a crowd
309.21	Separation anxiety	Fear of separation from well-known people
300.29	Simple phobia	Fear of an item
300.23	Social phobia	Fear of embarrassment or humiliation
313.21	Avoidant disorder of childhood (0–18 yr)	Fear of embarrassment leads to avoiding unfamiliar people
300.30	Obsessive-compulsive disorder	Recurrent obsessions or compulsions
300.02	Generalized anxiety disorder	Nonstressor related lasting $\geq$ 6 mo
313.00	Overanxious disorders	Nonstressor related under 18 yr of age
309.89	Post-traumatic stress disorder	Recurring thoughts of traumatic event
309.24	Adjustment disorder with anxious mood	Stressor-induced anxiety
300.00	Anxiety disorder not otherwise specified	

PSYCHOTIC ILLNESSES AND TREATMENT

See Table 16–9 for specific drug information.

TABLE 12–2.—SCHIZOPHRENIA: SYMPTOMS AND TREATMENT

DISORDER	MAJOR SYMPTOMS	TREATMENT PLAN
Schizophrenia	Bizarre delusions which may or may not have persecutory or jealousy content; auditory hallucinations; incoherence; decrease in level of functioning; symptoms present for 6 months at some time in life	See individual types
Catatonic	Mutism; negativism; rigid posture in inappropriate positions; may have motor excitement	Major tranquilizer; hospitalization; structured protective environment
Disorganized	Incoherent; delusions in fragments only; affect blunted, inappropriate, or silly	Major tranquilizer; structured environment
Paranoid	Delusions which are persecutory, grandiose, or jealous; hallucinations of same 3 types	Major tranquilizer; supportive but not overly friendly environment
Undifferentiated	Prominent delusions; incoherence; tangential thinking; hallucinations; grossly disorganized; other types excluded	Major tranquilizer; structured environment; routine medical follow-up; socialization groups
Residual	Emotional blunting; social withdrawal; eccentric behavior; illogical behavior; loose associations; past history of one of above types	Major tranquilizer; routine medical care

TABLE 12–3.—ORGANIC BRAIN SYNDROME

DISEASE	MAJOR SYMPTOMS	ETIOLOGY AND TREATMENT PLAN
Organic brain syndrome	Disturbance of attention, memory, intellect, and orientation; may have delusions or hallucinations	
Delirium	Clouded state of conciousness; disorientation; memory deficit; misinterpretations; illusions or hallucinations; incoherent; increased or decreased psychomotor activity	Systemic infections; metabolic disorders, including hypoxia; postop. state; substance abuse Tranquilizers PRN for agitation; structured environment
Dementia	Decrease intellectual ability leading to decrease in level of function; memory deficit; deficit in abstract thinking; impaired judgment; aphasia; agnosia; state of consciousness clear	Primary degenerative dementia (Alzheimer's); CNS infection; brain trauma; toxic metabolic disturbances; vascular diseases; normal pressure hydrocephalus; neurologic diseases
Amnestic syndrome	Long- and short-term memory deficit; clear state of consciousness; intellectual function intact	Head trauma; hypoxia; infarction; encephalitis; thiamine deficiency; alcohol abuse
Organic delusional syndrome	Delusions; intellect normal; state of consciousness clear; features resemble schizophrenia	Drug abuse; lesion in nondominant hemisphere
Organic hallucinosis	Persistent or recurrent hallucinations; intellect normal; state of consciousness clear; features resemble schizophrenia	Hallucinogen abuse; alcohol abuse; sensory deprivation Structured, supportive, protective environment

BORDERLINE PERSONALITY

TABLE 12–4.—BORDERLINE PERSONALITY

According to criteria set forth by the American Psychiatric Association in *DSM-III*, the patient must be over age 18 and show five of the following eight features as characteristic of their current and/or long-term functioning:

Impulsivity or unpredictability in at least two areas that are potentially self-damaging: spending money, sex, gambling, substance abuse, overeating, inflicting self-harm.

A pattern of unstable and intense interpersonal relationships.

Inappropriate, intense anger or lack of control of anger (temper).

Identity disturbance described many times by metaphors ("I feel like a robot") and that may involve poor self-image or gender identity confusion.

Marked shifts of mood lasting only a few hours and rarely a few days.

Self-destructive acts like self-imitation, frequent fights, or suicide gestures.

Chronic feelings of boredom, loneliness and emptiness.

Avoids being alone because of feelings of depression.

Treatment must be individualized but the cornerstone is surely patience, support, and limits. Psychotherapy must be weekly for about 2 years. Medications, though not useful for the long term, may be needed to control temporary crises.

State	Drug or Class
Emotional lability	Lithium carbonate
Anxiety states	Benzodiazepines
Psychotic episodes	Phenothiazines

ALCOHOLISM AND DETOXIFICATIONS

TABLE 12–5.—ALCOHOLISM

Scope of problem: Alcoholism is one of the leading causes of death and disability. It is certainly the nation's number one drug problem. Early recognition and treatment are important.

Presenting complaints and historical features that may be related to alcoholism:

Gastrointestinal bleeding
Recent auto accident
Unusual trauma or fracture
Blackouts with drinking
Abdominal pain
Hypertension
Heart disease
Sexual dysfunction
Amenorrhea

Weight loss
Family history of alcoholism
Seizures (especially a first seizure as an adult)
Insomnia
Anxiety
Depression
Marital discord
Legal problems
Job performance difficulties
Spouse's/other's complaints about drinking
Driving while intoxicated or an arrest record

TABLE 12–6.—PHYSICAL EXAMINATION FEATURES POSSIBLY
RELATED TO ALCOHOLISM*

Odor of alcohol on breath	Hepatomegaly
Anxiety	Splenomegaly
Depression	Testicular atrophy
Decreased level of consciousness	Cigarette burns
Tremors	Parotid gland enlargement
Hallucinosis	Hypertension
Spider nevus or angioma	Gynecomastia
Abdominal tenderness	Unexplained bruises

*From Scherger WE, Zachrich RL: *Med Times* August 1983, pp 30–
35. Reproduced by permission.

TABLE 12–7.—ALCOHOLISM SCREENING TESTS

A. Short Michigan Alcoholism Screening Test (SMAST)

	Yes	No
1. Do you feel you are a normal drinker? (By normal we mean do you drink less than or as much as most other people.)	(0 point)	(1 point)
2. Do others who are important to you ever worry or complain about your drinking?	(1 point)	(0 point)
3. Do you ever feel bad about your drinking?	(1 point)	(0 point)
4. Do friends or relatives think you are a normal drinker?	(0 point)	(1 point)
5. Are you always able to stop drinking when you want to?	(0 point)	(1 point)
6. Have you ever attended a meeting of Alcoholics Anonymous (AA) for yourself?	(3 points)	(0 point)
7. Has your drinking ever created problems between you and others who are important to you?	(1 point)	(0 point)

Continued.

TABLE 12–7.—Continued

8. Have you ever gotten into trouble at work because of your drinking?	(1 point)	(0 point)
9. Have you ever neglected your obligations, your family, or your work for two or more days in a row because you were drinking?	(1 point)	(0 point)
10. Have you ever gone to anyone for help about your drinking?	(3 points)	(0 point)
11. Have you ever been in a hospital because of your drinking?	(3 points)	(0 point)
12. Have you ever been arrested for drunken driving, driving while intoxicated, or driving under the influence of alcoholic beverages?	(1 point)	(0 point)
13. Have you ever been arrested, even for a few hours, because of other drunken behavior?	(1 point)	(0 point)

Scoring System
0–1 point—Normal
2 points—Possibly alcoholic
3 or more points—Probably alcoholic

B. C.A.G.E. Survey
   Are you . . .
   C utting down or feel the need to?
   A nnoyed when people criticize your drinking?
   G uilty about your drinking?
   E ye-opening with a drink in the morning?
   If yes to any question there is high probability of alcoholism.

TABLE 12–8.—ALCOHOL DETOXIFICATION ORDERS

Obtain current drinking history with emphasis on prior withdrawal experience; inquire specifically about other drug use (tranquilizers, sedatives, etc.) in addition to alcohol.
   Regular diet; between meal feeding as needed
   Up ad lib, with help first 24 hr
   Vital signs q4h
   Pajamas or hospital gown first 72 hr
   MOM 30 cc PO PRN
   Liquid antacid, 30 cc PO PRN
   Unless specified otherwise, the following medications:
      Gatorade with fructose, 0.5 gm/kg body weight on admission
      Multivitamin tablets, 1 PO b.i.d.
      $MgSo_4$, 2 cc of 50% solution IM
      Thiamine HCl, 50 mg IM
      ASA, 650 mg, or Tylenol, 650 mg

On admission the following lab tests: CBC with platelets, SMA 6/60 and 12/60, SGPT, GGT, PT, PTT, serum magnesium, folic acid, RPR, urinalysis, blood alcohol
PA and lateral chest X-rays and ECG
Detoxification regimen:
    Prophylaxis of delirium tremens:
        Diazepam (Valium) 10–20 mg q6h, or
        Chlordiazepoxide (Librium), 50–100 mg q6h
        If patient is already in detoxification, you may want to alternate these benzodiazepines with 30 mg of phenobarbital
        For imminent delirium tremens (which usually occurs 48–72 hr after blood pressure, pulse, and respirations increase): pentobarbital, 100–200 mg IM hourly until asleep or nystagmus and slurred speech

HOSTILE PATIENT

TABLE 12–9.—THE HOSTILE PATIENT

Patients may become hostile for a variety of reasons, including a long wait, offensive office personnel, failure to get better, etc. Two hostile persons cannot solve a problem. You will need to be the calm peacemaker despite your tendency to defend yourself, your practice, and your office staff. Confrontation can lead the patient to think in medicolegal terms and will leave everyone uneasy. Try to clarify the issues and then discuss alternative solutions.

If a patient is hostile and exhibiting psychotic symptoms you may need to request police help. Remember not to antagonize the patient. Offering a shot to help the patient relax and feel better may allow you the opportunity to administer a major tranquilizer.

Generally, state law permits involuntary hospitalization when the patient is either dangerous to himself or to others (including you). The police are often well versed in this procedure.

Rapid sedation may be achieved with one of the following drugs:

Drug	Dose	Time Interval	Total 24-hr Dose
Haloperidol (Haldol)	2.5–10 mg IM	q 30–60 min	100 mg
Chlorpromazine (Thorazine)	25–50 mg IM	q 60 min	75 mg (except for extremely unmanageable patients)

RELAXATION THERAPY

TABLE 12–10.—RELAXATION THERAPY

Relaxation therapy can be used to relieve stress and tension in some patients. It can be done in 5–10 minutes in the office and repeated by the patient several times a day. It is best introduced in a quiet uninterrupted atmosphere with the patient in a comfortable position. The patient should understand that he is not being hypnotized and will remain in control of his body. You will need to speak in a soft soothing monotone and continue talking until the therapy ends. You can use your own script or this sample: "You are going to relax to the best of your ability. Please close your eyes. As you relax you will feel tension leave your body, to be replaced by a calm soothing sensation. I want you to think of a pleasant landscape scene and see yourself relaxing there. Already you can feel your tense muscles relax. You may feel sleepy as relaxation takes over your body. With each breath you become more relaxed. Breathe in relaxation and exhale tension. Breathe in relaxation and exhale tension. With each breath you relax. Breathe in relaxation and breathe out all tension. Feel your arms and legs relax as we count to ten. 1 . . . 2 . . . 3 . . . 4 . . . 5 . . . 6 . . . 7 . . . 8 . . . 9 . . . 10. [You may ad lib here and discuss each area of the body.] Now feel how calm you are becoming and see yourself resting in that pleasant landscape scene. Every part of your body is relaxing now, your arms, your legs, your feet, your back, and your scalp. Breathe in relaxation and exhale tension. Now as we count backwards from 10 to 1 you will become more alert and more rested. 10 . . . 9 . . . 8 . . . 7 . . . 6 . . . 5 . . . . Breathe in relaxation and exhale tension. At zero you will be alert and well rested . . . 4 . . . 3 . . . 2 . . . 1 . . . 0 . . . . Open your eyes and feel how relaxed you are."

COUNSELING TECHNIQUES

TABLE 12–11.—COUNSELING THE FAMILY OR INDIVIDUAL*

COUNSELING FORMAT
Outline of counseling session
    Build a therapeutic relationship
    Assess the problem:
        Let each member describe the problem.
        Reflect the problem to make sure you understand it.
        Ask each member how it affects him/her.
        Allow ventilation and give support.
    Problem solve:
        How has it been dealt with in past?
        What can be done to change problem?
    Form a treatment plan
    Summarize the session: first the patient, then the counselor
COUNSELING TECHNIQUES
Engaging the family
    The process of beginning a trusting relationship is more difficult with the family than with an individual. Some guidelines are to talk to all members,

beginning the session by addressing each member with polite social questions. It is usually best to not address the patient first, particularly if it is a child. Make an attempt to pull in the member who seems the most reserved. Recognize the member whose opinion is valued—there probably is one—and make a point to honor this authority. Adopt the family's style of conversation so that everyone is at ease.

Initiating discussion of the problem

Open the discussion by asking a family member (other than the patient) how it came about that you are meeting today. Another approach is to ask what it is like being in this family these days. You may want to address this question to the youngest member since he/she is likely to be totally honest. When dealing with a child problem, it is best to ask the parent what problems the family needs to work on. Even though one member may have already given you details of the problem, it is better to let someone repeat it in front of the whole group. In supportive counseling sessions, such as grief, you may be the one to summarize the situation.

Structuring the session

The family or individual must perceive you as able to lead the session to feel secure enough to talk about painful material. There may be a struggle for control and leadership. You must win this struggle to be an effective counselor. Doherty and Baird suggest six core family counseling rules:

Each person has the right to speak without being interrupted.

When you have announced a procedure or plan of action, do not become sidetracked, e.g., if you say you want to hear everyone's opinion, do not let an argument interrupt that plan.

Steer the family back to the issues at hand when they stray.

Resist requests for solutions if requests seem premature or inappropriate, e.g., "I think the solution will come from you as a family. I will have ideas to help you."

Take charge of the physical arrangement of the session. Observe the seats they choose. Rearrange when needed. A circle is often good.

Take charge of who attends the session, make sure everyone knows who is expected to come to each meeting and insist that they be there.

Defining the problem

You may wish to define the problem by asking each member how he/she would like to see this relationship change. "What changes would you like to see?" You should encourage these to be specific, concrete, and positive.

History taking

This should occupy less than a third of the initial interview. The two most basic pieces of information are the onset of the problem, and how the family or person has attempted to cope with it.

Remaining neutral

To avoid casting family members in roles, you must believe that there are no villains or victims. Your support must be seen as distributed equally among the group.

Encouraging a collaborative set

Encourage the family to work on the problem together. Explain that they got to the problem together and now must pull together to get out.

Facilitate family discussion

Encourage the family to talk directly to one another during the session. They may resist and say that they feel silly, etc. If you have asked them to

Continued.

TABLE 12–11.—Continued

speak directly to each other, insist on it and don't back down. There are three good opportunities for this direct communication:
When a joint decision is being reached.
When a positive comment about a member is made to you, respond with "Why don't you *ask/tell* her that now."
If a member says another member will not listen, ask him if he will listen.
Generally, communications must be practiced in the session before being used by the family. Give support when dealing with stress, grief, or dislocation. To be an effective counselor you must provide support, and to do that you must genuinely want to support them. Here are five guidelines:
Listen, let people express their feelings.
Let them know that you are with them emotionally by reflecting the emotion you hear them expressing, e.g., "You still miss him a lot."
Do not move ahead of the family emotionally by promising that they will feel better soon or that it may not be as bad as they think.
Mobilize support systems for the family or individual.
Teach when you can clarify a situation. The art is to teach when information is needed and back out when the family processes that information.
Challenge the family
It is often best to let a member challenge the group. When a challenge is made a treatment plan should be in place.
Dealing with resistance
The two most common primary care counseling forms of resistance are tardiness or absenteeism and arguing with you. Schedule problems should be addressed to see if there is a hidden meaning in the tardiness. If not, you may want to confront them by saying "My time is important to me, and I would like you to respect it." If a member wants to argue with you, ask that he/she simply think about what you have said, or encourage him/her to describe how he/she sees the issues and how he/she would like to change things. You may gain valuable information by following their lead. Don't work hard to persuade the family that you are right, maybe you aren't.
MAKING BEHAVIORAL CONTRACTS
You should encourage all members to identify clearly the specific, concrete changes they are willing to make. This must be done in a cooperative, non-hostile group mood. Members must be willing to make the changes in good faith so that the others will make their changes. The family should plan to evaluate the contract to see if it is working.
AFTER-SESSION ASSIGNMENTS
It may be useful to follow through on some issues that arise during the session. For example, if sharing household tasks is an issue, you might help the family make specific assignments for the week. If the parents want to spend more time together, let them make specific plans for an event that week. Follow up on these assignments. Failure to follow through would be an important family dynamic to address.

*Adapted from Doherty WJ, Baird MA: *Family Therapy and Family Medicine*. New York, Guilford Press, 1983.

13 *Surgery*

Charles W. Smith, Jr., M.D.

SUTURES AND LACERATIONS

TABLE 13–1.—GUIDELINES FOR
SUTURE REMOVAL

SITE	NO. OF DAYS
Eyelid	3
Other head and neck	4–6
Extremities and trunk	7
Back and feet	10–14

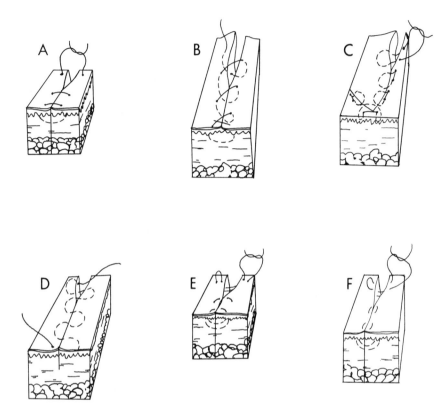

Fig 13–1.
Technique for suturing epidermis. Any of the techniques illustrated are acceptable. **A,** simple interrupted suture, good for irregular wounds. **B,** simple running suture, only for linear wounds (tends to invert), quick to do. **C,** half-buried mattress suture, good for flaps. **D,** subcuticular suture, good results (leaves no skin marks). **E,** vertical mattress suture, good for thick and thin skin (e.g., scalp, eyelid), good eversion. **F,** horizontal mattress suture, looks bad early but achieves good eversion later; must be applied loosely. (From Stuzin JM, Engrav LH, Buehler PK: *Postgrad Med* 1982; 71:81. Reproduced by permission.)

TABLE 13–2.—TYPES OF SUTURE MATERIAL*

MATERIAL	COMPOSITION	INDICATIONS FOR USE	COMMENTS
Absorbable			
Plain catgut	Sheep intestine connective tissue	Small blood vessels and subcutaneous fat	Causes marked inflammatory reaction in 1 wk
Chromic	Same, impregnated with chromic oxide	Same, especially if longer approximation is needed (e.g., bowel closure)	Causes less tissue reaction than catgut
Dexxon	Polyglycolic acid	Has almost replaced catgut	Less tissue reaction, lasts about 6 wk, stronger
Non-absorbable			
Silk	Silk	Artery ligation; use in infected fields	Strong, easy to use, low tissue reactivity
Cotton	Cotton	Same as silk	Not as strong as silk; maintains itself better in tissue than silk
Synthetic	Nylon Dacron Polypropylene	Internal surgery, when ease of use not critical; skin closure	Strong, low tissue reaction, somewhat hard to tie
Wire	Stainless steel wire	Closing abdomen and chest	Least tissue reactivity, very strong; hard to tie

*Adapted from McCredie JA, Burns GP: Operating room management, in McCredie J (ed): *Basic Surgery.* New York, Macmillan Publishing Co, 1977, pp 236–237.

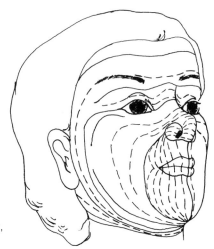

FIG 13–2.
Facial skin lines. (From Riley WB: Wound healing and problem scars, in Barrett BM (ed): *Manual of Patient Care in Plastic Surgery.* Boston, Little, Brown & Co, 1982, p 132. Reproduced by permission.)

TABLE 13–3.—TETANUS PROPHYLAXIS*

PATIENT	TETANUS-PRONE WOUND	NON-TETANUS-PRONE WOUND
Immunized patient, last toxoid <10 yr ago	0.5 cc of toxoid	None
Immunized, last toxoid >10 yr ago	0.5 cc of toxoid	0.5 cc of toxoid
Nonimmunized (or immunization history unknown)	0.5 cc of toxoid + 250 units of human tetanus antitoxin, then repeat toxoid in 6 wk and in 6 mo. to 1 yr	0.5 cc of toxoid; repeat in 6 wk and in 6 mo. to 1 yr

*Adapted from Litwin MS: Trauma: Management of the acutely injured patient, in Sabiston DC (ed): *Davis-Christopher Textbook of Surgery,* ed 12. Philadelphia, WB Saunders Co, 1981, p 417.

BURNS

TABLE 13-4.—DEPTH OF BURN INJURY*

DEPTH OF CLASSIFICATION	STRUCTURAL DAMAGE	CAUSAL AGENT	CLINICAL APPEARANCE	SENSATION
First-degree	Only superficial layers of epidermis devitalized; dilation of intradermal vessels	Ultraviolet exposure Very short flash	Erythema; blanches with pressure	Present
Second-degree (partial-thickness)	Destruction of epidermis to basal layer; deeper skin appendages preserved in dermal layer; clefting of epidermis with fluid collection	Spillage of scalding material Flash Some chemicals	Blister formation, erythema, weeping; superficial skin can be wiped away; erythematous areas should blanch with pressure	Present
Third-degree (full-thickness)	Destruction of all skin elements, epidermal and dermal; coagulation of subdermal blood vessels	Flame Immersion Some chemicals	Dry, pale white, charred, leathery, inelastic, visible thrombosed vessels; sometimes red from fixed hemoglobin and will not blanch	Absent
Fourth-degree (involvement of muscle, bone, and other deep structures)	Destruction of all skin elements along with necrosis of deeper structures	Electricity Flame occasionally	Deeply charred, shrunken, often with exposed bones; explosive appearing	Absent

*From Lewis ML: Thermal injuries, in Wilkins EW (ed): *MGH Textbook of Emergency Medicine*. Baltimore, Williams & Wilkins Co, 1983, p 626. Reproduced by permission.

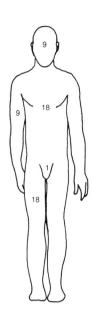

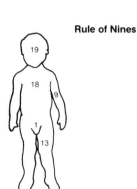

	Child	Adult
Head	19%	9%
Arms	9%	9%
Front Torso	18%	18%
Back Torso	18%	18%
Genitals	1%	1%
Legs	13%	18%
	100%	**100%**

Rule of Nines

FIG 13–3.
The rule-of-nines estimation of burned body area. (From Bass CB: Burns, in Barrett BM (ed): *Manual of Patient Care in Plastic Surgery.* Boston, Little, Brown & Co, 1982, p 292. Reproduced by permission.)

TABLE 13–5.—BURN TREATMENT

CRITERIA FOR HOSPITALIZING BURN PATIENTS
   Second-degree burns of more than 30% body surface area.
   Third-degree burn of face, hands, feet.
   Third-degree burn of more than 10% body surface area.
   Significant respiratory injury suspected.
   All electrical burns.
   Suspected child abuse.
FLUID REPLACEMENT IN BURN PATIENTS*
   First 24 hours: lactated Ringer's solution:
      4 cc × weight (kg) × % burn (total body surface area).
      Give ½ in first 8 hours; ¼ in 2nd 8 hours; remaining ¼ in 3rd 8 hours.
   24–48 hours:
      Decrease total amount by half.
      Add colloid (plasmanate or albumin, 7–8 cc/kg) to maintain plasma
         volume.
   48 hours to 10 days:
      Add oral liquids, advance as soon as possible to high-protein, high-calorie
         diet.
      Give additional colloid as needed.
      PRBCs to keep hematocrit >30%.

OUTPATIENT BURN MANAGEMENT[†]
Treat pain with appropriate dose of narcotic.
Apply cool compresses to burn or place in cool water.
Cleanse area with povidone-iodine solution.
Give appropriate tetanus prophylaxis.
Leave blisters intact (if large, evacuate aseptically and leave skin intact).
Cover burn with vaseline gauze, then a bulky dressing.
Wrap area with Kerlix or Kling dressing.
Change dressing every 3 days.
Debride all devitalized tissue every dressing change.
Continue until healing is complete.

  *Adapted from Bass CB: Burns, in Barrett BM (ed): *Manual of Patient Care in Plastic Surgery.* Boston, Little, Brown & Co, 1982, pp 296–297.
  [†]Adapted from Bass CB: Burns, in Barrett BM (ed): *Manual of Patient Care in Plastic Surgery.* Boston, Little, Brown & Co, 1982, p 313.

ASSESSMENT OF SURGICAL RISK

TABLE 13–6.—AMERICAN BOARD
OF ANESTHESIOLOGY CLASSIFICATION
OF PREOPERATIVE RISK*

CLASS	DESCRIPTION
I	No known risk
II	Mild to moderate disease (e.g., well-controlled diabetes)
III	Severe disease present (e.g., complicated diabetic)
IV	Life-threatening disease (e.g., severe angina)
V	Patient moribund (e.g., ruptured aortic aneurysm)

  *Adapted from Deutsch S: Anesthesia, in Papper S, Williams GR (eds): *Manual of Medical Care of the Surgical Patient,* ed 2, Boston, Little, Brown & Co, 1981.

TABLE 13–7.—PREOPERATIVE EVALUATION (FOR NONCARDIAC SURGERY)*

Obtain careful history and physical exam with focus on cardiac and respiratory.
Chest x-ray and ECG, urinalysis, BUN, creatinine.
If question of angina or if patient has several cardiac risk factors, perform graded exercise tolerance test.
Phonocardiogram if murmur or heart sounds are hard to characterize.
Echocardiogram if question of valvular heart disease.
Thallium scan (with exercise test) if ECG uninterpretable and in women suspected of having coronary disease.

Continued.

TABLE 13–7.—Continued

Gated pool scan if question of congestive heart failure not otherwise detectable.
Cardiac catherization if cerebral or major arterial surgery is planned in a patient with a history of significant coronary disease.
Maximize present cardiac function (i.e., blood pressure, rhythm, angina, and blood volume).
Arterial blood gas and spirometry if any history of pulmonary disease or in elderly patient.
IVP if surgery involves periureteral areas.

*Adapted from Deutsch S: Anesthesia, in Papper S, Williams GR (eds): *Manual of Medical Care of the Surgical Patient,* ed 2. Boston, Little, Brown & Co, 1981.

TABLE 13–8.—Weighting of Cardiac Risk Factors
for Noncardiac Surgery*

CRITERIA	POINTS[†]
Historical	
Age over 70 years	5
Myocardial infarction in previous 6 months	10
Examination	
S_3 gallop/jugular venous distention	11
Significant aortic valvular stenosis	3
ECG	
Premature atrial contractions or rhythm other than sinus	7
More than 5 premature ventricular contractions/min	7
General status	
Abnormal blood gases	3
K^+/HCO_3 abnormalities	3
Abnormal renal function	3
Liver disease/bedridden	3
Operation	
Emergency	4
Intraperitoneal/intrathoracic/aortic	3
Total possible	53

POINT TOTAL	LIFE-THREATENING COMPLICATIONS (%)	CARDIAC DEATHS (%)
0–5	0.7	0.2
6–12	5	2
13–25	11	2
26	22	56

*Adapted from Goldman L, Caldera DL, Nussbaum SR, et al: *N Engl J Med* 1977; 297:845.
[†]Use point total to estimate risk of complications, below.

TABLE 13–9.—DRUGS ASSOCIATED WITH PERIANESTHETIC PROBLEMS*

DRUG TYPE	EXAMPLES	PERIANESTHETIC PROBLEMS
Tricyclic antidepressants	Amitriptyline (Elavil) Desipramine (Pertofrane) Doxepin (Sinequan) Imipramine (Tofranil) Nortriptyline (Aventyl) Protriptyline (Vivactil)	Cardiovascular instability Tachycardia (anticholinergic effect) Orthostatic hypotension (central inhibition of vasomotor control; peripheral decrease in sympathetic tone) Dysrhythmia, if epinephrine is used
Monoamine oxidase inhibitors (MAOIs)	Isocarboxazid (Marplan) Nialamide (Niamid) Pargyline (Eutonyl) Phenelzine (Nardil)	Orthostatic hypotension (reduced release of sympathetic transmitter, false transmitter production)
Phenothiazines	Chlorpromazine (Thorazine) Fluphenazine (Permitil) Prochlorperazine (Compazine) Promazine (Sparine) Triflupromazine (Vesprin) Others	Orthostatic hypotension (peripheral α-sympathetic block) Dystonic syndrome Parkinson-like disorder
Antihypertensives	Methyldopa (Aldomet) Reserpine and related compounds Propranolol (see Beta blockers)	Cardiovascular instability secondary to essential hypotension
Diuretics	Chlorothiazide (Diuril) Hydrochlorothiazide (Esidrix, Hydrodiuril)	Hypokalemia Cardiac arrhythmias
Antidysrhythmic drugs	Quinidine (see also entries for propranolol and digitalis) Disopyramide (Norpace) Bretylium (Bretylol)	Dysrhythmias Muscle weakness Hypotension

Continued.

TABLE 13–9.—Continued

DRUG TYPE	EXAMPLES	PERIANESTHETIC PROBLEMS
Lithium carbonate		Prolonged action of both classes of neuromuscular blockers Cardiac arrhythmias
Antiparkinson drugs	L-dopa (Bendopa, Dopar, Larodopa) L-dopa/carbidopa (Sinemet)	Arrhythmias Orthostatic hypotension Chest wall rigidity
β-Blockers	Propranolol (Inderal) Pindolol (Visken)	Acute heart failure (decreased contractility) Bronchoconstriction Abrupt withdrawal may precipitate arrhythmia, angina, or infarction
Digitalis	Digoxin (Lanoxin) Many other preparations	Congestive failure Arrhythmias
Coronary vasodilators	Nitroglycerin tablets Amyl nitrate Isosorbide (Isordil) PETT (Peritrate) Nitroglycerin ointment (Nitro Bid, Nitrol)	Orthostatic hypotension Methemoglobinemia
Organophosphates	Echothiophate (Phospholine) Isoflurophate (Floropryl)	Prolonged apnea
Adrenal steroids	Hydrocortisone Prednisone Prednisolone Dexamethasone	Adrenal cortex suppression (unsuspected and unexplained hypotension)

*Adapted from Brunner EA, Eckenhoff JE: Anesthesia, in Sabiston DC (ed): *Davis-Christopher Textbook of Surgery*, ed 12. Philadelphia, WB Saunders Co, 1981, pp 210–212.

TABLE 13–10.—Cardiac Morbidity and Mortality due to Anesthesia and Surgery*

CARDIAC RISK CLASS[†]	CARDIAC DEATH RATE (%)	SERIOUS CARDIAC COMPLICATIONS (%)	WITHOUT SERIOUS COMPLICATIONS (%)
I	0.2	0.7	99
II	2.0	5.0	93
III	2.0	11.0	86
IV	56.0	22.0	22

*From Brunner EA, Eckenhoff JE: Anesthesia, in Sabiston DC (ed): *Davis-Christopher Textbook of Surgery,* ed 12. Philadelphia, WB Saunders Co, 1981, p 213. Reproduced by permission.
†Classification of cardiac risk:
I = healthy patient
II = slightly compromised (e.g., dyspnea on moderate exertion)
III = moderately compromised (e.g., dyspnea on mild exertion)
IV = severely compromised (e.g., dyspnea at rest)

LOCAL ANESTHESIA

TABLE 13–11.—COMMONLY USED LOCAL ANESTHETIC AGENTS*

TECHNIQUE	LOCAL ANESTHETIC	CONCENTRATION RANGE	DURATION OF ACTION	MAXIMAL SAFE DOSE
Topical anesthesia (mucous membranes)	Lidocaine	2–4%	15 min	100 mg
	Cocaine	4–10%	30 min	100–200 mg
	Tetracaine	1–2%	45 min	40 mg
	Benzocaine	2–10%	Several hr	—
Local infiltration	Procaine	0.5%	¼–½ hr	1000 mg
	Lidocaine	0.5–1%	½–1 hr	500 mg
	Mepivacaine	0.5–1%	½–1 hr	500 mg
	Tetracaine	0.025–0.1%	2–3 hr	75 mg
Major nerve block	Lidocaine	1–2%	1–2 hr	500 mg
	Mepivacaine	1–2%	1–2¼	500 mg
	Tetracaine	0.1– 0.25%	2–3 hr	75 mg
Epidural anesthesia	Procaine	1–2%	½–1 hr	1000 mg
	Lidocaine	1–2%	¾–1½ hr	500 mg
	Mepivacaine	1–2%	1–2¼ hr	500 mg
	Tetracaine	0.1– 0.25%	2–3 hr	75 mg
	Bupivacaine	0.25– 0.75%	2–4 hr	150 mg
Spinal anesthesia	Procaine	5%	½–1 hr	—
	Lidocaine	5%	¾–1½ hr	—
	Tetracaine	0.5%	1–2 hr	—
Intravenous regional anesthesia	Lidocaine	0.25–0.5%	Varies	100–150 mg

*From Brunner EA, Eckenhoff JE: Anesthesia, in Sabiston DC (ed): *Davis-Christopher Textbook of Surgery*, ed 12. Philadelphia, WB Saunders Co, 1981, p 197. Reproduced by permission.

PREOPERATIVE AND POSTOPERATIVE ORDERS

TABLE 13–12.—PREOPERATIVE AND POSTOPERATIVE ORDERS

ROUTINE PREOPERATIVE ORDERS
1. NPO (nothing by mouth) after midnight.
2. Bath before bedtime (head to toe, including shampoo).
3. Enema (may forego if patient can spontaneously evacuate).
4. Have patient void before leaving for operating room (alternatively, place Foley catheter).
5. Sedation (e.g., 15–30 mg of flurazepam or temazepam).
6. Change all PO medications to IV or IM.
7. Give preoperative medication (e.g., Demerol 75 mg, Phenergan 25 mg, and atropine 0.4 mg IM 30 minutes before surgery).
8. Bowel prep and IV fluids as appropriate.

ROUTINE POSTOPERATIVE ORDERS
1. Operation (state nature of procedure).
2. Vital signs (every 30 minutes for a few hours, then reduce as appropriate).
3. Diet (usually NPO until bowel sounds are present, then progress from clear to full liquids and solids as tolerated).
4. Activity (usually bed rest for 12–24 hours, then up with assistance and progress as appropriate).
5. Pain control (morphine 5–8 mg or Demerol 50–75 mg IM every 2–3 hours initially; change to oral, e.g., codeine or propoxyphene, as appropriate).
6. Antiemetics (e.g., Compazine 25 mg IM every 4–6 hours for postanesthetic nausea).
7. Respiratory (turn, cough, and deep breaths every 3–4 hours; add incentive spirometry, IPPB and/or mucolytic agents as indicated).
8. IV fluids as indicated.
9. Care of drains and tubes as indicated.
10. Continuation of prior medication as indicated.
11. Look for; notify surgeon if:
    Unstable vital signs (set limits).
    Unusual drainage on dressings or from tubes.
    Inability to void (set time limit).
    Other problem as appropriate.

TRAUMA

TABLE 13–13.—EVALUATION AND TREATMENT OF THE TRAUMA PATIENT*

Airway
Use nasotracheal, endotracheal, tracheostomy, or oral airway as indicated.
Assess arterial blood gases.
Assess chest wall stability.
Give O_2 at 2 L/min.
Vital signs
Monitor pulse, BP, and respirations every 10–15 minutes and record.
Insert nasogastric tube and Foley catheter; record intake and output.
Cardiovascular system
Start-16 gauge or larger IV line.
Give Ringer's lactate to keep urine output $\geq$ 30 cc/hr.
Apply MAST trousers and inflate if BP <80 mm Hg systolic.
Check all peripheral pulses.
Place on cardiac monitor.
Obtain chest x-ray.
Neurologic system
Assess level of consciousness and motor and sensory function.
If unconscious, treat as if patient had cervical spine injury.
If neck or head injury, obtain cervical spine x-ray.
Abdomen
Assess for tenderness, guarding, or rebound.
If patient is unconscious, peritoneal tap is indicated.
If hematuria is present, obtain IVP and cystogram.
Musculoskeletal
Splint fractures.
Clean wounds with saline; apply pressure dressings.
Other
Labs
Obtain CBC, coagulation profile, BUN, glucose,
type and hold, and urinalysis.
Arrange transfer as indicated
Send copies of all records.
History must be "ample."
A = allergies noted.
M = Medications and therapy given.
P = Past history.
L = Last meal.
E = Events leading to injury.

*Adapted from University of Iowa Hospitals and Clinics Emergency Treatment Protocols.

TABLE 13-14.—Glasgow Coma Scale

Evaluate and plot periodically to follow comatose patient. An initial score of ≥7 points indicates a poor prognosis in the trauma patient.

I. Best verbal response:

No response	1 point
Speech incomprehensible	2 points
Inappropriate speech	3 points
Confused speech	4 points
Oriented	5 points

II. Eye opening

Not open	1 point
Opens in response to pain	2 points
Response to speech	3 points
Spontaneous	4 points

III. Best motor response

No response	1 point
Extensor response	2 points
Abnormal flexion	3 points
Withdrawal	4 points
Localizes	5 points
Obeys commands	6 points

BREAST MASSES AND BREAST CANCER

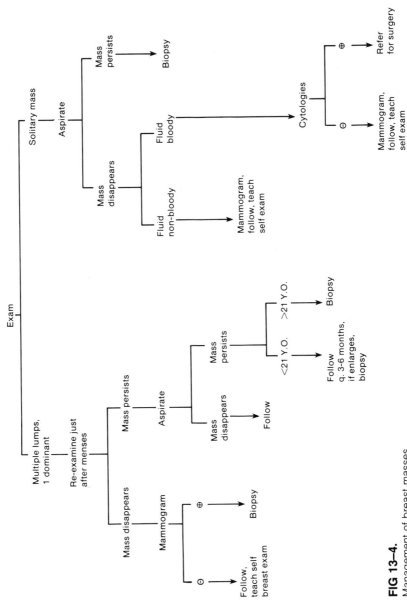

FIG 13–4.
Management of breast masses.

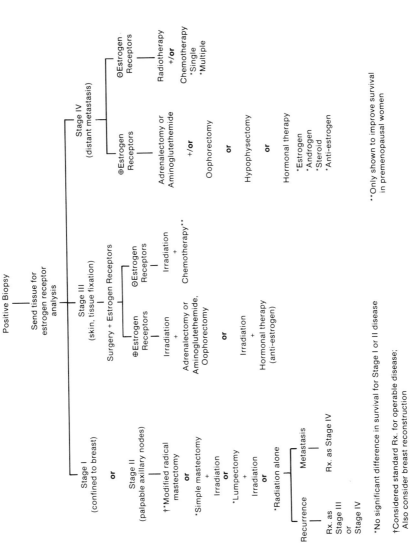

FIG 13–5.
Management of breast cancer.

INTESTINAL OBSTRUCTION AND ABDOMINAL PAIN

TABLE 13–15.—DIFFERENTIATING PARALYTIC ILEUS
FROM INTESTINAL OBSTRUCTION*

ASPECT	PARALYTIC ILEUS	MECHANICAL OBSTRUCTION
Symptoms		
Pain	Diffuse, mild aching pain, bloating sensation	Cramping, often severe, mid to lower abdominal pain
Vomiting	Occasional, mild vomiting episodes	Bilious or feculent vomiting
Physical signs		
Distention	Early marked distention, persistent	Moderate distention, worsens over time
Bowel sounds	Decreased or absent bowel sounds	Increased bowel sounds with rushes
Tenderness	Mild, diffuse tenderness to palpation	Mild, diffuse tenderness to palpation
X-ray signs		
Stomach gas	Usually increased	Sometimes present, normal amount
Bowel gas	Marked throughout small and large bowel	Only proximal to obstruction
Fluid in Bowel	Minimal	Large amount
"Stepladder" pattern	Occasionally seen	Often seen
Air/fluid levels in loop of bowel (upright film)	Same level across midabdomen	Different levels; "J-loops" seen

*Adapted from Condon RE, Brient B: Intestinal obstruction, in Condon RE, Nyhus LM (eds): *Manual of Surgical Therapeutics,* ed 2. Boston, Little, Brown & Co, 1972.

TABLE 13–16.—DIFFERENTIAL DIAGNOSIS OF BILIARY COLIC, ACUTE CHOLECYSTITIS, AND SUPPURATIVE COMPLICATIONS OF ACUTE CHOLECYSTITIS*

SYMPTOM	BILIARY COLIC	ACUTE CHOLECYSTITIS	SUPPURATIVE COMPLICATED CHOLECYSTITIS
Pain	Crampy	Steady	Steady
Nausea	Usually present	Usually present	Usually present
Vomiting	Occasional	Often present	Often present
Onset	Usually meal-related	Occasionally meal-related	Occasionally meal-related
Fever	Absent	99°–100° F	Usually 102° F or more
WBC count	<10,000	10,000–15,000	Usually >15,000
Bilirubin	Normal	1–4 mg/100 ml	Often >4 mg/100 ml
Course	Resolves 1–4 hr	Resolves 24–48 hr	Requires surgery acutely

*Adapted from Carey LC, Ellison EC: Acute cholecystitis, in Sabiston DC (ed): *Davis-Christopher Textbook of Surgery*, ed 12. Philadelphia, WB Saunders Co, 1981, p 1265.

DECUBITUS ULCERS

TABLE 13–17.—TREATMENT OF DECUBITUS ULCERS*

STAGE	DESCRIPTION	TREATMENT
I	Erythema, edema, punctate hemorrhages, superficial blisters or blebs	Remove pressure, eliminate shear forces, gentle cleaning every 6–8 hr; topical antibiotics and fine mesh gauze; Opsite® or Duoderm® is a good alternative
II	Full-thickness skin loss; erythematous halo; defects <3 cm	Consider excision and primary closure
III	Same as II, but defects >3 cm	Eliminate pressure, debride devitalized tissue; wet to dry dressings q6h until wound ready to graft, then use split-thickness skin graft
IV	Crater base with yellow-gray eschar; pus exudes from periphery surrounding red halo	Debride, in stages if needed; pack wound with damp gauze, covered with dry gauze at skin surface, q6h to q8h; graft with full-thickness graft after 2–3 wk
V	Cone-shaped defect; small skin opening with undermining and cavern formation	Extend wound and debride as above; treatment same as for stage IV
VI	Chronic ulcerative defect; often present months or years; bone often visible	Hospitalization; attention to nutrition, patient positioning; usually requires skin flap surgery

*Adapted from Agris J: Pressure ulcers, in Barrett BM (ed): *Manual of Patient Care in Plastic Surgery.* Boston, Little, Brown & Co, 1982, pp 347–363.

THYROID NODULES

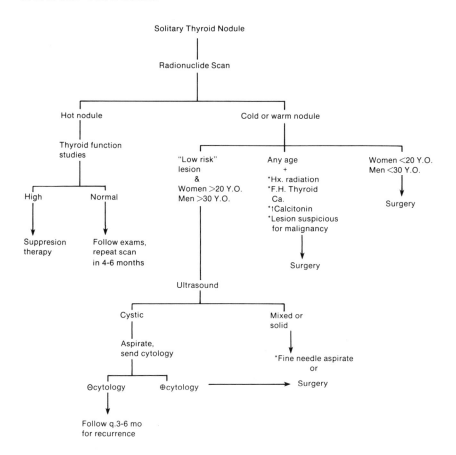

FIG 13–6.
Management of thyroid nodules.

TABLE 13–18.—Prevention of Wound Infection and Sepsis in Surgical Patients*

NATURE OF OPERATION	LIKELY PATHOGENS	RECOMMENDED DRUGS	ADULT DOSAGE BEFORE SURGERY[†]
CLEAN			
Cardiovascular			
Prosthetic valve and other open-heart surgery	*Staphylococcus epidermidis, S. aureus, Corynebacterium* sp., enteric gram-negative bacilli	Cefazolin *or* vancomycin[‡]	1 gm IV 1 gm IV
Arterial surgery involving the abdominal aorta, a prosthesis, or a groin incision	*S. aureus, S. epidermidis,* enteric gram-negative bacilli	Cefazolin *or* vancomycin[‡]	1 gm IM/IV 1 gm IV
Lower extremity amputation for ischemia	*S. aureus, S. epidermidis,* enteric gram-negative bacilli, anaerobes	Cefoxitin	1 gm IV
Orthopedic			
Total joint replacement, internal fixation of fractures	*S. aureus, S. epidermidis*	Cefazolin *or* vancomycin[‡]	1 gm IM/IV 1 gm IV
CLEAN-CONTAMINATED			
Head and neck Entering oral cavity or pharynx	*S. Aureus,* streptococci, oral anaerobes	Cefazolin	1 gm IM/IV
Gastroduodenal	Enteric gram-negative bacilli, gram-positive cocci	*High risk, gastric bypass, or percutaneous endoscopic gastrostomy only:* cefazolin *High-risk only:* cefazolin	1 gm IM/IV
Biliary tract	Enteric gram-negative bacilli, Group D strep, clostridia		1 gm IM/IV 1 gm IM/IV

	Likely Pathogens	Recommended Antimicrobials	Adult Dosage before Surgery[†]
Colorectal	Enteric gram-negative bacilli, anaerobes	*Oral:* neomycin plus erythromycin base	1 gm of each at 1 P.M., 2 P.M., and 11 P.M. the day before the operation[§]
		Parenteral: cefoxitin	1 gm IV
Appendectomy	Enteric gram-negative bacilli, anaerobes	Cefoxitin	1 gm IV
Vaginal or abdominal hysterectomy	Enteric gram-negative bacilli, anaerobes, Group B and D streptococci	Cefazolin	1 gm IM/IV
Cesarean section	Same as for hysterectomy	*High-risk only:* cefazolin	1 gm IV after cord clamping
Abortion	Same as for hysterectomy	*First trimester in patients with previous pelvic inflammatory disease:* aqueous penicillin G	1 million units IV
		Second trimester: cefazolin	1 gm IM/IV
DIRTY			
Ruptured viscus	Enteric gram-negative bacilli, anaerobes, Group D streptococci	Clindamycin plus gentamicin or tobramycin	600 mg IV q6h plus 1.5 mg/kg q8h IM/IV
		OR cefoxitin with or without gentamicin or tobramycin	1 gm q6h IV plus 1.5 mg/kg q8h IM/IV
Traumatic wound[‖]	S. aureus, Group A streptococci, clostridia	Cefazolin	1 gm q8h IM/IV

*From *Med Lett* 1987; 29:94. Reproduced by permission.

[†]Parenteral prophylactic antimicrobials for clean and clean-contaminated surgery can be given as a single dose just before the operation. For prolonged operations, additional intraoperative doses should be given q4–8h for the duration of the procedure. For dirty surgery, therapy should usually be continued for 5 to 10 days.

[‡]For hospitals in which methicillin-resistant *S. aureus* and *S. epidermidis* frequently cause wound infection, or for patients with penicillin or cephalosporin allergy.

[§]After appropriate diet and catharsis (RL Nichols in GL Mandell et al [eds]: *Principles and Practice of Infectious Diseases*, ed 2. New York, John Wiley & Sons, 1985, p 1641).

[‖]For bite wounds, in which likely pathogens may also include oral anaerobes, *Eikenella corrodens* (humans), and *Pasteurella multocida* (dogs and cats), some *Medical Letter* consultants recommend use of amoxicillin-clavulanic acid (Augmentin) or ampicillin/sulbactam (Unasyn).

14 *Pediatrics*

Edward T. Bope, M.D.

IMMUNIZATIONS

TABLE 14–1.—Immunizations: General Principles

It is more important that every child receive every immunization than that a rigid schedule is followed. Absolute contraindications to immunizations are:
Immune deficiency in child or family member
γ-Globulin within 3 months
Relative contraindications to immunizations are:
A febrile illness
Febrile convulsions or neurologic disorders
If a scheduled dose of DPT or TOPV is missed, it is not necessary to repeat the series, no matter how long the interval.
Premature infants can be started on immunizations when they weigh > 10 lb.
Live virus vaccines, e.g., TOPV and MMR, should be given 1 mo. apart.

TABLE 14–2.—Recommended Schedule for Active Immunization of Infants and Children

AGE	IMMUNIZATION
2 mo.	Diptheria-tetanus-pertussis (DTP) #1, trivalent oral polio (TOPV) #1
4 mo.	DTP and TOPV #2
6 mo.	DTP #3
12 mo.	Hematocrit and tuberculin PPD tine
15 mo.	Measles-mumps-rubella (MMR), DTP #4, OPV #3
18 mo.	*Hemophilus* B conjugate vaccine
5 yr	Diphtheria-tetanus pediatric type (DT), TOPV #4, MMR #2
>5 yr, every 10 yr	Diphtheria-tetanus adult type (Td)

TABLE 14–3.—IMMUNIZATION SCHEDULE FOR CHILDREN WHO DID NOT START IMMUNIZATIONS IN EARLY INFANCY*

TIME LINE	GENERAL SCHEDULE	MEASLES IN COMMUNITY	RAPID DPT	POOR COMPLIANCE AT 15 MO.
First visit	DPT #1 TOPV #1 PPD	MMR PPD	DPT #1 TOPV #1 PPD	DPT #1 TOPV #1 MMR PPD
1 mo.	MMR (insert in schedule at 15 mo.)	DPT #1 TOPV #1 *PRP-D (insert at 18 mo.)	MMR	DPT #2 PRD-D (Up to age 5)
2 mo.	DPT #2 TOPV #2	DPT #2 TOPV #2	DPT #2 DPT #3 TOPV #3	DPT #3 TOPV #3
3 mo.	PRP-D (insert at 18 mo.)		PRP-D (insert at 18 mo.)	
4 mo.	DPT #3 TOPV #3 (where polio may be imported)		TOPV #3 (where polio may be imported)	TOPV #3 (where polio may be imported)
5 mo.		DPT #3 TOPV #3 (where polio may be imported)		
10–16 mo. after last dose	DPT #4 TOPV #3 or #4	DPT #4 TOPV #3 or #4	DPT #4 TOPV #3 or #4	DPT #4 TOPV #3 or #4
Preschool	DPT #5 TOPV #4 or #5	DPT #5 TOPV #4 or #5	DPT #5 TOPV #4 or #5	DPT #5 TOPV #4 or #5
14–16 yr	Td	Td	Td	Td

*DPT = diphtheria, pertussis, tetanus; TOPV = trivalent oral polio vaccine; MMR = measles, mumps, rubella; HibVax = Hemophilus influenzae B vaccine; Td = tetanus, diphtheria adult. Repeat MMR at school entry.

TABLE 14–4.—Immunization Usage Guidelines

IMMUNIZATION*	AGENT	SIDE EFFECTS	USAGE GUIDELINES
Diphtheria Pertussis Tetanus	Toxoid	Fever, pain, erythema, induration, nodule	Seizure disorder or previous CNS symptoms are contraindications to further pertussis doses; can be given during afebrile gastrointestinal or respiratory disease
Polio	Three strains of live attenuated polio virus	None common	May be given to pregnant mothers if exposed to polio; if parents have not been immunized, give adults 2–3 doses of IPV (inactivated polio virus) before immunizing children
Measles	Live attenuated rubeola virus	Fever, rash	MMR must be given after age 15 mo.
Mumps	Live attenuated mumps virus	None	MMR may be used prophylactically if exposed to disease, although not guaranteed to prevent disease
Rubella	Live attenuated rubella virus	Fever, rash, arthralgia, arthritis, neuropathy	All must be satisfied in postmenarchal female: Not pregnant Absence of rubella titer Prevent pregnancy for 3 mo. Give consequences of pregnancy Warn of side effects
Hemophilus	Purified capsular polysaccharide	Mild febrile and local reaction	May be used at 18 mo. for high risk or day care children

*Abbreviations expanded in Table 14–3.

EVALUATION OF THE NEWBORN

TABLE 14–5.—EVALUATION OF THE NEWBORN

Apgar score—The newborn is evaluated at 1 and 5 minutes after birth. Points are given to each of the five criteria and added for a total score. The 5-minute score is the one most useful in predicting neonatal and long-term prognosis.

CONDITION	APGAR SCORE
Best condition	8–10
Moderately depressed	5–7
Severely depressed	≤4

TABLE 14–6.—DETERMINING THE APGAR SCORE*

| ASPECT | POINTS | | |
	0	1	2
Heart rate	Absent	Slow (<100)	>100
Respiratory effort	Absent	Slow, irregular	Good, crying
Muscle tone	Limp	Some flexion of extremities	Active motion
Response to catheter in nostril (tested after oropharynx is clear)	No response	Grimace	Cough or sneeze
Color	Blue or pale	Body pink; extremities blue	Completely pink

*Adapted from Apgar V: *JAMA* 1958; 168:1985.

TABLE 14–7.—Conditions of High Risk for the Newborn*

Antenatal	Natal	Postnatal
Maternal age > 35	Breech delivery or other	Respiratory
Maternal diabetes	abnormal	distress
Maternal hypertension	presentation	Birth asphyxia
Maternal hemorrhage	Premature delivery	Hypothermia
Maternal infection	Multiple births	Meconium
Prolonged rupture of	Maternal hypotension	staining
membranes	Prolonged labor	Preterm infant
Maternal drug therapy	Prolapsed cord	Small-for-dates
Reserpine	Heavy sedation of	infant
Lithium carbonate	mother	HIV infection
Magnesium	Cesarean section	
Alcohol	Abnormal fetal heart	
Adrenergic blocking	rate	
drugs	Meconium-stained fluid	
Maternal drug dependency	Polyhydramnios	
Heroin	Maternal infection,	
Methadone	herpes, HIV, etc.	
Maternal anemia or		
isoimmunization		

*Adapted from McIntyre KM, Lewis AJ: *Textbook of Advanced Cardiac Life Support.* Dallas, American Heart Association, 1983.

TABLE 14–8.—Drugs Used in Resuscitation of the Newborn*

DRUG	INDICATION	DOSAGE
Atropine sulfate	Bradycardia	0.02 mg/kg
Sodium bicarbonate	Metabolic acidosis	2.0 mEq/kg initially
10% Calcium chloride	Low cardiac output	0.3 ml/kg
10% Calcium gluceptate	Low cardiac output	0.5ml/kg
10% Calcium gluconate	Low cardiac output	1.0 ml/kg
Dextrose	Low glucose stores	2.0 ml/kg 25%
Epinephrine hydrochloride	Bradycardia	0.1 ml/kg, 1:10,000 solution
Albumisol	Low blood volume	10–15 ml/kg, 5% solution
Naloxone	Respiratory depression secondary to narcotics	0.01 mg/kg q2–3 min

*Adapted from McIntyre KM, Lewis AJ: *Textbook of Advanced Cardiac Life Support.* Dallas, American Heart Association, 1983.

GROWTH AND DEVELOPMENT

TABLE 14–9.—Developmental Assessment and Guidance*

AGE	GROSS MOTOR	VISUAL MOTOR	LANGUAGE	SOCIAL	GUIDANCE
1 mo.	Raises head slightly from prone, makes crawling movements	Has tight grasp, follows to midline	Alert to sound (e.g., by blinking, moving, startling)	Regards face	Car seats, fever control, thermometers, talking to baby, sleeping, stimulating mobiles
2 mo.	Holds head in midline	No longer clenches fist tightly, follows object past midline	Smiles after being stroked or talked to	Acts increasingly alert	
3 mo.	Supports self on forearms in prone, holds head up steadily	Holds hands open at rest, pulls at clothing	Coos (produces long vowel sounds in musical fashion)	Reaches for familiar people or objects; anticipates feeding	Car seats, diet, stimulating safe toys, babysitters
4 mo.	Sits well when propped	Moves arm in unison to grasp, touches cube placed on table	Orients to voice 5 mo.—turns head toward bell, says "ah-goo"	Enjoys looking around environment	
6 mo.	Rolls from back to front, sits well, puts feet in mouth in supine position	Reaches with either hand, transfers, uses raking grasp	Babbles 7 mo.—waves bye-bye 8 mo.—"dada/mama" inappropriately	Recognizes strangers, plays pat-a-cake	Car seats, stair gates, electric cord and outlet covers, crawling, stranger anxiety, peek-a-boo, banging toys

Continued.

TABLE 14-9.—Continued

AGE	GROSS MOTOR	VISUAL MOTOR	LANGUAGE	SOCIAL	GUIDANCE
9 mo.	Creeps, pulls to feet, likes to stand	Uses overhand pincer grasp, probes with forefinger, holds bottle, finger-feeds	Imitates sounds 10 mos.—"dada/ mama" appropriately 11 mo.—one word	Starts to explore environment	Car seats, water bath safety, finger-foods, cup weaning, teeth care, first book, appropriate discipline, Ipecac
12 mo.	Walks alone or with hand held, pivots when sitting, cooperates with dressing	Uses pincer grasp, throws objects, lets go of toys	Follows one-step command with gesture, uses two words 14 mo.—uses three words	Imitates actions comes when called, cooperates with dressing	Car seats, books, water safety, burns, scalds, diet, decreased appetite, riding toys, pull toys, temper tantrums, nightmares, toilet training
15 mo.	Walks well, creeps upstairs	Builds tower of 2 blocks in imitation of examiner, scribbles in imitation	Follows one-step command without gesture, uses 4–6 words and immature jargon (runs several unintelligible words together)		

Age	Gross Motor	Fine Motor/Adaptive	Language	Personal-Social	Anticipatory Guidance
18 mo.	Runs, throws toy from standing without falling	Turns 2–3 pages at a time, fills spoon and feeds self	Knows 7–10 words, points to one body part when named, uses mature jargoning, includes intelligible words	Copies parent in tasks (e.g., sweeping, dusting), plays in company of other children	Car seats, books, playground, safety babysitter, giving up blanket etc., appropriate discipline, learning to play with others
21 mo.	Squats in play, goes up steps	Builds tower of 5 blocks, drinks well from cup	Points to 3 body parts, uses two-word combination	Asks to have food and to go to toilet	
24 mo.	Walks up and down steps without help; jumps with both feet off floor, throws ball overhand	Turns pages one at a time, removes shoes, pants, etc.; unbuttons; holds pencil in adult fashion	Uses 50 words, two-word sentences three pronouns; names objects in pictures; uses plurals, past tense and pronoun "I" correctly most of the time.	Tells first and last names when asked, gets drink without help	
3 yr	Pedals tricycle, can alternate feet when going up steps	Dresses and undresses partially, dries hands if reminded	Tells story about experiences, knows his/her sex	Shares toys, takes turns, plays well with others	

Continued.

TABLE 14-9.—Continued

AGE	GROSS MOTOR	VISUAL MOTOR	LANGUAGE	SOCIAL	GUIDANCE
4 yr	Hops, skips, alternates feet going downstairs	Buttons clothing fully, catches ball	Knows all colors, says song or poem from memory	Tells "tall tales"; plays cooperatively with a group of children	Consideration should be given to discussing "private" areas and setting limits for those areas.
5 yr	Skips, alternating feet; jumps over low obstacles	Ties shoes, spreads with knife	Prints first name, asks what a word means	Plays competitive games, abides by rules, likes to help in household tasks	

*Adapted from *The Harriet Lane Handbook*, ed. 10. Chicago, Year Book Medical Publishers, Inc.,

NEWBORN RESUSCITATION
PHASE I: RESPIRATORY SUPPORT

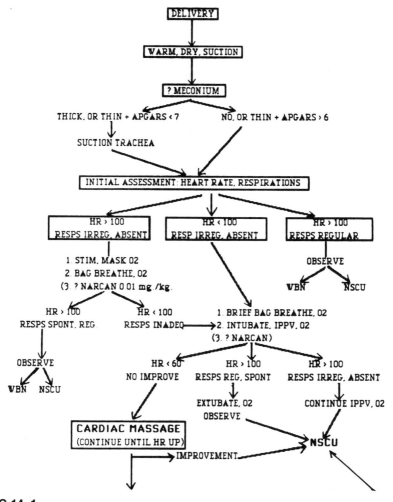

FIG 14–1.
Newborn resuscitation phase I: respiratory support. (Courtesy of Patrick Wall, MD, Riverside Methodist Hospitals, Columbus, Ohio.)

NEWBORN RESUSCITATION
PHASE II: DRUG SUPPORT

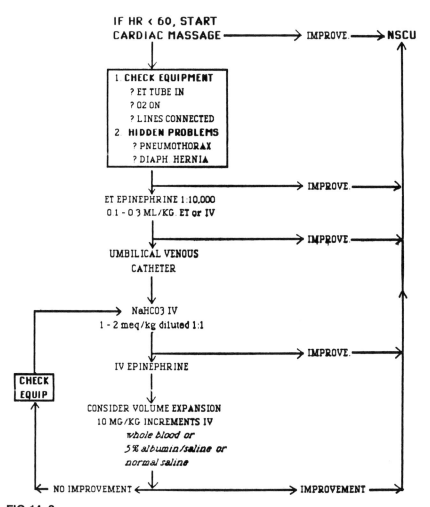

FIG 14–2.
Newborn resuscitation phase II: drug support. (Courtesy of Patrick Wall, MD, Riverside Methodist Hospitals, Columbus, Ohio.)

TABLE 14–10.—TIME OF APPEARANCE OF SEXUAL CHARACTERISTICS: AMERICAN GIRLS*

ASPECT	DESCRIPTION	AGE
Pelvis	Female contour assumed and fat deposition begins	8–10 yr
Breasts	First hypertrophy or budding	8–11 yr
	Further enlargement and pigmentation of nipples	12–13 yr
	Histologic maturity	12–17 yr
Vagina	Secretion begins and glycogen content of epithelium increases with change in cell type	8–13 yr
Pubic hair	Initial appearance	8–13 yr
	Abundant and curly	9–15 yr
Axillary hair	Initial appearance	9–15 yr
Acne	Varies considerably	9–17 yr

*Adapted from Watson EH, Lowrey GH: *Growth and Development of Children,* ed. 5. Chicago, Year Book Medical Publishers, 1967.

TABLE 14–11.—TIME OF APPEARANCE OF SEXUAL CHARACTERISTICS: AMERICAN BOYS*

ASPECT	DESCRIPTION	AGE
Breasts	Some hypertrophy, often assuming a firm nodularity	11–15 yr
	Disappearance of hypertrophy	12–16 yr
Testes and penis	Increase in size begins	10–12 yr
	Rapid growth	12–15 yr
Pubic hair	Initial appearance	10–14 yr
	Abundant and curly	13–17 yr
Axillary hair	Initial appearance	11–15 yr
Facial and body hair	Initial appearance	12–16 yr
Acne	Varies considerably	11–18 yr

*Adapted from Watson EH, Lowrey GH: *Growth and Development of Children,* ed 5. Chicago, Year Book Medical Publishers, 1967.

TABLE 14–12.—DENTAL DEVELOPMENT*

| | DECIDUOUS TEETH | | | | PERMANENT TEETH | |
| | Eruption | | Shedding | | Eruption | |
	Maxillary	Mandibular	Maxillary	Mandibular	Maxillary	Mandibular
Central incisors	6–10 mo.	5–8 mo.	7–8 yr	6–7 yr	7–8 yr (4)	6–7 yr (3)
Lateral incisors	8–12 mo.	7–10 mo.	8–9 yr	7–8 yr	8–9 yr (6)	7–8 yr (5)
Cuspids	16–20 mo.	16–20 mo.	11–12 yr	9–11 yr	11–12 yr (12)	9–11 yr (7)
1st premolar	—	—	—	—	10–11 yr (8)	10–12 yr (9)
2nd premolar	—	—	—	—	10–12 yr (10)	11–13 yr (11)
1st molars	10–18	10–18 mo.	9–11 yr	9–12 yr	6–7 yr (1)	6–7 yr (2)
2nd molars	20–30 mo.	20–30 mo.	10–12 yr	11–13 yr	12–14 yr (13)	12–13 yr (14)
3rd molars	—	—	—	—	17–30 yr (15)	17–30 yr (16)

*Note: Sexes are combined, although girls tend to be slightly advanced over boys. Averages are approximate values derived from various studies. Numbers in parentheses give order of eruption.

HYPERBILIRUBINEMIA

TABLE 14–13.—Common Causes of Jaundice in the First Week of Life*

Due to immaturity of the infant liver, many babies become jaundiced during the first week of life. The most common diagnosis is physiologic jaundice, which appears after 24 hours. The bilirubin, mostly indirect, may rise to 12 mg/100 ml in the term infant and higher in the premature infant with physiologic jaundice.

DIAGNOSIS	CLINICAL AND LABORATORY DATA
Physiologic jaundice	Observed 2–4 days after birth. Elevated indirect serum bilirubin. Peak, 12–14 mg.
Hemolytic disease Rh incompatibility	Onset usually within 24 hours. Hepatosplenomegaly. Petechiae. Rh negative mother; Rh positive infant. Anemia with reticulocytosis. Positive Coombs test. Elevated indirect serum bilirubin. Nucleated red cells in peripheral blood smear.
ABO incompatibility	Jaundice appears within 24 hours. Mild anemia and hepatosplenomegaly. Mother—O blood group; infant—either A or B group. Anemia with reticulocytosis. Peripheral blood smear reveals microcytosis and nucleated red cells. Elevated indirect serum bilirubin.
Congenital spherocytosis	Anemia and splenomegaly. Spherocytes on peripheral blood smear. Elevated indirect serum bilirubin. Coombs test negative.
Jaundice associated with breast feeding	Jaundice appears between fourth and seventh day of life. May reach very high levels during second or third week. Disappears rapidly when breast feeding is discontinued, however this is usually unnecessary.

*From Rakel RE: *Textbook of Family Practice,* ed 3. Philadelphia, WB Saunders Co, 1984, p 547. Reproduced by permission.

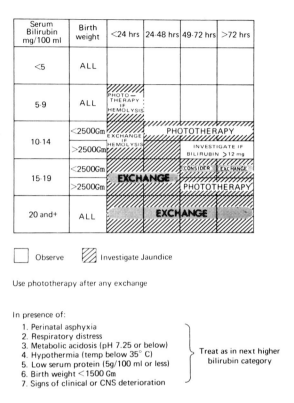

Serum Bilirubin mg/100 ml	Birth weight	<24 hrs	24-48 hrs	49-72 hrs	>72 hrs
<5	ALL				
5-9	ALL	PHOTO— THERAPY IF HEMOLYSIS			
10-14	<2500Gm	EXCHANGE IF HEMOLYSIS	PHOTOTHERAPY		
	>2500Gm			INVESTIGATE IF BILIRUBIN >12 mg	
15-19	<2500Gm	EXCHANGE		CONSIDER EXCHANGE	
	>2500Gm			PHOTOTHERAPY	
20 and+	ALL	EXCHANGE			

☐ Observe   ▨ Investigate Jaundice

Use phototherapy after any exchange

In presence of:

1. Perinatal asphyxia
2. Respiratory distress
3. Metabolic acidosis (pH 7.25 or below)
4. Hypothermia (temp below 35° C)
5. Low serum protein (5g/100 ml or less)
6. Birth weight <1500 Gm
7. Signs of clinical or CNS deterioration

} Treat as in next higher bilirubin category

FIG 14–3.

Guidelines for management of neonatal hyperbilirubinemia. (From Avery GB [ed]: *Neonatology*. Philadelphia, JB Lippincott Co 1975. Reproduced by permission.)

TABLE 14–14.—Ruling Out Physiologic Jaundice*

Criteria which rule out the diagnosis of physiologic jaundice[†]
  1. Clinical jaundice in the first 24 hr of life.
  2. Total serum bilirubin concentrations increasing by more than 5 mg/dl (85 μmol/L) per day.
  3. Total serum bilirubin concentration exceeding 12.9 mg/dl (221 μmol/L) in a full-term infant or 15 mg/dl (257 μmol/L) in a premature infant.
  4. Direct serum bilirubin concentration exceeding 1.5–2 mg/dl (26–34 μmol/L).
  5. Clinical jaundice persisting for > 1 wk in a full-term infant or 2 wk in a premature infant.

*From Avery GB (ed): *Neonatology,* ed 2. Philadelphia, JB Lippincott Co, 1975. Reproduced by permission.
[†]The absence of these criteria does not imply that the jaundice *is* physiologic. In the presence of any of these criteria, the jaundice must be investigated.

SPECIFIC FORMULAS FOR SPECIFIC PROBLEMS

TABLE 14–15.—Specific Formulas for Specific Problems*

PROBLEM	FORMULA
Lactose intolerance	ProSobee, Isomil, Mullsoy (lactose-free formulas)
Malabsorption of fat	Portagen, Osmolite (contains medium-chain triglycerides)
Protein	Nutramigen (hydrolyzed protein)
	Pregestimil (hydrolyzed protein and medium-chain triglycerides)
Inborn errors:	
Amino acid	Lofenalac (low phenylalanine content)
Galactosemia	Nutramigen (galactose free)
	Soy formulas (galactose free)
Fructose	Similac, Enfamil, SMA (fructose free)

*From Rakel RE: *Textbook of Family Practice,* ed 3. Philadelphia, WB Saunders Co, 1984, p 550. Reproduced by permission.

COMMON INFECTIOUS DISEASES

TABLE 14–16.—COMMON INFECTIOUS DISEASES

DISEASE	INCUBATION	PRODROME	SIGNS AND SYMPTOMS	ISOLATION	TREATMENT
Chickenpox (varicella)	10–21 days	Minimal	Mixture of macules, papules, vesicles; spreads from trunk to extremities for 5–20 days	Until all lesions are crusted; infectious 2 days before appearance	Symptomatic
Diphtheria	2–6 days	Rapid onset of signs and symptoms	Moderate fever, malaise, sore throat; gray, tenacious membrane in throat; respiratory distress	Until two negative nose and throat cultures 24 hours apart	Antitoxin penicillin
Fifth disease (erythema infectiosa)	6–14 days	None	Maculopapular rash on face with circumoral pallor (slapped cheek) and spreading to extremities; rash lasts a few days to a few weeks and is brought out by warmth	Not needed	None

Hepatitis A	15–20 days	Rapid onset	Fever, anorexia, headache, abdominal pain, liver enzyme elevation, jaundice	Stool, urine, and blood for 1 month	Bed rest, fluids, immune serum γ-globulin to contacts
Hepatitis B	6 wk to 6 mo.	Insidious onset	Slight fever and mild gastrointestinal upset jaundice, hepatomegaly, elevated liver enzymes	Body excretions until surface antigen negative	Bed rest, fluids, hepatitis B immune globulin to intimate contacts, ISG to others
Herpangina (coxsackie group A)	?	None	High fever, vomiting, ulcers of oral mucosa for 5–6 days	2–6 days	Symptomatic
Meningococcal meningitis	1–7 days	URI, fever, headache, diarrhea	Meningitis, purpuric or petechial rash; septic arthritis	Until 24 hr after first antibiotic	Penicillin or chloramphenical
Mononucleosis	2–8 wk	None	Fatigue, anorexia, exudative tonsillitis, lymphadenopathy, splenomegaly; maculopapular rash not unusual	Avoid saliva contact for 3 mo.	Symptomatic

Continued.

TABLE 14-16.—Continued

DISEASE	INCUBATION	PRODROME	SIGNS AND SYMPTOMS	ISOLATION	TREATMENT
Mumps	14–21 days	None	Asymptomatic in 30%–40%; swelling and pain of the salivary glands; fever	Communicable from 7 days before to 9 days after occurrence of swelling	Symptomatic
Poliomyelitis	7–14 days usual; 5–35 days max.	Fever, lassitude, GI upset	Paralysis heralded by nuchal rigidity and stiffness of back; pain and tenderness in affected muscles	Secretions 1 wk, stool 6 wk	Supportive, bed rest
Roseola (exanthum subitum)	1–15 days	3–4 days of sustained high fever	Fine pink rash begins at defervescense and lasts 2 days; seen from 6 mo. to 3 years of age	Unknown	Fever control

Rubella, German measles, 3-day measles	14–21 days	Lymphadenopathy, fever, headache, malaise	Maculopapular discrete rash appears on face and rapidly spreads to trunk and proximal extremities, lasting 1–3 days; postauricular and suboccipital lymphadenopathy	Communicable from 7 days before until 5 days after rash appears	None
Rubeola (measles)	10–12 days	High fever, cough, coryza, and conjunctivitis for 3 days	Koplik spots appear 1–2 days before maculopapular rash; rash is confluent and spreads from hairline to face, then body; lasts 4–5 days	From 5th day of incubation to 5th day after rash appears	Symptomatic care of cough, coryza, conjunctivitis
Whooping cough (pertussis)	5–10 days, 21 days max.	1–3 wk of cough, coryza, and occasional emesis	Short paroxysmal cough ending with inspiratory "whoop"	5–10 days on treatment	Erythromycin

TABLE 14-17.—Respiratory Disorders

	BRONCHIOLITIS	ASTHMA	PNEUMONIA	EPIGLOTTITIS	LARYNGOTRACHEOBRONCHITIS
	Onset: 3 mo.–3 yr	Onset: infancy to adulthood	Onset: all ages	2–7 yr	<3 yr
	Previous history negative	Previous history often positive	Previous history often negative	Previous history often negative	Previous history of rhinorrhea and cough
	Frequent in winter Afebrile or mildly febrile	Frequent all seasons Usually afebrile	Frequent in winter Febrile	Any season 39.4°C (103°F)	Late fall and winter 39–40°C (102–104°F)
	Prolonged expiration Inspiratory and expiratory obstruction	Prolonged expiration Expiratory obstruction	No prolonged expiration Obstructive respiratory usually lacking	Normal expiration Inspiratory stridor	Normal expiration Inspiratory obstruction barking cough
	Respiratory distress marked Usually hyperresonant Wheezing, rales, or rhonchi	Respiratory distress mild to marked Usually hyperresonant Wheezing	Respiratory distress mild marked Usually hyperresonant Rales	Respiratory distress marked No wheezing	Respiratory distress mild to marked Wheezing may be present
	Chest findings bilateral Lymphocytosis	Chest findings bilateral Eosinophilia	Chest findings either unilateral or bilateral Lymphocytosis or "viral" or "bacterial" white count and differential, polymorphonuclear leukocytosis	Bilateral Elevated WBC count (>18,000/mm³)	Bilateral Normal WBC count
	Hyperaeration	Hyperaeration	Pneumonic infiltrate or consolidation	Normal chest x-ray; abnormal neck x-ray	Normal neck and chest x-rays
	Antibiotic in severe cases	Bronchodilatation, epinephrine	Appropriate antibiotic if bacterial	Ampicillin and chloramphenicol	Cool mist, observe

OTITIS MEDIA

TABLE 14–18.—OTITIS MEDIA

Diagnosis
  Hyperemic tympanic membrane.
  Opacity of tympanic membrane.
  Bulging and poor mobility of tympanic membrane.
  Fever not always present, and when present, should remind you to look for
    concomitant disease, e.g., pneumonia, URI.
  Earache (variable).
Etiology
  Newborns
    Gram-negative bacilli.
  Infants
    Streptococcus pneumoniae 40%.
    Hemophilus influenzae 20%.
    Group A β-hemolytic *Streptococcus*.
Treatment
  See Table 14–19 and Fig 4–4.

TABLE 14–19.—TREATMENT OF OTITIS MEDIA*

ANTIBIOTIC	DOSE (mg/kg/day)	DOSES/ DAY	DURATION (DAYS)
Ampicillin	50–200	q.i.d.	10
Amoxicillin	30–50	t.i.d.	10
Amoxicillin–Clavulanate K	40	t.i.d.	10
Cefaclor	40	b.i.d.	10
Erythromycin/sulfisoxazole	50/150	q.i.d.	10
Trimethoprim/sulfamethoxazole	10/50	b.i.d.	10

*Other treatment modalities include analgesia, heat, and antipyretics.

PARASITIC INFECTIONS

TABLE 14-20.—PARASITIC INFECTIONS

PARASITE	DIAGNOSIS	DRUG (USE ONE)	DOSAGE
Pinworm (*Enterobius vermicularis*)	Demonstration under microscope, ova on tape applied and removed from anus, or visualization of pinworm (white and looks like an eyelash)	Mebendazole Pyrantel pamoate	100 mg single dose 11 mg/kg in a single dose, max 1 gm; repeat in 2–3 wk
Giardiasis (*Giardia lamblia*)	Multiple stool examinations	Quinacrine HCL Metronidazole Furazolidone	2 mg/kg t.i.d. pc × 5d max 300 mg/d 5 mg/kg t.i.d. × 5d 1.25 mg/kg q.i.d. × 7–10d
Roundworm (*Ascaris lumbricoides*)	Adult worm vomited or passed in stool	Mebendazole Pyrantel pamoate	100 mg b.i.d. × 3d for children >2 yr 11 mg/kg once (max. 1 gm)
Visceral Larva migrans (*toxocara canis, T. cati*)	Generally by history of exposure to cats and dogs; may be anemic; signs: fever, hepatomegaly	Diethylcarbamazine Thiabendazole	2 mg/kg t.i.d. × 7–10d 25 mg/kg b.i.d. × 5d (max. 3 gm/d)
Tapeworm (*taenia saginata, T. solium*)	Demonstration of worm segments or eggs in stool	Niclosamide	For children 11–34 kg, single dose of 1 gm; for children >34 kg, 1.5 gm; for teenagers and adults, 2 gm

FEBRILE SEIZURES

TABLE 14–21.—Febrile Seizures

Definition
  Tonic-clonic seizure <15 min.
  Occur in children aged 3 mo. to 5 yr
  Fever present
  No evidence of intracranial infection, by sign or symptom; spinal tap should be
    done if there is any suspicion of infection of the CNS
Risk factors
  Family history
  Abnormal neurodevelopmental status
  Atypical seizures
  Past history of febrile seizures—about one third who have one seizure and are
    not treated prophylactically will have more episodes
Treatment (generally only prophylactic, once seizure is over)
  Temperature control is needed
  Phenobarbital, 3–6 mg/kg in 3 to 4 doses per day; blood level 15–20 ng/dl
  Valproic acid, 15–60 mg/kg in 3 doses per day

MENINGITIS

TABLE 14–22.—Meningitis

Fever, headache, nuchal rigidity, irritability, nausea, vomiting and altered mental
status are all symptoms of meningitis. The two most common types are aseptic
and bacterial. The spinal fluid should be cultured for TB, fungus, and viruses as
well.

CSF	ASEPTIC MENINGITIS	BACTERIAL MENINGITIS
Gram stain	Negative	May be positive
Opening pressure	Elevated	Elevated
WBC count	50–4,000/mm^3	100–60,000/mm^3 mostly PMN
Protein	NL or increased	Elevated
Glucose	NL or increased	Decreased

TABLE 14–23.—GRAM STAIN–DIRECTED THERAPY FOR MENINGITIS

STAIN MORPHOLOGY	LIKELY ORGANISM	FIRST CHOICES	ALTERNATE THERAPY
Gram (+) cocci in chains or pairs	*Streptococcus*	Penicillin G + gentamicin for 24 hr	Chloramphenicol Cefotaxime Ceftriaxone
Gram (+) cocci in clusters	*Staphylococcus* β-Lactamase + β-Lactamase −	Nafcillin, penicillin G	Vancomycin
Gram (−) cocci Gram (−) coccobacilli	*Neisseria meningitidis* *Hemophilus influenzae* β-Lactamase − β-Lactamase +	Penicillin G Ampicillin Chloramphenicol	Chloramphenicol Chloramphenicol Cefotaxime, ceftriaxone
Gram (−) enteric rods	*E. coli* *Klebsiella* *Salmonella* *Serratia* *Pseudomonas*	Cefotaxime Ceftriaxone or ceftizoxime Ceftazidime + IV aminoglycoside	Trimethoprim-sulfamethoxazole Azlocillin, mezlocillin Carbenicillin or pipercillin + IV aminoglycoside
Gram (+) rods	*Listeria monocytogenes*	Ampicillin, penicillin + gentamicin	Trimethoprim-sulfamethoxazole

TABLE 14–24.—PRESUMPTIVE THERAPY FOR BACTERIAL MENINGITIS*

AGE GROUP	PATHOGENS	THERAPY

<1 mo.	Group B *Streptococcus*
	Gram-negative enteric
	   bacilli
	Listeria monocytogenes
	Hemophilus influenzae
	Streptococcus
	   pneumoniae
	Neisseria meningitidis
	Staphylococcus aureus
	   (predominantly in
	   premature infants)
		Ampicillin plus gentamicin or
		   ampicillin + cefotaxime;
		   20% of *H. influenzae* is
		   ampicillin resistant

1–3 mo.	*H. influenzae*
	N. meningitidis
	S. pneumoniae
	Group B *Streptococcus*
		Ampicillin + cefotaxime;
		   20% *H. influenzae* is
		   ampicillin resistant

3 mo.–9 yr	*H. influenzae*
	S. pneumoniae
	N. meningitidis
		Cefotaxime or ceftriaxone or
		   ampicillin +
		   chloramphenicol; 20% of
		   H. influenzae is ampicillin
		   resistant

>9 yr	*N. meningitidis*
	S. pneumoniae
	H. influenzae
		Penicillin G,
		   chloramphenicol,
		   ceftriaxone, cefotaxime,
		   or cefuroxime

*Adapted from Rakel RE: *Conn's Current Therapy*. Philadelphia, W.B. Saunders Co, 1989.

TABLE 14–25.—CSF CHARACTERISTICS IN THE NORMAL CHILD AND SOME NEUROLOGIC DISORDERS*

DISEASE	INITIAL PRESSURE (mm H$_2$O)	APPEARANCE	CELLS	PROTEIN (mg/dl)	SUGAR (mg/dl)	OTHER TESTS	COMMENTS
Normal	<180	Clear	0–5 (some accept up to 10) mononuclear cells; in neonates, up to 30	15–35 (lumbar)	50–80 (two thirds of blood glucose)	CSF IgG index: <0.7 units = CSF IgG/serum IgG; CSF albumin/serum albumin lactate dehydrogenase (LDH), 2–30 IU/L	CSF protein in first month may be up to 170 mg/dl in small-for-dates or premature infants; 20–50 red cells in the first days of life
Bloody tap	Normal or low	Bloody (sometimes with clot)	One white cell for each 700 red cells	1 mg protein for each 800 erythrocytes above "normal"	Normal		Spin down fluid; supernatant will be clear and colorless
Acute bacterial meningitis	200–750+	Opalescent to purulent	100 to many thousands, mostly PMNs; fewer cells possible early	50 to many hundreds	Decreased; may be none	Smear and culture mandatory for identification; LDH > 30 IU/L	Blood, nose, and throat cultures; very early, sugar may be normal
Partially treated bacterial meningitis	Usually increased	Clear or opalescent	Usually increased, PMNs usually predominate	Elevated	Normal or decreased	LDH > 30 IU/L.	Smear and culture often negative
Postmeningitic hydrocephalus	Variable	Clear	0–10	Variable; may be low	Often low	Smear and bacterial cultures negative	Low CSF glucose may be due to disturbed transport mechanism
Tuberculous meningitis	150–750+	Opalescent	250–500; monocytes predominate	45–500; parallels cell count	Decreased; may be none	Smear for acid-fast organism; culture and inoculation of CSF	Very early, PMNs may predominate; skin test almost always positive; chest x-ray
Fungal meningitis	Increased	Variable; often clear	10–500; early, mostly PMNs; late, mostly monocytes	Elevated and increasing	Decreased	India ink preparations, culture, inoculations, immunofluorescence tests	Often superimposed in patients who are debilitated or on immunosuppressive or tumor therapy
Brain abscess	Normal or increased	Usually clear	5–500 in 80%; mostly PMNs	Usually slightly increased	Normal; occasionally decreased		Cell count related to proximity to meninges; findings as in purulent meningitis if abscess perforates

Condition	Pressure	Appearance	Cells	Protein	Sugar	Special Tests	Remarks
Acute poliomyelitis	Usually normal	Clear or slightly opalescent	10–500+, mostly monocytes; PMNs early	Normal to 350; often progressive increase	Normal		Stool virus and serum antibody studies
Polyneuritis: Early Late	Normal and occasionally increased	Normal Xanthochromic if protein high	Normal; occasionally slight increase	Normal 45–1500	Normal	Bacterial cultures negative; γ-globulin may be elevated	Try to find etiology; viral infections, toxins, lupus, infectious mononucleosis, diabetes, etc.
Aseptic meningoencephalitides	Normal or slightly increased	Clear unless cell count is above 300	0 to few hundred, mainly monocytes; PMNs predominate early	20–125	Normal; may be low in mumps	CSF, stool, throat wash for viral cultures; LDH < 30 IU/L	Acute and convalescent serum antibody studies; in mumps marked pleocytosis (up to 1,000 lymphocytes);
Neurosyphilis	Normal to 400	Clear unless protein is very high	10–100, mainly monocytes	25–150; higher in meningitis	Normal	Positive CSF serology; CSF IgG index increased	Blood serology positive in untreated cases; Treponema pallidum immobilization test positive
Parainfectious encephalomyelitis (measles, varicella, vaccinia)	80–450, usually increased	Usually clear	0–50, mainly monocytes	15–75	Normal	CSF γ-globulin IgG index normal or increased; oligoclonal bands absent	No organisms; fulminant cases resemble bacterial meningitis
Supratentorial tumors	150–800+, usually increased	Usually clear	Usually normal	Usually normal; increased proximal to obstruction	Normal	Radiodiagnostic studies	
Brain stem tumors	Usually normal	Clear	Usually normal	Usually normal	Normal	Radiodiagnostic studies	
Cerebellar and fourth ventricle tumors	150–800+, usually increased	Usually clear	0–150; normal in 80%; occasionally, cytologic identification of tumor cells	Normal or slightly elevated	Normal	Radiodiagnostic studies	Lumbar tap contraindicated; ventricular CSF may be normal

Continued.

TABLE 14–25.—Continued

DISEASE	INITIAL PRESSURE (mm H2O)	APPEARANCE	CELLS	PROTEIN (mg/dl)	SUGAR (mg/dl)	OTHER TESTS	COMMENTS
Spinal cord tumors with block	Normal or low; quantitative, manometric studies	Clear to yellow	0–100, mainly monocytes	Normal in 15%; 45–3,500 in 85%	Normal	Myelography; CT spine scan	Color related to amount of protein; very high protein; fluid may clot
Meningeal carcinomatosis	Often elevated	Clear to opalescent	Cytologic identification of tumor cells	Often mildly to moderately elevated	Often depressed		Most commonly seen in childhood in leukemia; also in medulloblastoma, meningeal melanosis
Encephalopathies (lead, anoxic, uremic, toxic)	Increased	Clear to slightly yellow	Normal, occasionally increased; mainly monocytes	Normal or increased	Normal		Increased lead in blood and urine; increased coproporphyrins in urine; BUN high
Cerebral concussion Cerebral contusion	Normal Increased or normal	Clear Xanthochromic or bloody	Normal Few to several thousand red cells	Normal	Usually normal; below 50 in 15%.	Normal Supernatant fluid xanthochromic	The occasional reduction of sugar is probably related to the presence of blood; protein is increased in relation to admixture
Subdural hematoma	Increased	Clear in 30%, xanthochromic in 70%	Normal (if fluid is clear)	Often normal in acute subdural hematoma if CSF is not bloody	Normal	Radiodiagnostic studies	Blood in CSF due to coexisting other injury

						Radiodiagnostic studies	
Epidural hematoma	Above 200 in two-thirds of cases	Clear	See Comments				Lumbar tap contraindicated if this diagnosis very likely; fluid may be xanthochromic if contusion coexists; cells, protein, and sugar assumed to be normal
Cerebral hemorrhage	Usually high	Xanthochromic	Amount and type depend on severity of hemorrhage	Normal to 2000; usually high	Usually normal; occasionally high or low	Supernatant fluid xanthochromic; radiodiagnostic studies	
Subarachnoid hemorrhage	Usually high	Xanthochromic or grossly bloody	Presence of all cellular elements of blood	Increase related to amount of blood	Usually high; see Comments	Supernatant fluid xanthochromic	CSF glucose may be low 7–14 days after initial bleeding
Demyelinating diseases	Variable; more often elevated in some leukodystrophies	Clear	0–100, mainly monocytes	Slightly elevated in 25%	Normal	Increased CSF IgG index (>0.7 units); oligoclonal bands present; consider CT brain scan	Schilder's disease, leukodystrophies, neuromyelitis optica, multiple sclerosis, etc.

*From Kempe CH, Silver HK, O'Brien D, et al: *Current Pediatric Diagnosis and Treatment*, ed 8. Los Altos, Calif, Lange Medical Publications, 1984. Reproduced by permission.

DIARRHEA AND STOOLING DISORDERS

TABLE 14–26.—Noninfectious Causes of Intractable Diarrhea*

CONDITION	FIRST-STEP SCREENING	SECOND-STAGE SCREENING	SPECIFIC DIAGNOSTIC STUDIES
Hirschsprung's disease (1)†	Abdominal radiograph	Barium enema	Rectal biopsy
Stenosis of bowel (1)	Abdominal radiograph	Gastrointestinal series	Exploratory laparotomy
Milk protein sensitivity (1)	Cow's milk elimination	Rechallenge with cow's milk	Consistent response to cow's milk protein
Agammaglobulinemia (Swiss type) (1)	Peripheral blood smear (lymphocytes)	Serum protein electrophoresis	Biopsy of lymph nodes
Disaccharide intolerance (1,2)	Stool pH—test for reducing substances	Tolerance test for sugars	Trial carbohydrate elimination; may use fructose
Cystic fibrosis (1,2)	Sweat test		Repeat sweat test
Celiac disease (2)	History	Trial of gluten-free diet	Intestinal biopsy
Ulcerative colitis (3)	Stool guaiac	Sigmoidoscopy, barium enema	
Ova and parasites	Stool cultures		

*Adapted from Avery GG, et al: *Pediatrics* 1968; 41:781.
†Age at onset: (1) infant, (2) toddler, (3) toddler or older child.

TABLE 14–27.—Stooling Disorders With Constipation*

CLINICAL	HIRSCHSPRUNG'S DISEASE	ENCOPRESIS
Age	Birth or soon thereafter	After 2 yr; usually older
Toilet training	Usually successful	Usually successful initially
Constipation	Yes	Yes
Toilet use	Usually	Infrequent
Soiling	Rarely	Constant
Rectal ampula	Usually empty	Stool present
Stool size	Usually normal; pellet or ribbon-like	Very large
Resolution	Surgery	Psychotherapy

*Adapted from Rakel RE: *Textbook of Family Practice,* ed 3. Philadelphia, WB Saunders Co, 1984, p 562.

RABIES

TABLE 14–28.—Guidelines for Postexposure Rabies Prophylaxis*

ANIMAL SPECIES	CONDITION OF ANIMAL AT TIME OF ATTACK	TREATMENT
Domestic dog or cat	Healthy and available for 10 days of observation	None, unless animal develops rabies
	Suspicious	HRIG and HDCV; discontinue after 5 days if animal is healthy
	Rabid	HRIG and HDCV
	Unknown	Consult public health officials; if treatment is indicated, give HRIG and HDCV
Wild animals; skunk, bat, fox, coyote, raccoon, bobcat and other carnivores	Regard as rabid unless proven negative by laboratory test	HRIG and HDCV

Continued.

TABLE 14–28.—Continued

| Other animals; livestock, rodents, rabbits, and hares | Consider individually. Provoked bites of squirrels, hamsters, guinea pigs, gerbils, chipmunks, rats, mice and other rodents or rabbits and hares which almost never call for antirabies prophylaxis. Local or state public health officials should be consulted concerning questions that arise about the need for rabies prophylaxis. |

*HRIG = human rabies immune globulin; HDCV = human diploid cell vaccine. Regimen is day O HRIG + HDCV, day 3, 7, 14, and 28 HDCV alone. HRIG dosage is 20 IV/kg ½ dose IM and ½ dose in wound edge. HDCV dose is 1 ml each injection if HDCV has ever been given previously for bite or preexposure. Vaccination HRIG is not used in this regimen.

ATTENTION DEFICIT

TABLE 14–29.—Attention Deficit Hyperactivity Disorder (ADHD)

Hyperactivity is a syndrome of behavior, not a psychiatric disease. It affects 5%–15% of school-aged children. The diagnosis is made by observing the child and eliciting a history of several of the following behaviors from the child's parents and teachers:

Increased motion activity	Impulsiveness
Distractibility	Antisocial behavior
Short attention span	Learning disabilities
Restlessness	Poor academic performance

Treatment may involve only reassurance of teachers and parents and manipulation of the environment such as a definite home routine, and structured rather than open classroom with frequent breaks. When this behavior interferes with academic and social performance, drug therapy should be considered.

TABLE 14–30.—Drug Therapy for Attention Deficit Hyperactivity Disorder (ADHD)

DRUG	AGE (YR)	INITIAL DOSE	SUBSEQUENT DOSE
Methylphenidate (Ritalin)	6–8	5 mg in A.M.	Increase daily dose by 5 mg each week to max of 60 mg/day
	9–12	10 mg in A.M.	
Pemoline (Cylert)	6	37.5 mg in A.M.	Increase daily dose by 18.75 each week to max of 112.5 mg/24 hr.
Dextroamphetamine (Dexedrine)	3–5	2.5 mg qd	Raise daily dose 5 mg each week until desired response. (Max 40 mg/d).
	7–6	5 mg qd	
Imipramine (Tofranil)	6–8	10 mg in A.M.	Divide dose and each week increase by 10 mg daily until desired response. (max 75 mg/d).
	7–8	25 mg in A.M.	

RHEUMATIC FEVER

TABLE 14–31.—The Diagnosis of Rheumatic Fever—Jones Criteria Revised*

There is a high probability of acute rheumatic fever if two major criteria or one major and two minor criteria are present, supported by evidence of recent Group A streptococcal infection such as scarlet fever, increased ASO titer, or positive throat culture.

MAJOR CRITERIA	MINOR CRITERIA
Carditis	Arthralgia
Chorea	Fever
Erythema marginatum	Previous rheumatic fever or rheumatic heart disease
Polyarthritis	
Subcutaneous nodules	Prolonged PR interval
	Elevated sed rate or C-reactive protein or leukocytosis

*Adapted from *Circulation* 1984; 69:204A–208A.

TABLE 14–32.—DIFFERENTIAL DIAGNOSIS OF RHEUMATIC FEVER, RHEUMATOID
ARTHRITIS, AND SYSTEMIC LUPUS ERYTHEMATOSUS*

ASPECT	RHEUMATIC FEVER	RHEUMATOID ARTHRITIS	SYSTEMIC LUPUS ERYTHEMATOSUS
Age trend	5 yr	5 yr	5 yr
Sex ratio	Equal	Girls 1.5:1	Girls 5:1
Joint findings			
Pain	Severe	Moderate	. . .
Swelling	Nonspecific	Nonspecific	Nonspecific
Tenderness	Severe	Moderate	. . .
Bone x-ray	None	Frequent	Occasional
Morning stiffness	Yes	Yes	Yes
Rash	Erythema marginatum	Rheumatoid arthritis rash	Malar flush
Chorea	Yes	No	Rarely
Clinical carditis	+	Rare	Late
Laboratory tests			
WBC	Normal to high	Normal to high	Decreased to normal
Latex	–	+ (10%)	+ occasionally
Sheep cell agglut	–	+ (10%)	–
LE cell prep.	–	+ (5%)	+
Biopsy			
Skin rash	Nonspecific	Nonspecific	Diagnostic
Nodules	Nonspecific	Nonspecific	Nonspecific
Response to sallicylates	Rapid	Slow, usually	Slow or none

*From Brewer EJ Jr: *Juvenile Rheumatoid Arthritis.* Philadelphia, WB Saunders Co, 1970, p 91. Reproduced by permission.

15 *Orthopedics*

Edward T. Bope, M.D.

ARTHROCENTESIS

TABLE 15–1.—ARTHROCENTESIS

Indications
    Analysis of joint fluid.
    Relief of pain by drainage of an effusion.
    Installation of medication (see Table 15–2).
    Drainage of hemarthrosis.
Contraindications
    Infection in skin or soft tissue.
    Coagulation disorder.
General technique
    Identify landmarks and mark site with indelible ink.
    Use aseptic technique.
    Provide generous local anesthesia of the overlying skin and subcutaneous tissues.
    Choose syringe appropriate for effusion size: 3–50 cc.
    Advance needle with negative pressure.
    Remove effusion.
    Apply sterile bandage.
Technique (site approach)
    Shoulder (anterior approach)
        Seat patient with hand in lap.
        Palpate the glenohumeral joint (between the coracoid process and humeral head).
        Internally rotate shoulder and feel the joint groove lateral to the coracoid.
        Direct the needle (20–22 gauge) dorsally and medially into the joint space. A slight superior direction will avoid the neurovascular bundle.
    Shoulder (posterior approach)
        Rotate the patient's arm internally by having the patient place the hand on the opposite shoulder.
        Palpate the acromion process.
        Insert the needle 1 cm below the posterior tip of the acromion.
        Direct it anteriorly and medial to the humeral head.

Continued.

TABLE 15–1.—Continued

Wrist (dorsal approach)
 Patient should be sitting with pronated palm flexed slightly over a rolled towel.
 Mark the bony process of the distal radius and ulna.
 Direct the needle into the groove between the two bony processes just lateral to the extensor pollicis longus tendon.
Elbow
 Place patient's relaxed arm in lap or on pillow 45° from complete extension.
 Turn palm toward abdomen or pillow.
 Palpate the lateral epicondyle.
 The shallow depression distal to it represents the joint.
 Enter perpendicular to joint with a 22-gauge needle.
Ankle (medial approach)
 Place foot at 45° plantar flexion with heel on table.
 Palpate medial malleolus.
 Insert the needle 1.2 cm proximal and volar to the distal end of medial malleolus.
 Direct the needle 45° posteriorly, slightly upward and medial.
Knee (medial approach)
 Patient should be supine with a relaxed knee (patella freely moveable).
 Mark the inferior plane of the patella (the underside).
 Direct the needle (18 gauge) parallel to the inferior plane of the patella.
 Compression of the suprapatellar pouch may help aspiration.

TABLE 15–2.—ASSESSMENT OF SYNOVIAL FLUID*

PRESUMPTIVE DIAGNOSIS	APPEARANCE	MUCIN CLOT/ VISCOSITY	CELL COUNT (WBCs/cu mm)	% POLYS (PMNs)	PROTEIN (gm/dl)	ALBUMIN (gm/dl)	GLUCOSE % OF SERUM	CRYSTALS	COMMENTS
Normal	Clear, straw-colored	Good/high	30–150	<20	1–4	1–2	90	None	· · ·
Noninflammatory									
Trauma	Clear, turbid red or xanthochromic	Good/high	750–20,000	<30	1.3–5.0	2.5	90	None	Many RBCs, few cartilage fragments
Osteoarthritis	Clear, straw-colored	Fair to good/high	1,000–7,500	20–60	2.9–5.5	2.5	90	None	Many cartilage fragments
Systemic lupus erythematosus	Clear or turbid	Good/high	1,000–5,000	<20	1.5–4.0	2.5	90	None	LE cells
Inflammatory									
Rheumatoid Arthritis	Turbid, greenish yellow	Poor/low	5,000–100,000	60–95	3–6	2.5–3.7	80	None	Latex positive, ragocytes, low complement
Gout	Turbid, white	Poor/low	1,000–70,000	50–95	2.5–5.0	1.5–3.5	90	Sodium urate	Strongly negative birefringence
Pseudogout	Clear turbid	Fair/low	500–80,000	30–95	· · ·	· · ·	90	Calcium pyrophosphate	Weakly positive birefringence, many RBCs
Rheumatic fever	Slightly turbid	Good/low	300–100,000	60–90	1.5–5.0	2.5	90	None	—
Reiter's disease	Turbid	Fair/low	700–45,000	>60	2.5–6.0	2.0–3.6	· · ·	None	PMNs in macrophages
Infectious									
Bacterial	Turbid, gray or yellow	Poor/low	5,000–5,000,000 (>75,000)	>90	2.8–6.8	1.5–3.8	20	None	Bacteria on Gram stain, culture positive
Tuberculous	Turbid, gray or yellow	Poor/low	2,500–100,000	50	4–6	2.8–4.2	50	None	Acid-fast on smear 20% culture—80%; biopsy—90%

*Adapted from Ekhoyan G: *Medical Procedures Manual*. Chicago, Year Book Medical Publishers, 1981, pp 88–89.

ANTINUCLEAR IMMUNOFLUORESCENCE

TABLE 15–3.—Patterns of Antinuclear Immunofluorescence*

DISEASE	DIFFUSE (HOMOGENEOUS)	PERIPHERAL (RIM)	SPECKLED	NUCLEOLAR	% ANA POSITIVITY
Aging (> 60 yr)	Variable	Variable	Variable	Variable	20
Chronic liver disease	Variable	Variable	Variable	Variable	20
Drug-induced SLE	Common	Common	Less common	Less common	>90
Idiopathic pulmonary fibrosis	Variable	Variable	Variable	Variable	10
Lupus	Most common	Most common	Common	Less common	>90
Mixed connective tissue disease	Less common	Less common	Common	Less common	>90
Polymyositis	Variable	Variable	Variable	Variable	20
Pneumoconiosis	Variable	Variable	Variable	Variable	10
Rheumatoid arthritis	Common	Less common	Variable	Less common	30–50
Scleroderma	Less common	Less common	Common	Common	>70
Sicca syndrome	Less common	Less common	Common	Common	50–70

*Adapted from Beary JF III, et al (eds): *Manual of Rheumatology and Outpatient Orthopedic Disorders.* Boston, Little, Brown & Co, 1981, p 16.

ORTHOPEDIC MANEUVERS

TABLE 15–4.—ORTHOPEDIC MANEUVERS/TESTS

Knee Valgus Stress Test: To test medial collateral ligament.
Patient: Supine, leg extended and supported by examiner.
Examiner: Beside extremity tested with one hand on distal lateral femur and other on medial tibia below the joint line.
Technique: Apply medial pressure on femur while distracting tibia laterally. Note amount of opening of medial knee. It should be minimal. Compare with other leg.

Knee Varus Stress Test: To test lateral collateral ligament.
Patient: Supine, leg extended and supported by examiner.
Examiner: Beside extremity tested with one hand on distal medial femur and other on the lateral tibia below the joint line.
Technique: Apply lateral pressure on the femur while distracting the tibia medially. Note amount of opening of lateral knee. It should be minimal. Compare to other leg.

Straight Leg Raise: To test for protrusion of disk causing radicular pain.
Patient: Supine
Examiner: Gently hold leg at knee and ankle.
Technique: Slowly raise the leg through 60° of motion. Pain will be felt if positive between 30° and 60° in back, hip, and leg.

Spurling Test: To test for cervical restriction or foramen restriction.
Patient: Seated on stool.
Examiner: Standing with hands on patient's head.
Technique: Apply downward pressure with neck straight, left, left posterior, right, right posterior. Elicited pain or neurologic symptom is positive test.

McMurray Sign: To test for tears in medial and lateral menisci.
Patient: Supine and relaxed with knee completely bent.
Examiner: Standing at the side of the injured limb.
Technique: Grasp the heel and rotate the foot externally while abducting the leg and extending the knee. A click or pain is significant for lateral tear. Opposite maneuver can be positive for medial tear and is done by rotating the foot internally and abducting the leg while extending the knee.

Apprehension Test: To test for patella subluxation.
Patient: Seated
Examiner: Hand on affected patella.
Technique: Gently push the patella laterally. A start of apprehension is positive. If negative, examiner can extend the knee and then passively flex the knee while gently pushing the patella laterally.

Continued.

TABLE 15–4.—Continued

Anterior Drawer Sign: To test the anterior cruciate.
    Patient: Supine, hip flexed 45°, knee flexed 90°.
    Examiner: Sitting on patient's ipsilateral foot.
    Technique: Place hands around the tibia just below the joint line. Apply anterior force and note the amount of anterior motion. Always compare with other knee.
Lachman Test: When the knee can't be flexed.
    Patient: Supine, hip and knee extended.
    Examiner: Standing beside patient.
    Technique: Grasp the femur with one hand and the tibia below the joint line. Apply a distracting force to the tibia and note the excursion.
Posterior Drawer Sign: To test the posterior cruciate.
    Patient: Supine, hip flexed, 45°, knee flexed 90°.
    Examiner: Sitting on patient's ipsilateral foot.
    Technique: Same as anterior drawer sign, except apply posterior force on tibia.

INTRA-ARTICULAR INJECTION

TABLE 15–5.—INTRA-ARTICULAR STEROID INJECTIONS

Mix 1% lidocaine and steroid:
    For elbow or ankle, 10–40 mg of methylprednisolone acetate in 0.5 ml of 1% lidocaine.
    For knee or shoulder, 40–80 mg of methylprednisolone acetate in 1 ml of 1% lidocaine.
Use the approaches listed in Table 15–1 to enter the joint.
Aspirate to be sure you are not in a vessel.
Inject and apply a sterile bandage.
Advise patient that there may be an initial irritation from the steroid lasting less than 24 hours.
This may need to be repeated in severe inflammation.
Bursae overlie these joints and can be injected with the same preparation.

AVERAGE RANGES OF JOINT MOTION

TABLE 15–6.—AVERAGE RANGES OF
JOINT MOTION

JOINT	DEGREES
Shoulder	
Horizontal flexion	135
Horizontal extension	—
Neutral abduction	170
Forward flexion	158
Backward extension	53
Inward rotation	70
Outward rotation	90
Elbow	
Flexion	146
Extension	0
Forearm	
Pronation	71
Supination	84
Wrist	
Flexion	73
Extension	71
Radial deviation	19
Ulnar deviation	33
Hip	
Beginning position flexion	—
Flexion	113
Extension	28
Abduction	48
Adduction	31
Inward rotation	45
Outward rotation	45
Knee	
Beginning position flexion	—
Flexion	134
Ankle	
Flexion (plantar)	48
Extension (dorsiflexion)	18
Fore part of the foot	
Inversion	33
Eversion	18

*From *Manual of Orthopaedic Surgery.*
Chicago, American Orthopedic Association,
1966. Reproduced by permission.

SCOLIOSIS SCREENING

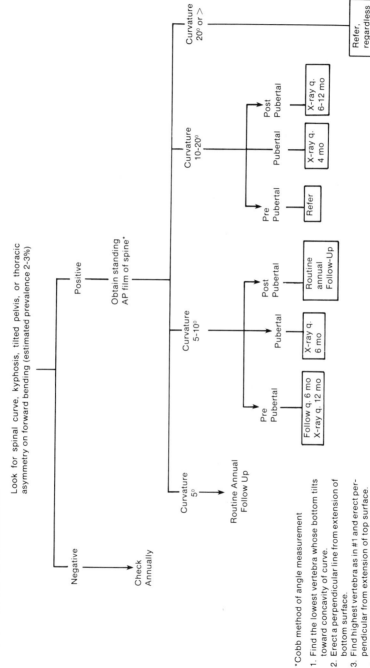

Look for spinal curve, kyphosis, tilted pelvis, or thoracic asymmetry on forward bending (estimated prevalence 2-3%)

*Cobb method of angle measurement

1. Find the lowest vertebra whose bottom tilts toward concavity of curve.
2. Erect a perpendicular line from extension of bottom surface.
3. Find highest vertebra as in #1 and erect perpendicular from extension of top surface.
4. Measure intersecting angle = angle of scoliosis

FIG 15–1.
Scoliosis screening and follow-up.

DISEASES WITH POLYARTHRITIS

TABLE 15–7.—Differential Diagnosis of Diseases With Polyarthritis*

ASPECT	RHEUMATOID ARTHRITIS	GONOCOCCAL ARTHRITIS	RHEUMATIC FEVER	JOINT MANIFESTATIONS OF INFECTIOUS DISEASES	OSTEOARTHRITIS	GOUT
Age	Adults under 40	Young adults	Children and young adults	Children, mainly	Middle age	Middle age
Etiology	Nonspecific or infectious	Gonococcus	Probably allergic from hemolytic streptococcus	Allergic or specific infectious	Metabolic disturbance; senescence	Disturbance of purine metabolism
Mode of onset	Usually insidious; occasionally acute	Acute	Acute	Acute	Insidious	Acute
Involvement	Periarticular and synovial; no effusion	Periarticular and synovial; moderate effusion	Periarticular and synovial; very little effusion	Periarticular and synovial; rarely, purulent effusion	Spurring and lipping of bones at joints	Accumulation of sodium monourate in joint spaces and ends of bones
Joints affected	Many, large and small	Often multiple, sometimes monarticular; knees, ankles, wrists, elbows, feet	Multiple and migratory; mainly large joints	Usually multiple	Mainly weight-bearing joints and distal phalangeal joints of fingers	Frequently multiple; sometimes monarticular; toes and fingers often

Continued.

425

TABLE 15–7.—Continued

ASPECT	RHEUMATOID ARTHRITIS	GONOCOCCAL ARTHRITIS	RHEUMATIC FEVER	JOINT MANIFESTATIONS OF INFECTIOUS DISEASES	OSTEOARTHRITIS	GOUT
Result	General debility; joint ankylosis and deformity	Little general effect; may go on to ankylosis	No residual joint trouble; residual cardiac involvement	Usually no residual joint involvement; occasionally suppurative arthritis	General health good; no ankylosis; mainly pain	Swellings due to deposits of urates (tophi); urates may be discharged through skin
Diagnostic aids	Increased sedimentation rate of RBC; presence of streptococcus agglutinins in blood	Presence of genitourinary gonorrhea; positive complement fixation test; gonococci in joint fluid; therapeutic test	Severe acute infectious manifestations; cardiac involvement; relief of pain by salicylates	Manifestations of the disease of which the arthritis is a complication	Absence of evidence of infection	High blood uric acid; increased urate content of urine; presence of urate crystals in discharging crystals
X-ray findings	Rarefaction of ends of bones; thinning of joint space	Soft tissue swelling when acute; "moth-eaten" bone ends when chronic	Negative	Negative	Spurring and lipping of bones	Punched-out areas at ends of bones after years of disease
Course	Chronic with acute exacerbations	Acute or chronic	Acute with recurrences	Acute	Chronic	Chronic with acute exacerbations

*From Yater, WM: *Fundamentals of Internal Medicine.* New York, Appleton-Century-Crofts. Reproduced by permission.

RHEUMATOID ARTHRITIS

TABLE 15–8.—Diagnostic Criteria for Rheumatoid Arthritis*

Classic rheumatoid arthritis: Requires 7 of the following criteria. Criteria 1–5 must be continuously present for at least 6 weeks.

Definite rheumatoid arthritis: Requires 5 of the following criteria. Criteria 1–5 must be continuously present for at least 6 weeks.

Probable rheumatoid arthritis: Requires 3 of the following criteria. One of criteria 1–5 must be continuously present for at least 6 weeks.

    Criteria
1. Morning stiffness
2. Pain on motion or tenderness in at least one joint[†]
3. Soft tissue swelling in at least one joint[†]
4. Swelling of at least one other joint within past 3 months[†]
5. Symmetric joint swelling[†]—same joint both sides of body; distal phalangeal joint does not count
6. Subcutaneous nodules[†]
7. X-ray changes: decalcification adjacent to affected joint
8. Positive rheumatoid factor
9. Poor mucin precipitate from synovial fluid
10. Histologic changes in synovium
11. Histologic changes in nodules

Possible rheumatoid arthritis: Requires 2 of the following criteria and joint symptoms continuously present for at least 6 weeks.
1. Morning stiffness
2. Pain on motion or tenderness recurring or persisting for 3 weeks[†]
3. History or observation of joint swelling
4. Subcutaneous nodules[†]
5. Elevated sedimentation rate or C-reactive protein
6. Iritis

*Adapted from Schumacher HR (ed): *Primer on the Rheumatic Diseases,* ed 9. Atlanta, Arthritis Foundation, 1988, p 316.
[†]Observed by physician

TABLE 15–9.—Rheumatoid Factor

    Rheumatoid factor is an antibody found in many disease states but in high titer in rheumatoid arthritis. It can occur in 5% of normal patients less than 60 years old and in 30% of normal patients over 80 years old.

    Other diseases associated with elevated levels of rheumatoid factor are:

Ankylosing spondylitis	Leprosy
Chronic active hepatitis	Psoriatic arthritis
Cirrhosis	Sarcoidosis
Dermatomyositis	Sjögren's syndrome
Enteropathic arthritis	Subacute bacterial endocarditis
Idiopathic pulmonary fibrosis	Systemic lupus erythematosus
Juvenile chronic arthritis	

TABLE 15–10.—Juvenile Rheumatoid Arthritis

SYNDROMES	% OF CASES OF JRA	SIGNS AND SYMPTOMS	PROGNOSIS
Systemic onset disease Male > female; median age at onset, 5 yr	25	Fever, rash, arthritis, myalgia and distinctive extra-articular manifestations such as lymphadenopathy, splenomegaly, hepatomegaly, pericarditis, pneumonitis, pleuritis; ANA and RF are negative	One third become disabled; chronic, progressive
Polyarticular disease Seronegative: Female > male; median age at onset, 2 yr	25	Insidious onset, initially involves small joints of hands and feet; RF negative, 25% are ANA positive	One sixth become disabled
Seropositive: female > male; median age at onset, 12 yr	10	Insidious onset, initially involves hands and feet; RF positive, ANA negative, nodules, tendonitis, HLA-B27 present in 75%	Rapidly progressive
Pauciarticular Female > male; median age at onset, 2–4 yr	30	Involves one or a few joints, most commonly knees and ankles; 50% have chronic iridocyclitis; RF negative, ANA positive in 50%	Good prognosis, mild disability

OSTEOARTHRITIS AND OTHER JOINT DISORDERS

TABLE 15–11.—Joint Disorders

Osteoarthritis (degenerative joint disease)
  Loss of joint cartilage and bone hypertrophy.
  Present in 85% of people >70 years old.
  Symptoms begin in fifth and sixth decades.
  Joint pain with use of weight-bearing.
  Heberden's nodes found on dorsolateral aspect of base of distal phalanx.
  Sedimentation rate is normal.
  Rheumatoid factor negative.
Systemic lupus erythematosus (SLE)
  Diagnosis: Patient must have four of the following manifestations, not neces-
    sarily at the same time:
  Malar rash
  Discoid rash
  Photosensitivity
  Oral or nasopharyngeal ulcers
  Arthritis (2 or more joints)
  Pleuritis or pericarditis
  Urine casts or proteinuria >0.5 gm/24 hr
  Seizures or psychosis
  Hematologic disorder:
    hemolytic anemia
    or leukopenia <4,000/mm^3 on 2 occasions
    or lymphopenia <1,500/mm^3 on 2 occasions
    or thrombocytopenia <100,000/mm^3
  Immune disorder
    LE cells
    or anti-DNA
    or anti-smooth muscle
    or false positive serologic test for syphilis for 6 months
  Antinuclear antibody

Continued.

TABLE 15–11.—Continued

Acute gouty arthritis
   Arthritis Foundation Classification Criteria:
      One or more of the following:
         Urate crystals in joint fluid
         Tophus containing urate crystals.
      Six of the following:
         More than one attack
         Maximum inflammation in one day
         Attack of monoarticular arthritis
         Observed joint erythema
         First metatarsophalangeal joint painful or swollen
         Unilateral attack at first metatarsophalangeal joint
         Unilateral attack at tarsal joint
         Suspected tophus
         Hyperuricemia
         X-ray evidence of asymmetric swelling within a joint
         X-ray evidence of subcortical cysts without erosions
         Negative joint fluid culture during attack
Raynaud phenomenon: A common disorder with female predominance (5:1)
   manifested as episodic transient pallor of the fingers when exposed to cold.
   The pallor is followed by cyanosis and finally by rubor and pain. Episodes may
   last from minutes to hours. In 50%–90% of cases there is no associated sys-
   temic disease.
Pseudogout (calcium pyrophosphate deposition disease)
   Three forms
      1. Acute arthritis
      2. Chondrocalcinosis
      3. Progressive oligoarticular disease
   10% of patients also have hyperparathyroidism or hemochromatosis.
   Synovial fluid (see Table 15–3)
   X-ray films may reveal calcifications in menisci or hyaline cartilage.
   There is a hereditary form (autosomal dominant).
   Treatment: Anti-inflammatory agents

SHOULDER PAIN

TABLE 15–12.—EVALUATION AND TREATMENT OF SHOULDER PAIN*

ENTITY	CHARACTER OF PAIN, HISTORY	PHYSICAL FINDINGS	X-RAY FINDINGS	TREATMENT
Glenohumeral osteoarthritis	Dull, aching, not severe	Crepitus, ↓ ROM	Degenerative changes of joint	Conservative†
Rotator cuff injury	Chronic pain, history of weakness in arm elevation	Pain in active abduction, 70°–100° positive "drop arm" sign	Normal, or degenerative changes of greater tuberosity	Surgery if total, otherwise conservative†
Bicipital tendonitis	Pain, anterior shoulder; radiates to biceps and forearm; limited abduction	Tender to palpation in bicipital groove; pain on resisted elbow flexion or wrist supination	Irregularity of bicipital groove (requires special views)	Conservative† plus steroid injection over bicipital groove
Adhesive capsulitis (frozen shoulder)	Pain and stiffness often follows prior shoulder condition, i.e., prolonged immobility	Restricted active and passive ROM, all planes	Localized osteopenia; otherwise normal	Prevention: Early mobilization of shoulder injuries; steroid injection plus conservative†
Calcific tendinitis/subacromial bursitis	Sudden, severe, diffuse pain, radiates to deltoid; can't sleep on side	Severe pain on active abduction; tender over upper deltoid and teres major	Calcification of supraspinatus tendon	Conservative;† treat pain; intrabursal steroid injection; rest, but mobilize ASAP

Continued.

431

TABLE 15–12.—Continued

Thoracic outlet syndrome	Pain in shoulder and/or arm, plus fullness or numbness	↓ sensation, muscle weakness, ↓ radial pulse; positive Adson's maneuver (↓ pulse plus reproduces symptoms)	Cervical rib on chest x-ray film	Postural training; surgery if recurrent
Referred shoulder pain	Many types, usually diffuse and vague; consider neck, arm, hand pain	Exam of shoulder should be normal	Normal	Diagnose underlying cause, e.g., nerve root compression, lung/plueral disease, MI, subphrenic abscess

*Adapted from Kozin F, in McCarty DJ (ed): *Arthritis and Allied Conditions*, ed 9. Philadelphia, Lea & Febiger, 1979, p 1100.
†Conservative treatment: sling, ASA or NSAID, cold packs for acute, hot packs for chronic pendulum q.i.d.

LOW BACK PAIN

TABLE 15–13.—LOW BACK PAIN*

Differential diagnosis
  Mechanical low back pain:
    Ligament sprain
    Acute or chronic muscle pain
  Herniated nucleus pulposis
  Degenerative joint disease
  "Facet syndrome"
  Congenital spinal anomalies
  Rheumatic disease (RA, anklyosing spondylitis)
  Referred pain (GI, GU, GYN)
  Metastatic bone lesions
Symptoms
  Stiffness (muscular component)
  Ache in A.M. (inflammation)
  Numbness, weakness, paresthesia, ↑ with Valsalva, radiation (neurologic
    component, radiculopathy)
  Bladder, bowel or sexual dysfunction (sacral radiculopathy, cord tumor)
Examination
  Observe lordosis: Loss of lordosis represents body's attempt to remain rigid
    and protect a sore back.
  Palpate for trigger points.
  With the patient supine, flex the hip by lifting the extended leg. If pain is pro-
    duced, note the position. This indicates pain with nerve stretching.
  Check reflexes:

Test	Nerve Root	Nerve
Knee jerk	L2, L3, L4	Femoral
Ankle jerk	L5, S1, S2	Posterior tibial

  Check motor strength:

Test	Nerve	Muscle
Squat	L2, L3, L4	Quadriceps
Toe walk	L4, L5	Anterior Tibialis
Great toe extension	L5	Extensor Hallicus Longus

Continued.

TABLE 15–13.—Continued

Further testing when needed:

Test	Implication
EMG	Confirms or quantifies neurologic defect
CT scan or myelogram	Evaluates for herniated disc, spinal stenosis, or extradural masses
Lumbosacral x-rays	Evaluates for disc space narrowing, DJD facet joints, tumor, anomalies
Sed. rate	Screens for rheumatic diseases
Urinalysis	Infection, proteinuria

Acute treatment
    Strict bed rest for pain of all etiologies.
    Anti-inflammatory medications for DJD and acute injury.
    Analgesics.
    Heat for mild to moderate stiffness.
    Point specific ice massage in severe pain.
    Muscle relaxants.
Chronic Treatment
    Weight loss.
    Corset for short-term immobilization.
    Physical therapy for stretching and long-term muscle conditioning program.
    Surgical consult if documented neurologic defect and failure to respond to conservative therapy.

*Courtesy of Paul Dusseau, MD, Riverside Family Practice Center, Columbus, Ohio.

MONORADICULAR SYMPTOMS

TABLE 15–14.—MONORADICULAR SYMPTOMS AND THEIR ETIOLOGY*

AFFECTED NERVE ROOT	PAIN	TENDERNESS	PARESTHESIAS AND SENSORY DEFICIT	WEAKNESS, FASCICULATION, AND ATROPHY	REFLEX CHANGES
6th Cervical	Radiation from neck into lateral arm and forearm; interscapular pain	Lower cervical spine, brachial plexus, median nerve	Dorsal and lateral aspect of thumb	Biceps	Diminished biceps reflex
7th Cervical	Same as 6th cervical	Lower cervical spine, brachial plexus	Index finger and usually middle finger	Triceps	Depressed or absent triceps reflex
8th Cervical	Radiation from neck into medial arm and forearm; interscapular pain	Lower cervical spine, brachial plexus, ulnar nerve	5th and ulnar half of 4th finger ulnar side of hand	Intrinsic hand muscles	None
4th Lumbar	Back pain radiation into anterior thigh	Midlumbar spine, femoral nerve	Anterior thigh just above knee	Quadriceps	Depressed or absent knee reflex
5th Lumbar	Back pain radiating into buttocks and posterior aspect of thigh	Low lumbar spine, sciatic and occasionally superficial peroneal nerves	Dorsum of foot and great toe	Dorsiflexors of foot and great toe	None
1st Sacral	Same as 5th lumbar	Lumbosacral junction, sciatic nerve	Lateral aspect foot and small toe	Plantar flexors of foot (calf)	Depressed or absent ankle reflex

*From Blacklow RS: Signs and Symptoms, ed 6. Philadelphia, JB Lippincott Co, 1983, p 233. Reproduced by permission.

SPORTS INJURIES

TABLE 15–15.—COMMON SPORTS INJURIES

INJURY/CONDITION	HISTORY	SPECIAL TESTING/HISTORY	TREATMENT	RESUMPTION OF SPORTS
Ligamentous injuries of the knee	Twisting injuries with pain and swelling	Testing is specific for ligament injured	Treatment is dependent on grade of injury	
Medial collateral Lateral collateral Anterior cruciate Posterior cruciate	Lateral force Medial force "Pop" or "snap" heard in 50%	Valgus stress test Varus stress test Anterior drawer sign Posterior drawer sign	Grade I (pain, swelling, stable): ice, compression dressing; grade II (pain, swelling, moderate unstable): cylinder cast 4–6 weeks; grade III (marked instability): usually surgical but may improve with immobilization	When knee is minimally painful, stable, range of motion is good, and patient can run in place, hop on affected leg, run figure-of-8 in both directions, start and stop quickly
Meniscus tear	Twisting injury followed by swelling, locking, pain and negative ligament stress test	Arthroscopy; knee locking or "giving way" is typical	Surgical resection, often through arthroscope	Minimal pain, good range of motion
Patella subluxation	Generally bilateral knee pain, squatting, climbing stairs	Clicking on squatting and pain on climbing stairs	Quadriceps strengthening; patellar cut-out brace	When comfortable

Condition	Symptoms	Diagnosis	Treatment	Return to Play
Corns, calluses, blisters	Painful hypertrophic skin changes	May need x-ray to see if there is underlying structural deformity	Padding, reduction of source of friction	When comfortable
Subungual hematoma	Traumatic hematoma with pain	Trauma	Evacuation of hematoma with perforation of nail by hot paper clip or needle	When comfortable
Stress fractures	Repetitive stress like running; sudden or gradual onset of pain and swelling	Most common in shafts of first, second, third metatarsals	Short leg cast for 3–4 weeks then weight-bearing but protected	Gradually when asymptomatic
Plantar fasciitis	Burning ache along fascia, worse with activity	X-ray may show calcaneal spurs	Ice, Achilles tendon stretch, anti-inflammatory drug	With good warm-up after improving
Achilles tendinitis	Repeated stress to the Achilles tendon, pain and swelling	None	Limit running while acute; anti-inflammatory drug	When asymptomatic with aggressive Achilles tendon stretch program
Shin splints	Aching pain in posteromedial aspect of lower leg after running	None	Ice and rest; tendon stretching	When asymptomatic, tendon stretch program; avoid hard surfaces
Hamstring pull	Pain in back of thigh or at hamstring origin in pelvis	X-ray may show avulsion injury	Ice, rest, stretch program	When asymptomatic, good warm-up needed to avoid reinjury
Brachial plexus injury	Hyperextension of neck with counter traction of arm	Numbness in arm and fingers lasting ≤5 min	Protect shoulder	If lasting <5 min, may resume

TABLE 15–16.—SPORTS MEDICINE HEAD INJURIES

Mild concussion
No loss of consciousness
Brief headache
Dazed behavior, mental confusion
Lack of coordination
Ringing in ears
Return to play: when symptoms are clear. Obtain neurosurgical consultation after 3 mild concussions.
Moderate concussion
Loss of consciousness <5 min
Headache
Change in behavior
Numbness
Weakness
Return to play: after 24 hours of observation and symptoms are clear. Obtain neurosurgical consultation after 2 moderate concussions.
Severe concussion
Loss of consciousness >5 min
Headache
Change in behavior
Lack of coordination
Weakness
Return to play: after emergency treatment, hospitalization, and neurosurgical evaluation.

TABLE 15–17.—HEAT ILLNESS

Heat injuries include syncope, cramps, exhaustion, and stroke. These are all preventable, and an unlimited water supply must be readily available for the athletes. Sling psychrometer and wetbulb reading are useful guides for practice precautions.
<66°F: No precautions necessary.
67–77°F: Unlimited water available and all athletes must be encouraged to drink whether thirsty or not.
78–94°F: Alter practice schedule to a lighter routine and lighter clothing, withhold heat illness susceptible athletes.
>95°F: No practice.
Weight loss of individual athletes after practice during conditioning will identify susceptible or "at risk" athletes.

General Guidelines After Practice Weight Loss
3% loss: Safe.
5% loss: Susceptible to heat illness.
7% loss: Dangerous because subsequent sweating capability is severely limited, and heat stroke is likely.

PHYSICAL THERAPY MODALITIES

TABLE 15–18.—PHYSICAL THERAPY MODALITIES

MODALITY	ACTION	INDICATIONS	CONTRAINDICATIONS	HOW TO ORDER
Moist heat:				
Hot packs	Circulation Muscle relaxation	Muscle spasm Joint contracture	Sensory loss Malignant tumor Open lesions	20 min
Whirlpool	Cleansing Muscle relaxation	Open lesions Muscle spasm	Poor heat tolerance Cortisone withdrawal	20 min
Therapeutic pool	Decrease gravity to aid in exercise	To aid exercise and ambulation training	Cardiovascular disease	Temp 94°–96°; progress from shallow to deep water; continue exercise after leaving water
Dry heat:				
Diathermy	Circulation Muscle relaxation	Muscle spasm Chronic pain Adhesive capsulitis	Metallic implants Coagulation defects Sensory loss Open lesions Malignancy	20 min, 3 times/week, for 1– 2 weeks
Infrared		Muscle spasm Relief of pain Promotes healing of open lesions	Sensory loss Excessive scar tissue	Buy infrared bulb, keep 20″ from skin; direct it perpendicular to skin for 30 min; may repeat after cooling skin 1 hour

Continued.

TABLE 15–18.—Continued

MODALITY	ACTION	INDICATIONS	CONTRAINDICATIONS	HOW TO ORDER
Deep heat: Ultrasound	Muscle relaxation	Joint pain Contractures	Application to eyes Pregnancy, malignancy Caution S/P laminectomy	10–15 min
Cold packs, ice massage		Acute trauma	Raynaud phenomena Cryoglobulinemia	Freeze water in paper cups; peel away paper at open end; massage affected area with circular movement
Intermittent traction	Spine distraction	Cervical DJD Lumbar DJD Herniated disk	Unstable vertebrae Malignancy Pregnancy Spinal cord disease	50–60 lb (max. of 10 for neck); intermittently; need PT instruction
Paraffin baths	Minimizes pain Heats joint capsule	Arthritis	Sensory loss which could lead to burns	5–10 min per treatment; home units and MITS are available with PT instruction

CASTING TECHNIQUES

TABLE 15–19.—CASTING TECHNIQUES*

General principles
  The hotter the water, the faster the plaster will set.
  Stockinette should be the first layer applied.
  Next, line the extremity with padding (e.g., Webril).
  Extra padding or felt should be applied to bony prominences.
  Wear gloves (protection and smoothing of plaster).
  Soak plaster until bubbling stops, squeeze gently, then apply.
  Start plaster at either end.
  Advance plaster about ⅓–½ width of roll per turn.
  Six or seven layers are the usual thickness needed.
  Turn stockinette onto plaster and incorporate into cast to form smooth soft
    edge.
  Sculpt plaster with both hands while applying.
  Do not pull plaster tight as you roll it.
  Check capillary filling and for paresthesias q1–2 h for first 24 hours while
    awake; office f/u in 24–48 hours.
Short arm cast: For nondisplaced fractures of the forearm and wrist
  Have an assistant hold patient's arm in 90° flexion with arm partially extended
    while applying case.
  Extend cast to, not beyond, MCP joints.
  Include thumb, if for navicular fracture.
  Hold wrist in 15°–20° extension.
  If thumb spica, hold thumb in "neutral" position.
  Use 4″ plaster (2″ may be used for hand and thumb).
Short leg cast: For nondisplaced fractures of the lower leg and ankle
  Apply with patient on end of table, knee at 90° flexion.
  Keep ankle in neutral position avoiding plantar flexion.
  Use 6″ plaster (4″ may be used around ankle).
  After applying one or two layers, fold four 4″ splints longitudinally and place
    one on each side and front and back of ankle.
  Apply one additional layer and trim as needed.
  If walking cast is desired, fill arch of foot with splints to make a flat surface;
    apply rubber "walker" and secure with a plaster bandage.

---

*Adapted from Iverson LD, Clawson DK: *Manual of Acute Orthopedic Therapeutics,*
ed 2. Boston, Little, Brown & Co, 1982, pp 66–77.

16 *Drug Therapy*

Barry L. Carter, Pharm.D.

SELECTED DRUG CATEGORIES

TABLE 16–1.—ANTIARRHYTHMIC AGENTS

DRUG (HOW SUPPLIED)	DOSAGE	ADVERSE REACTIONS	COMMENTS
1A agents			
Quinidine sulfate (various) Tabs., caps.: 100, 200, 300 mg Tabs. (sustained-release) (Quinidex): 300 mg Inj.: 200 mg/ml Quinidine gluconate (Duraquine, Quinaglute) Tabs.: 324, 330 mg (sustained-release)	200–300 mg 3–4 × daily, then individualize Sustained-release: 300–600 mg q8–12h (max 1,800 mg/day) Parenteral: 300–600 mg IM or IV; inject IV *slowly* (1 ml/min of diluted solution) Therapeutic range: 2–6 µg/ml	Nausea, diarrhea, cinchonism (tinnitus, headache, vertigo), hypotension, syncope, thrombocytopenia, fever, dysrhythmias, angioedema, asthma	Monitor BP, ECG, QT prolongation, serum levels Sulfate = 83% quinidine; gluconate = 62% quinidine *Interactions:* Quinidine ↑ digoxin levels, warfarin response; ↓ quinidine effect with phenobarbital, phenytoin, rifampin, thiazides, urinary alkalinization; ↑ quinidine effect with cimetidine Warnings: digitalize first in patients with atrial fibrillation/flutter; avoid IV administration; caution with heart block *Contraindications:* digoxin toxicity, severe conduction defects, CHF, poor renal function

Continued.

TABLE 16–1.—Continued

DRUG (HOW SUPPLIED)	DOSAGE	ADVERSE REACTIONS	COMMENTS
Disopyramide (Norpace and Various) Caps.: 100 mg, 150 mg Controlled release (Norpace-CR): 100, 150 mg	Load: 300 mg (200 mg if < 50 kg); maintenance: 400– 800 mg/day in 4 doses (q12h with sustained release) *Children:* < 1 yr, 10–30 mg/ kg/day, 1–4 yr, 10–20; 4– 12 yr, 10–15; 12–18 yr, 6– 15 mg/kg/day *Renal Impairment:* CrCl: 30–40 ml/min, 100 mg q8h; 15–30, 100 mg q12h; < 15, 100 mg q24h	Dry mouth, urinary retention, constipation, blurred vision, congestive heart failure, enhanced AV conduction, heart block, ventricular arrhythmias	Capsule contents can be mixed in cherry syrup High anticholinergic Avoid in patients with history of CHF, WPW, bundle-branch block, or those taking β-blockers or verapamil Contraindicated: shock, sick sinus, AV block Digitalize before using in atrial fibrillation Monitor ECG for QRS or QT prolongation, discontinue or lower dose if >25%–30% widening; monitor serum levels
Procainamide (Procan, Pronestyl, various) Tabs., Caps.: 250, 375, 500 mg Tabs. (sustained): 250, 500, 750, 1,000 mg Inj.: 100, 500 mg/ml	Oral: load 1 gm, maintenance dose is 50 mg/kg/day (given 3gh), then adjust (q6h for sustained release) IV bolus: 100 mg q5min (slowly at 50 mg/min), up to 1 gm or suppression of dysrhythmia or toxicity IV infusion: 20–25 mg/min for 30 min, then 2–5 mg/min	Anorexia, nausea, urticaria, SLE syndrome, blood dyscrasias, QRS and QT interval prolongation, dysrhythmias, fever, neutropenia, hypotension	Monitor BP, ECG, QT interval, procainamide and NAPA serum levels, ANA *Contraindications:* procain allergy, 2d- or 3d-degree AV block, myasthenia gravis Procan-SR or Pronestyl SR given q6H—wax matrix may be found in stool but no drug remains

1B Agents

Lidocaine (Xylocaine, various) Inj.: Various Cream, soln., jelly	See Chapter 7 for parenteral dosage regimens.	Numbness, twitching, euphoria, dysphoria, drowsiness, convulsions, bradycardia, hypotension, rash, urticaria	*Contraindications:* hypersensitivity, Adams-Stokes, WPW, severe nodal block ↓ Metabolism in CHF and liver disease ↑ Levels with propranolol and cimetidine (Tagamet) Additive effects with procainamide Levels ↑ after 24 hr following acute MI
Phenytoin	See individual drug section (Table 16–11)		
Tocainide (Tonocard) Tabs: 400, 600 mg	400 mg every q8h, range (1,200–1,800 mg) well controlled patients q12h	Up to 50%, have nausea, vomiting, dizziness, tremor, confusion, paresthesias, and other CNS reactions, pulmonary fibrosis, blood dyscrasias; increase rate in atrial fib/flutter	*Cautions:* CHF, heart block Monitor: CBC Food may decrease side effects
Mexiletine (Mexitil) Caps.: 150, 200, 250 mg	Load: 400 mg; maintenance: 200 mg q8h (max 1,200 mg day); some controlled every 12 h; reduce dose with liver disease or severe CHF	High percentage nausea, vomiting, dizziness, tremor, increased LFTs, rash, seizures	*Cautions:* conduction disturbance, liver damage *Contraindications:* 2d- or 3d-degree heart block

Continued.

445

TABLE 16–1.—Continued

DRUG (HOW SUPPLIED)	DOSAGE	ADVERSE REACTIONS	COMMENTS
1C agents			
Encainide (Enkaid) Caps.: 25, 35, 50 mg	25 mg q8h, increase in 3–5 days if necessary to 50 mg q8h (recommend that drug be started in hospital)	Proarrhythmias, dizziness, tremor, headache, GI, CHF	Complex kinetics are phenotypically determined Contraindications: 2d- or 3d-degree block Caution: CHF, SSS
Flecainide (Tambocor) Tabs: 100 mg	Initial: 100 mg q12h (max 600 mg/day) (recommend that drug be started in hospital)	CNS common, proarrhythmias, CHF, heart block, rash, blood dyscrasias (rare)	Contraindications: 2d- or 3d-degree block Caution: CHF, liver disease, SSS, propranolol, verapamil
II agent			
Propranolol	See Table 16–2 for beta blockers		
III Agents			
Bretylium (Bretylol) Inj.: 50 mg/ml	5–10 mg/kg IV, repeat if needed; maintenance: 1–2 mg/min	Hypotension, nausea, vomiting, proarrhythmias	Monitor BP, arrythmias
Amiodarone (Cordarone) Tabs: 200 mg	Due to the extreely complex kinetics, severe adverse reactions, and multiple drug interactons, this drug should be used only by those with experience with this agent.		
IV agents			
Verapamil Digoxin	See calcium channel blocker table See individual drugs		

TABLE 16–2.—BETA BLOCKERS

DRUG	DOSAGE	ADVERSE REACTIONS	COMMENTS
Beta-blockers	See individual agents for dosing (Table 16–11) *Receptors Blocked:* / *Daily Doses:*	Drowsiness, dizziness, fatigue, nightmares, bronchospasm, bradycardia, heart failure, heart block, cold extremities, GI disturbances, impotence. Labetalol has higher incidence of nasal stuffiness, orthostatic dizziness, dry mouth, and impotence due to α-blockade	β_1 selective agents will inhibit β_2 in higher doses
Acebutolol	β_1 (partial agonist) 2		All may aggravate asthma, COPD, CHF, and block symptoms of hypoglycemia in insulin-dependent diabetics; avoid using
Atenolol	β_1 1		Reduce dose over 1–2 wk when discontinuing
Labetalol	$\beta_1, \beta_2, \alpha_1$ 3–4		Food increases absorption of propranolol and metoprolol
Metoprolol	β_1 1–2		Epinephrine → marked hypertension may occur from vasoconstriction
Nadolol	β_1, β_2 1		↑ incidence of bradycardia and conduction disturbances with verapamil and diltiazem
Pindolol	β_1, β_2 (partial agonist) 2		
Propranolol	β_1, β_2 2–4		
Timolol	β_1, β_2 2		

447

TABLE 16–3.—CALCIUM CHANNEL BLOCKERS*

PROPERTY	NIFEDIPINE (PROCARDIA, ADALAT)	VERAPAMIL (ISOPTIN, CALAN)	DILTIAZEM (CARDIZEM)
Half-life	2–5 hr	10–18 hr (chronic dosing)	3–5 hr
Daily doses	3–4 (once with sustained)	2–3 (once with sustained)	3–4 (twice with sustained)
Heart rate	Increase	0, decrease	0, decrease
Vasodilation	+ + +	+ +	+
AV conduction	0	Decrease	Decrease
Cost	+ + +	+ +	+ + +

*See individual agents for additional information.

TABLE 16–4.—COMMON DRUGS FOR HYPERLIPIDEMIAS*†

DRUG‡	CHOLESTEROL	LDL	HDL	TRIGLYCERIDES
Cholestyramine	↓	↓	0, ↑	0, ↑
Colestipol	↓	↓	0, ↑	0, ↑
Niacin	↓	↓	↑	↓
Gemfibrozil	↓	↓	↑	↓
Lovastatin	↓ ↓	↓ ↓	↑	↓
Probucol	↓	↓	↓	0

*Adapted from *Drug Facts and Comparisons, 1988 Edition.* St Louis, Facts and Comparisons, Division of JB Lippincott Co, 1988, p 171f.
†See individual drugs for dosing and availability.
‡The only agents that have been shown to lower cardiovascular morbidity include cholestyramine, niacin, and gemfibrozil.

TABLE 16–5.—ORAL CONTRACEPTIVES

	ESTROGEN (μg)	PROGESTERONE (mg)	ANDROGENIC ACTIVITY IN PROGESTERONE
Low estrogen, low progest.			
Loestrin 1/20	E-20	NA-1	+ +
Ovcon-35	E-35	N-0.4	+ +
Brevicon/Modicon	E-35	N-0.5	+ +
Ortho Novum 10/11	E-35	N-0.5 × 10 days 1.0 × 11 days	+ +
Norinyl/Ortho Novum 1/35	E-35	N-1	+ +
Norinyl/Ortho Novum 1/50	M-50	N-1	+ +
Low estrogen, moderate to high progest.			
Nordette	E-30	L 0.15	+ + +
LoOvral	E-30	Norgest. 0.30	+ + +
Loestrin 1.5/30	E-30	NA 1.5	+ +
Demulin 1/35	E-35	ED 1.0	+ +
Ovral	E-50	Norgest. 0.5	+ + +

KEY:
Estrogen:
E—ethinyl estradiol
M—mestranol

Progesterones:
N—norethindrone
NA—norethindrone acetate
L—levonorgestrel
Norgest.—Norgestrel
ED—ethynodiol diacetate
Noreth.—Norethynodrel

NOTE: The overall estrogen/progesterone balance for a given estrogen dose will depend on the progestin and dose, i.e., Norethynodrel contains estrogenic activity which will add to overall estrogenic content, while norgestrel is antiestrogenic

Continued.

TABLE 16-5.—Continued

	ESTROGEN (µg)	PROGESTERONE (mg)	ANDROGENIC ACTIVITY IN PROGESTERONE
Moderate estrogen, low to high progest.			
Norlestrin 1/50	E-50	NA 1.0	++
Ovcon -50	E-50	N 1.0	++
Norlestrin 2.5/50	E-50	NA 2.5	++
Demulen	E-50	ED 1.0	++
Norinyl/Ortho Novum 1/80	M-80	N 1.0	++
High estrogen, low to high progest.			
Enovid-5	M-75	Noreth. 5.0	0
Enovid-E	M-100	Noreth. 2.5	0
Norinyl/Ortho Novum 2 mg	M-100	N 2.0	++
Ovulen	M-100	ED 1.0	++

	Progestin	Antiestrogen	Estrogen
N	+	++	+
NA	+	+++	+
L	+++	+++	0
Norgest.	+++	+++	0
ED	++	+	+
Noreth.	+	0	+++

Estrogen excess: nausea, edema, leukorrhea, breast tenderness, migraine, hypertension

Estrogen deficiency: irritability, nervousness, hot flashes, decreased menstrual flow, early or midcycle breakthrough

Progesterone excess: increased appetite, weight gain, fatigue, oily scalp, acne, hair loss, hirsutism, depression

Progesterone deficiency: late breakthrough, spotting, heavy menstrual flow, amenorrhea

Serious adverse reactions: thromboembolic disorders, MI, liver tumors, hypertension, gallbladder disease, congenital abnormalities
Contraindications: thromboembolic disorders, MI, history of DVT, coronary artery disease, breast carcinoma, undiagnosed vaginal bleeding, pregnancy, liver tumors
Warnings: smoking, age over 40, diabetes, hypertension, migraine
Interaction: pill failures reported with rifampin, ampicillin, tetracycline, barbiturates, phenytoin, carbamazepine; OC ↓ effects of anticonvulsants, antihypertensives, antidiabetics

Progesterone only

Micronor/Nor-QD	N 0.35	+ +
Ovrette	Norgest. 0.075	+ + +

Triphasics*

	Phase I	Phase II	Phase III
TriNorinyl	0.5 mg N	1 mg N	0.5 mg N
	35 μg EE	35 μg EE	35 μg EE
Ortho Novum	0.5 mg N	0.75 mg N	1 mg N
7/7/7	35 μg EE	35 μg EE	35 μg EE
Tri-Levlen and Triphasil	0.05 mg L	0.075 mg L	0.125 L
	30 μg EE	40 μg EE	30 μg EE

*The triphasic pills have lower progestin doses; however, advantages are yet to be determined.

TABLE 16-6.—CORTICOSTEROIDS

DRUG (HOW SUPPLIED)	DOSAGE			ADVERSE REACTIONS	COMMENTS
	Relative potency	Equivalent dose (mg)	Usual dose (mg/day)		
GLUCOCORTICOIDS				Sodium retention, hypokalemia, nausea, vomiting, associated with peptic ulcer, pancreatitis, impaired wound healing, hirsutism, acne, excitement, euphoria, psychosis, muscle weakness, menstrual irregularities; Cushing's; hyperglycemia, glaucoma, cataracts	Take with meals
Short-acting					Avoid abrupt withdrawal after long-term treatment; tapering not necessary with 7–10-day treatment.
Hydrocortisone Tab.: 5, 10, 20 mg Inj.: 25, 50 mg/ml	1.0	20.0	20–240		Administer in A.M. if single dose
Cortisone Tab.: 5, 10, 25 mg Inj.: 25, 50 mg/ml	0.8	25.0	20–300		May mask signs of infections
Intermediate					Avoid in pregnancy and lactation
Prednisone Tab.: 1, 2.5, 5, 10, 20, 25, 50 mg Syrup: 5 mg/5 cc	4.0	5.0	5–100		TOPICAL STEROID POTENCY
Prednisolone Tab.: 1, 5 mg	4.0	5.0	5–100		*Low Potency* Hydrocortisone 0.5% 1.0% 2.5% 0.25%
Methylprednisolone (Medrol) Inj. Tab.: 2, 4, 8, 16, 24, 32 mg	5.0	4.0	20–120		Methylprednisolone (Medrol) Dexamethasone (Decaderm) 0.1%
Triamcinolone (Kenalog) Tab.: 1, 2, 4, 8, 16 mg Syrup: 2, 4 mg/5 cc Inj.: 10, 25, 40 mg/ml	5.0	4.0	4–60		Methylprednisolone (Medrol) 1.0% Betamethasone (Celestone) 0.2% Clocortolone (Cloderm) 0.1%
Long-acting Dexamethasone (Decadron) Tab.: 0.25, 0.5, 0.75, 1.5, 2, 4, 6 mg Inj.:	25.0	0.75	0.75–9		Hydrocortisone valerate (Westcort) 0.2% Betamethasone valerate (Valisone) 0.01%

Betamethasone (Celestone) Tab.: 0.6 mg Inj.	25.0	0.6	7.2–12.0

Flurandrenolide (Cordran) 0.025%

Triamcinolone acet (Kenalog) 0.025%

Intermediate Potency

Halcinonide (Halog) 0.025%

Betamethasone valerate (Valisone) 0.1%

Desonide (Tridesilon) 0.05%

Flurandrenolide (Cordran) 0.05%

Triamcinolone acetonide (Kenalog) 0.1%

High Potency

Betamethasone dipropionate (Diprosone) 0.05%

Triamcinolone acetonide 0.5%

Amcinonide (Cyclocort) 0.1%

Fluocinolone (Synalar) 0.2%

Diflorasone (Florone) 0.05%

Halcinonide (Halog) 0.1%

Fluocinonide (Lidex) 0.05%

TABLE 16-7.—THYROID HORMONES*

DRUG (HOW SUPPLIED)	DOSE EQUIVALENT / DOSAGE	ADVERSE REACTIONS	COMMENTS
Thyroid USP Thyroglobulin Levothyroxine (T₄) Liothyronine (T₃)	65 mg (1 gr) 65 mg 0.1 mg 25 μg	See levothyroxine	See levothyroxine
Thyroid USP Tabs.: 16, 32, 65, 98, 130, 195, 260, 325 mg	Initial: 65 mg/day increase by 65 mg q30d if necessary Myxedema: initial 16 mg/day × 2 wk, then 32 mg/day × 2 wk, then 65 mg/day *Children:* same as adults		
Levothyroxine (T₄) (Levothyroid, Synthroid, various) Tabs.: 0.025, 0.05, 0.1, 0.125, 0.15, 0.175, 0.2, 0.3 mg Inj.: 0.1, 0.2, 0.5 mg	*Usual Adult:* 0.1–0.2 mg/day; myxedema or cardiac disease; begin with 0.025 mg/day and increase by 0.025 mg/day at 3–4-week intervals *Children:* Age — μg/kg/day 0–6 mo. — 8–10 6–12 mo. — 6–8 1–5 yr — 5–6 6–12 yr — 4–5 Parenteral (IV or IM): 0.2–0.5 mg (without heart disease)	Palpitations, tachycardia, angina, nervousness, sweating, diarrhea, tremors, heat intolerance	Bioavailability differences exist between products; do not interchange without monitoring Half-life 6–7 days; full effect seen 3–4 weeks after dosage change Monitor T₄, T₃RI, and TSH 0.1 mg T₄ = 65 mg thyroid USP Many drugs can alter thyroid function tests (see *Med. Lett. Drugs Ther.* 1981; 23:30–2) Cholestyramine can bind thyroid and ↓ effects.

*Information on thyroid USP and levothyroxine is included since levothyroxine is most appropriate and thyroid USP is still used.

TABLE 16–8.—ANTIDEPRESSANTS*†

	NE	SE	ANTIACH	SED	ORTHO
Tertiary amines					
Amitriptyline (Elavil etc)	+ +	+ + + +	+ + + +	+ + +	+ +
Imipramine (Tofranil etc)	+ + +	+ + + +	+ + +	+ +	+ + +
Doxepine (Adapin etc)	+	+ +	+ + +	+ + +	+ +
Trimipramine (Surmontil)	+	+	+ + +	+ + +	+ +
Secondary amines					
Nortriptyline (Pamelor etc)	+ + +	+ +	+ +	+ +	+
Desipramine (Norpramin etc)	+ + + +	+ +	+ +	+ +	+ +
Protriptyline (Vivactil)	+ + +	+ +	+ + +	+	+ +
Tetracyclic					
Maprotiline (Ludiomil)	+ + +	+	+ +	+ +	+ +
New drugs					
Trazodone (Desyrel)	0	+ +	0	+ + +	+ + +
Fluoxetine (Prozac)	0	+ + +	0	0	+

*Adapted from *Drug Facts and Comparisons, 1988 Edition.* St Louis, Facts and Comparisons, Division of JB Lippincott Co, 263a.
†See individual drugs for dosing. NE = norepineprhine, SE = serotonin; ANTIACH = anticholinergic; SED = sedation; ORTHO = orthostatic hypotension. 0 = none; + = slight; + + = moderate; + + + = high; + + + + = very high.

TABLE 16–9.—PROPERTIES OF COMMON ANTIPSYCHOTICS*†

DRUG	EPS	SED	ANTIACH	ORTHO
Aliphatic				
Chlorpromazine (Thorazine, etc.)	+ +	+ + +	+ +	+ + +
Promazine (Sparine, etc.)	+ +	+ +	+ + +	+ +
Piperidine				
Mesoridazine (Serentil)	+	+ + +	+ +	+ +
Thioridazine (Mellaril)	+	+ + +	+ + +	+ + +
Piperazine				
Prochlorperazine (Compazine)	+ + +	+ +	+	+
Fluphenazine (Prolixin)	+ + +	+	+	+
Trifluoperazine (Stelazine, etc.)	+ + +	+	+	+
Thioxanthene				
Thiothixene (Navane, etc.)	+ + +	+	+	+
Butyrophenone				
Haloperidol (Haldol)	+ + +	+	+	+

*From *Drug Facts and Comparisons, 1988 Edition.* St Louis, Facts and Comparisons, Division of JB Lippincott Co, p 265. Reproduced by permission.

†See individual agents for dosing. EPS = extrapyramidal effects; SED = sedation; ANTIACH = anticholinergic; ORTHO = orthostatic hypotension. + = slight; + + = moderate; + + + = high.

TABLE 16–10.—Cephalosporins

DRUG	DOSE	COMMENTS
CEPHALOSPORINS (1ST GENERATION)		
Cefaclor (Ceclor) Caps.: 250, 500 mg Susp.: 125, 250 mg/5 cc	*Adults:* 250–500 mg t.i.d. *Children:* Otitis—40 mg/kg/day in 3 doses; other infections—20–40 mg/kg/day, up to 1 gm	Spectrum: more active against gram (+) than other cephs. *Staph.*, *S. pneumoniae*, *S. pyogenes*, *E. coli*, *H. influenzae*, *Klebsiella*, *Proteus mirabilis* Adverse effects: nausea, vomiting, diarrhea, rash, candidiasis 5%–8% have cross-sensitivity to penicillins Do not adequately penetrate for meningitis

Cefadroxil (Duricef, Ultracef)
Caps.: 500 mg
Tabs.: 1000 mg
Susp.: 125, 250, 500 mg/5 cc
	Adults: 1–2 gm once or twice daily
	Children: 30 mg/kg/day given q12h; alter dosing interval in renal impairment
	See comments
		See above spectrum and side effects
		CrCl: 25–50 ml/min: q12 h
		         10–25 ml/min: q24h
		         0–10 ml/min: q36h

Cephalexin (Keflex) Caps.: 250, 500 mg Tabs.: 1000 mg Susp.: 125, 250 mg/5 cc; 100 mg/1cc	*Adults:* 250–500 mg q.i.d. *Children:* 25–100 mg/kg/day in 4 doses	See above spectrum and side effects.

Cephradine (Anspor, Velosef)
Caps.: 250, 500 mg
Tabs.: 1,000 mg
Susp.: 125, 250 mg/5 cc
Inj.: various
	Adults: Oral: 250–500 mg q.i.d.; parenteral: 0.5–1 gm q6h, up to 8 gm/day
	Children: Oral: 25–50 mg/kg/day, up to 4 gm/day; parenteral: 50–100 mg/kg/day in 4 doses; alter interval with renal impairment. See comment
		See above spectrum and side effects
		CrCl: >20 ml/min: q6–12h
		    15–19 ml/min: q12–24h
		    10–14 ml/min: q24–40h
		    5–9 ml/min: q40–50h
		    <5 ml/min: q50–70h

Continued.

TABLE 16-10.—Continued

DRUG	DOSE	COMMENTS		
Cefazolin (Ancef, Kefzol) Parenteral: various	*Adults:* 250 mg–1.5 gm q6–8h, up to 12 gm/day *Children:* 25–100 mg/kg/day given in 3–4 doses	See above spectrum and side effects Higher serum levels and longer half-life compared to cephalothin (Keflin) or cephapirin (Cefadil) Renal impairment:		
		CrCl (ml/min)	% of Normal Dose	Interval
		40–70	60%	12 hr
		20–40	25%	12 hr
		5–20	10%	24 hr
Cephalothin (Keflin) Parenteral: various	*Adults:* 500 mg–1 gm q4–6h, up to 12 gm/day *Children:* 80–160 mg/kg/day in 4–6 doses	See above spectrum and side effects IM is very painful Renal impairment:		
		CrCl (ml/min)	Max. Adult dose	
		50–80	2 gm q6h	
		25–50	1.5 gm q6h	
		10–25	1 gm q6h	
		2–10	0.5 gm q6h	
		<2	0.5 gm q8h	
Cephapirin (Cefadyl) Parenteral: various	*Adults:* 500 mg–1 gm q4–6h, up to 12 gm/day *Children:* 40–80 mg/kg/day in 4 doses; renal impairment: 7.5–15 mg/kg every 12 hr	See above spectrum and side effects Serum levels similar to cephalothin (Keflin)		

CEPHALOSPORINS (2ND GENERATION)

Drug	Dose	
Cefamandole (Mandol) Parenteral: various	*Adults:* 500 mg–2 gm q4–8h (12 gm max.) *Children:* 50–150 mg/kg/day in 3–6 doses; do not exceed adult dose. *Renal impairment:*	Spectrum: *S. aureus, S. pneumoniae, S. pyogenes, E. coli, Hemophilus influenzae, Proteus mirabilis*, other *Proteus* species, *Providencia*, some anaerobes
		Cefamandole more active than cefoxitin against *Hemophilus, Enterobacter*
	CrCl (ml/min)	Dose
	50–80	0.75–2 gm q6h
	25–50	0.75–2 gm q8h
	10–25	0.5–1.25 gm q8h
	2–10	0.5–1 gm q8–12h
	<2	0.25–0.75 gm q12h
		Cefotetan and cefoxitin have good anaerobic coverage
		Adverse reactions: similar to first-generation, plus bleeding abnormalities; Antabuse reactions reported with cefamandole
Cefonicid (Monocid) Parenteral	0.5–2 gm q24h; reduce dose with renal impairment	
Ceforanide (Precef) Parenteral	0.5–1 gm q12h; reduce dose with renal impairment	
Cefotetan (Cefotan) Parenteral	0.5–3 gm q12h; increase dosing frequency with renal impairment.	Good anerobic coverage, including *B. fragilis*; may cause bleeding and disulfiram reactions

Continued.

TABLE 16–10.—Continued

DRUG	DOSE	COMMENTS
Cefoxitin (Mefoxin) Parenteral: various	Adults: 1–2 gm q6–8h (3–12 gm/day); Children (>3 mo.): 80–160 mg/kg/day in 4–6 doses Renal Impairment:	See cefamandole spectrum. Cefoxitin more active against some anaerobes (e.g., Bacteroides) Causes more pain and phlebitis on injection

CrCl (ml/min)	Dose
30–50	1–2 gm q8–12h
10–29	1–2 gm q12–24h
5–9	0.5–1 gm q12–24h
<5	0.5–1 gm q24–48h

| Cefuroxime (Zinacef) Parenteral | Adults: 750 mg–1.5 gm q6–8h; meningitis: up to 3 gm q8h Children (over 3 mo.): 50–100 mg/kg/day in 3–4 doses; meningitis: 200–400 mg/kg/day in 3–4 doses Renal Dysfunction: | Not active against Serratia, Pseudomonas, or Bacteroides Indicated for meningitis caused by susceptible strains of Staphylococcus, Strep. pneumoniae, Hemophilus, N. meningitis |

CrCl (ml/min)	Dose
10–20	750 mg q12h
<10	750 mg q24h

| Cefuroxime (Ceftin) Tabs: | Children: 125 mg BID, (250 mg BID for otitis in child > 2 yr). Adults: 250–500 mg BID. | |

CEPHALOSPORINS (3RD GENERATION)

Spectrum: Less active than first-generatioin agents against gram-positives, and less active than some second-generation agents against anaerobes.
Adverse reactions: in addition to those of first-generation agents, there are more GI reactions and superinfections; see individual agents also. (Do to cost of these agents, they should generally be reserved for more severe infections.

Drug / Route	Dosage	Spectrum / Comments
Cefoperazone (Cefobid) Parenteral	*Adults:* 1–2 gm b.i.d. (max. 12 gm); no alteration with renal dysfunction; hepatic disease: 4 gm max.	Bleeding abnormalities, Antabuse reactions and suprainfections reported. Excreted into bile, half-life ↑ 2–4 × in hepatic disease (max. dose 4 gm)
Cefotaxime (Claforan) Parenteral	*Adults:* 1–2 gm q4–6h (max. 12 gm/day). *Infants:* 0–1 week, 50 mg/kg q8h; 1 mo.–12 yr, 50–180 mg/kg/day in 4–6 doses	See spectrum above; many isolates of *Pseudomonas* and *Bacteroides* are resistant
Ceftazidime (Fortaz, etc.) Parenteral	250 mg–2 gm q8–12h	Approved for meningitis due to susceptible organisms. Most active agent against *Pseudomonas* but resistance may develop rapidly; reserve for patients likely to have *Pseudomonas*
Ceftizoxime (Cefizox) Parenteral	*Adults:* 500 mg to 4 gm q8–12h. *Renal Impairment:* Reduce dosage	See spectrum above
Ceftriaxone (Rocephin) Parenteral	1–2 gm q12–24h; no dosage adjustment in renal impairment.	Indicated for meningitis and most gonorrhea infections; can be given once daily for less severe infections. See Chapters 5 and 10 for dosing for gonorrhea.
Moxalactam (Moxam)	*Adults:* 1–2 gm q8h; serious infection: up to 4 gm q8h. *Children:* 50 mg/kg q6h. *Neonates:* 0–1 week, 50 mg/kg q12h; 1–4 weeks, 50 mg/kg q8h	See above for spectrum. Indicated for meningitis due to susceptible *E. coli, Klebsiella, Hemophilus*. May cause bleeding abnormalities and Antabuse reactions

INDIVIDUAL DRUGS

TABLE 16–11.—Individual Drugs

DRUG	DOSAGE	ADVERSE REACTIONS	COMMENTS
Acebutolol (Sectral) Caps: 200, 400 mg	200–400 mg 1–2 × daily (max. 1,200 mg/day)	See beta-blocker Table 16–2	See Table 16–2
Acetaminophen (Liquiprim Tempra, Tylenol Various) Tabs.: 160, 325 mg, 500 mg Caps.: 325 mg, 500 mg Chew tab.: 80 mg Liq.: 120, 160, 325 mg/5 cc Drops: 100 mg/1 cc 120 mg/2.5 cc Supp.: 125, 325, 650 mg	*Adults:* 325–650 mg PO q4– 6h up to 4 gm daily (acute) or 2.6 gm (chronic) *Children:* <1 yr: 60 mg 1–3 yr: 60–120 mg 3–6 yr: 120–180 mg 6–12 yr: 160–325 mg given q4–6h	*Rare:* Skin eruptions urticaria, anaphylactoid reactions, leukopenia, thrombocytopenia, neutropenia Poisoning	
Acyclovir (Zovirax) Top. Oint. 5% Vials 500 mg Oral 200-mg capsules	*Topical:* Apply q3h (6 times daily) × 7 days *IV* (infuse over 1 hour): *Adults:* 5 mg/kg q8h × 7 days *Children:* 250 mg/m² q8h; increase dosage interval with renal impairment *Oral:* 200 mg 5 times daily for 5–7 days	*Topical:* Stinging, burning, pruritus, rash *Systemic* transient increase in serum creatinine, renal dysfunction, encephalopathy, headache, arthralgia, rash, hives	Topical effective for primary infection only Adequate hydration is necessary with IV Resistance has been reported.

Drug	Dose	Side Effects	Notes
Albuterol (Proventil, Ventolin) Tabs.: 2, 4 mg Syr.: 2 mg/5 cc Inhaler: (200 inhalations)	*Children:* <6 yr: 0.1 mg/kg/dose given q8h (max. 12 mg/day) 6–11 yr: 2 mg TID (max. 24 mg/day) *Adults:* 2–4 mg TID to QID (max. 32 mg/day) Inhalation: 2 puffs Q4–6 h	Restlessness, nervousness, headache, tachycardia, palpitations, tremor	Duration 3–6 hr, Excessive use may indicate life-threating asthma *Warnings:* diabetes, hyperthyroid, heart disease, MAO inhibitors. Inhaled is more effective than oral.
Allopurinol (Lopurin, Zyloprim) Tabs.: 100 mg, 300 mg	*Acute gout:* 100 mg once daily; increase weekly by 100 mg/day up to 800 mg/day or urate < 6 mg/dl *Maintenance:* 100–300 mg/day; reduced renal function: CrCl 10–20: 200 mg/day < 10: 100 mg/day < 3: 100 mg 5–6 days/week	Maculopapular skin rash, urticaria, purpura, exfoliative dermatitis, toxic epidermal necrolysis (discontinue if rash appears); nausea, vomiting, diarrhea, abdominal pain, blood dyscasias, alopecia	Urine output should be maintained at 2–3 L/day *Interactions:* (1) → metabolism of azothioprine (Imuran) and mercaptopurine (Purinethol), reduce dose of antineoplastics to 25% of usual dose; (2) ↑ response to warfarin (Coumadin); (3) ↑ skin rash with ampicillin; (4) May ↑ incidence of marrow suppression with cyclophosphamide (Cytoxan)
Alprazolam (Xanax) Tabs.: 0.25, 0.5, 1.0 mg	0.25–0.5 mg TID (max. 4 mg/day *Elderly:* 0.25 mg 2–3 × daily	Sedation, ataxia, drowsiness, dependence, paradoxical reactions such as anger, or hostility	*Half-life:* 12–15 hr; early and intense withdrawl may occur Avoid use in pregnancy *Interactions:* cimetidine, disulfiram, erythromycin, propranolol, oral contraceptives, rifampin

Continued.

TABLE 16–11.—Continued

DRUG	DOSAGE	ADVERSE REACTIONS	COMMENTS
Amikacin (Amikin) Vials: 100 mg/2 cc 500 mg/2 cc 1,000 mg/4 cc Syr.: 500 mg/2 cc	Individualize based on creatinine clearance; see Table 16–12	Nephrotoxicity, ototoxicity, purpura, drug fever, rash, neuromuscular blockade	Monitor serum creatinine; keep peak serum levels < 30 and trough levels < 5 Inactivated by penicillins when combined in IV solution Synergistic with β-lactam agents
Amiloride (Midamor) Tabs.: 5 mg Tabs.: 5 mg plus 50 mg hydrochlorothiazide (Moduretic)	Add 5 mg/day to usual thiazide; usual dose 5–10 mg/day; max. 15–20 mg/day	Hyperkalemia (10%), headache, nausea, vomiting, abdominal pain	Should not be used alone—add to a thiazide in patients with hypokalemia; do not use in renal impairment
Aminophylline (various) Inj.: 250 mg/10 cc 500 mg/20 cc Tabs.: 100, 200 mg	Must be adjusted for age, smoking, CHF See long-acting theophylline. See Chapter 8 for dosing schedules.	Nausea, vomiting, diarrhea, tremor, restlessness, insomnia, seizures, dysrhythmias	Tablets—short serum half-life Aminophylline is 79% theophylline Serum levels: 1–2 days to reach steady state; draw any time with constant infusion, or 1 hr after oral Interactions: ↓ levels with smoking, barbiturates, phenytoin, ↑ levels with erythromycin, cimetidine, flu vaccine, oral contraceptives, ciprofloxacin, norfloxacin.

Drug (forms)	Dosage	Side effects	Comments
Amitriptyline (Elavil, various) Tabs.: 10, 25, 50, 75, 100, 150 mg Inj.: 10 mg/ml	*Initial:* 50–75 mg hs; increase q3–4d by 25 mg/day; max. 150–200 mg; reduce dose in elderly or adolescents *IM:* 20–30 mg q.i.d. See Table 16–8 for comparison	Sedation, dry mouth, blurred vision, urinary hesitancy, constipation, orthostatic hypotension, tachycardia, rash	Due to long half-life can be given once daily; 3–4 weeks is adequate trial *Contraindications:* recent MI, concomitant MAO inhibitors, seizure disorders
Amoxicillin (Amoxil, Larotid, various) Chew tabs.: 125, 250 mg Caps.: 250, 500 mg Susp.: 50 mg/ml, 125 mg/5 cc, 250 mg/5 cc	*Adults:* 250–500 mg q8h PO *Children:* 30–50 mg/kg/day given q8h PO *Uncomplicated cystitis:* 3 gm single dose	Rash, urticaria, anaphylaxis, GI irritation, candidiasis, diarrhea less frequent than with ampicillin	May reduce effectiveness of oral contraceptives; effective against most gram-positive strep. (*pyogenes* and *pneumoniae*), *E. coli;* most *S. aureus* species are resistant
Amoxicillin plus clavulanate (Augmentin) Tabs.: 125, 250mg Chew tabs.: 125, 250 mg Susp. 125, 250 mg/5 cc	Same as amoxicillin on a mg/kg basis	Same as amoxicillin but a much higher incidence of GI side effects	Covers same organisms as amoxicillin plus *H. influenzae, B. catarrhalis,* and staphylococci that produce β-lactamase
Ampicillin (various) Caps.: 250, 500 mg Susp.: 100 mg/cc, 125 mg, 250 mg, 500 mg/5cc Vials: 125, 250, 500, 1,000, 2,000 mg	*Adults:* 250–500 mg q6h PO *Children:* 50–100 mg/kg/day in 4 doses PO *Parenteral (mild infections):* 50–100 mg/kg/day (2–4 gm) *Parenteral (severe infections):* 200–300 mg/kg/day (6–12 gm).	Rash, diarrhea, urticaria, anaphylaxis, GI irritation, candidiasis	≤100% rash in patients with mononucleosis Same as amoxicillin comments

Continued.

465

TABLE 16–11.—Continued

DRUG	DOSAGE	ADVERSE REACTIONS	COMMENTS
Aspirin (various) Tabs.: 60, 325, 500 mg Caps.: 325, 500 mg Supp.: 65, 325, 650 mg	*Adults:* 325–650 mg q4–6h; rheumatic conditions, 3–6 gm/day *Children:* 65 mg/kg/24 hr in 4–6 doses *Juvenile rheumatoid arthritis:* 90–130 mg/kg/24 hr in 4–6 doses	Nausea, dyspepsia, GI bleeding, tinnitus, allergy, anaphylaxis, asthma Poisoning	Monitor serum levels (20–30 mg/dl) for anti-inflammatory effect; in anti-inflammatory doses metabolism is saturated and q8h dosing is sufficient *Interactions:* (1) caution with warfarin (Coumadin); (2) ↑ risk of hemorrhage with alcohol, steroids or anti-inflammatories
Atenolol (Tenormin) Tabs.: 50, 100 mg	25–100 mg once daily Renal dysfunction: CrCl 15–35: 50 mg/day CrCl < 15: 50 mg every other day	See Table 16–2	Reduce dose over 1–2 weeks when discontinued; excreted renally
Atropine Tabs.: 0.3, 0.4, 0.6 mg Inj.: 0.05 mg/ml, 0.1 mg/ml, 0.3 mg/ml, 0.4 mg/ml, 1 mg/ml	*Adults:* 0.4–0.6 mg PO q4–6h; bradycardia: 0.5 mg q20min up to 2 mg total *Children:* 0.01 mg/kg/dose q4h PRN up to 0.4 mg total *Resuscitation:* 0.01–0.03 mg/kg once, repeat in 20 min	Blurred vision, flushing, tachycardia, palpitations, nervousness, drowsiness, nausea, vomiting, dyspepsia, dry mouth, urinary retention	Contraindicated in narrow angle glaucoma, GI obstruction

Azlocillin (Azlin) Vials: 2 gm, 3 gm, 4 gm for IV administration	*Adults:* 100–200 mg/kg/day (2–3 gm q6h) Serious infections: 225–300 mg/kg/day (16–24 gm/day) *Children* (Do not use in neonates): for cystic fibrosis, 450 mg/kg/day (75 mg/kg q4h) up to 24 gm/day *Renal dysfunction:* CrCl 10–30: 1.5 gm q12h to 2 gm q8h CrCl < 10: 1.5–3 gm q12h	Hypersensitivity, rash, anaphylaxis, fever High doses (especially with renal dysfunction): neurotoxicity, edema, platelet dysfunction with bleeding abnormality	Spectrum not as broad as with piperacillin Contains 2.2 mEq/gm sodium (0.4–0.9 gm/day) Inactivates aminoglycosides when combined in IV solution Infuse IV over 5–30 min Reserve for serious infection and usually should combine with an aminoglycoside
Beclomethazone Aerosol (Beclovent, Vanceril) Nasal inhaler (Beconase, Vancenase)	*Adults* (inhaled): 2 puffs 3–4 × daily, 20 puffs max.; nasal: 1 spray in each nostril 2–4 × daily *Children:* 6–12 yr (inhaled): 1–2 puffs 3–4 × daily, 10 puffs max.; nasal: not recommended in children <12 years	*Inhaled:* dry mouth, hoarseness, oral candida, bronchospasm, rash, adrenal suppression. *Nasal:* rare	200 doses per inhaler If using inhaled bronchodilators, these should be used 10 min before beclomethazone Taper oral steroids while converting to inhaler
Betaxolol (Betoptic) Soln.: 5.6 mg/cc	Glaucoma: 1 drop BID	Potentially same as other β-blockers but fewer systemic side effects than topical timolol	May cause brief sting or discomfort. Could potentially interact with other systemic cardioactive drugs.

Continued.

TABLE 16–11.—Continued

DRUG	DOSAGE	ADVERSE REACTIONS	COMMENTS
Brompheniramine (Dimetane, various) Tabs.: 4 mg; 8, 12 mg timed release Elix.: 2 mg/5 cc Inj.: 10 mg/ml	*Adults:* Initial, 4 mg 2–3 × day; max., 24 mg/day *Children* 6–12 yr; 2–4 mg, 2–3 × day; max. 24 mg *Children* 2–6 yr: 1–2 mg, 2–3 × day	Drowsiness, dizziness, dry mouth, GI distress, anticholinergic	Long duration may make sustained release unnecessary Begin with low dose and titrate to maximum dose for allergic rhinitis *Contraindications:* narrow angle glaucoma, prostatic hypertrophy, acute asthma, newborn infants, stenosing peptic ulcers, GI obstruction, MAO inhibitors
Bumetanide (Bumex) Tabs.: 0.5, 1.0 mg Inj.: 0.25 mg/ml	*Oral:* 0.5–2.0 mg single daily dose; max. 10 mg *Parenteral:* 0.5–1.0 mg IV or IM (IV over 1–2 min); may repeat × 2; do not exceed 10 mg/24 hr Use in children < 18 yr not established	Nausea, vomiting, diarrhea, tinnitus, hearing loss, (ototoxicity), hypokalemia, hyperglycemia, hyperuricemia, hyponatremia, azotemia, dehydration, elevations in liver function tests, rash	Contraindicated in hepatic coma or severe electrolyte depletion. Discontinue if renal function deteriorates Interactions: ↓ natruresis with probenecid; ↑ lithium serum levels; may ↑ ototoxicity and nephrotoxicity from aminoglycosides; indomethacin (other nonsteroidals?) may ↓ urine sodium and volume

| Buspirone (BuSpar) Tabs.: 5, 10 mg | Initial: 5 mg TID.; increase by 5mg/day to a max. of 60 mg daily | Dizziness, headache, lightheadedness, insomnia, nervousness | May require 2–3 weeks for efficacy. Rarely causes sedation and does not have additive effects with alcohol Cannot be used prn Appears to have no abuse potential Use for chronic anxiety disorder |
| Captopril (Capoten) Tabs.:: 12.5, 25, 50, 100 mg | *Initial:* 12.5 mg 2 × daily; increase to 50 mg 3 × daily; if necessary, add low-dose thiazide diuretic; max. dose 100–150 mg daily but can increase to 450 mg daily, reduce dose with renal impairment Infants: 0.5–0.6 mg/kg daily | Skin rash (7%), allergy, altered or lost taste (7%), proteinuria, renal insufficiency, blood dyscrasias, GI irritation, hypotension, cough. Patients on severe salt restrictions or diuretics or with renal artery stenosis may have precipitous hypotension or increase in BUN | Discontinue other antihypertensives before starting if possible Take 1 hr before meals Skin rash may disappear with lower dosage Monitor neutrophils and urine protein Caution with severe renal impairment, or renal artery stenosis Avoid using potassium-sparing diuretics or potassium supplements |

Continued.

TABLE 16–11.—Continued

DRUG	DOSAGE	ADVERSE REACTIONS	COMMENTS
Carbamazepine (Tegretol) Chew tabs.: 100 mg Tabs.: 200 mg	*Adults:* Initial—200 mg 2 × daily; increase by 200 mg/day to max. of 1.2 gm/day; use minimum effective dose *Children:* <6 yr: 10–20 mg/kg/day; 6–12 yr, initial 100 mg 2 × daily; increase by 100 mg/day at 6–8-hr intervals; Do not exceed 1,000 mg	Drowsiness, dizziness, nausea, vomiting, blood dyscrasias, abnormal liver function tests, seizures (abrupt withdrawal), nystagmus, ataxia, rashes	Monitor serum levels; therapeutic levels usually 4–12 µg/ml. Monitor CBC, liver function Contraindicated with history of bone marrow suppression or concomitant MAO inhibitors Interactions: ↑ warfarin metabolism; ↑ levels with erythromycin, diltiazem, verapamil, cimetidine, isoniazid; ↓ levels with other anticonvulsants
Carbenicillin Tabs. (Geocillin): 382 mg Inj. (Geopen, Pyropen): numerous	*Adults:* 250–500 mg/kg/day (15–40 gm/day) IV *Children:* UTI: 50–100 mg/kg/day; serious infections: 250–500 mg/kg/day Reduce dose with renal dysfunction Oral (UTI or prostatitis): 382–764 mg 4 × day	Hypersensitivity, rash, anaphylaxis, fever, hypokalemia, sodium retention, edema High doses (especially with renal dysfunction): neurotoxicity, edema, platelet dysfunction with bleeding abnormality	Tablets—low serum levels, only use in UTI or prostatitis Injection contains about 5 mEq sodium/gm (3.5–4.7 gm/day) Inactivates aminoglycosides when mixed in same IV solution Usually combined with aminoglycoside for serious infections (e.g., *Pseudomonas*)

Cephalosporins (see Table 16–10)

Drug	Dosage	Side Effects	Comments
Chlordiazepoxide (Librium, various) Caps.: 5, 10, 25 mg Tabs.: 5, 10, 25 mg Inj.: 100 mg/ampule	Anxiety: usual 5–10 mg 3–4 × daily; alcohol withdrawal: up to 300 mg/day *Elderly:* 5 mg, 2–4 × daily *Children* >6 yr: 5–10 mg 2–3 × daily	Drowsiness, ataxia, confusion, lethargy, paradoxical excitement, hypotension, respiratory depression	Do not give parenterally in patients with shock, coma, intoxication Use with extreme caution in elderly due to delayed elimination Congenital malformations have been reported Avoid alcohol or other CNS depressants ↑ levels with cimetidine (Tagamet) Dependence may occur
Chlorothiazide (Diuril, various) Tabs.: 250, 500 mg Susp.: 250 mg/5cc Inj.: 500 mg/20cc	*Adults:* 250 mg 1–2 × daily; if greater diuresis necessary, give 250 mg t.i.d. or q.i.d. *Children:* 10 mg/lb/day in 2 doses	See hydrochlorothiazide	Absorption is saturated above 250 mg; 250 mg b.i.d. produces greater diuresis than 500 mg once daily Generally, hydrochlorothiazide is a better choice: see Hctz for other comments
Chlorpheniramine (Chlortrimeton, various) Tabs.: 2, 4 mg Tabs. (timed release): 8, 12 mg Caps. (timed release): 8, 12 mg Syrup: 2 mg/5 cc Inj.: 10, 100 mg/cc	*Adults:* 4–8 mg b.i.d.; allergic rhinitis: 4 mg b.i.d., increase by 4 mg/day every 2–3 days until 24 mg/day or symptoms subside *Children* 6–12 yr: 2–4 mg 2–3 ×/day; <6 yr: 0.35 mg/kg/day in 2–3 doses	Drowsiness, sedation, dry mouth, dizziness, GI distress, urinary hesitancy, constipation; paradoxical excitement especially in children	Long duration of action sustained release is unnecessary—can be given b.i.d. or t.i.d. Dosage titration decreases potential for adverse effects Begin titration 2 weeks before allergic season to prevent symptoms; effective dose may be higher than those recommended

Continued.

TABLE 16–11.—Continued

DRUG	DOSAGE	ADVERSE REACTIONS	COMMENTS
Chlorpromazine (Thorazine, various) Tabs.: 10, 25, 50, 100, 200 mg Caps. (timed release): 30, 75, 150, 200, 300 mg Syrup: 10 mg/5 cc 30 mg/cc 100 mg/cc Supp.: 25 mg/100 mg Inj.: 25 mg/cc	*Adults:* 25 mg t.i.d. initially, gradually increase; max. 1,000 mg/day; use low dose in elderly; nausea: 10–25 mg q4–6h *Children:* 10–25 mg t.i.d., max. 100–200 mg; IM: 5–12 yr, 75 mg/day, max.; < 5 yr: 40 mg/day max.; nausea: 0.25 mg/lb q4–6h PO; 0.5 mg/lb q4–6h PR; 0.25 mg/lb q4–6h IM	Dry mouth, sedation, blurred vision, constipation, urinary retention, orthostatic dizziness, tachycardia, ECG changes, pseudoparkinsonism, dystonia, tardive dyskinesia, akathisia, photosensitivity, rash, jaundice, heat stroke, neuroleptic malignant syndrome, blood dyscrasias, lowered seizure threshold	Bioavailability difference may occur with different brands Once daily dosing sufficient for chronic use—sustained release unnecessary Periodically evaluate long-term therapy to limit adverse effects See Table 16–9 for comparison of antipsychotics
Chlorpropamide (Diabinese, various) Tabs.: 100, 250 mg	Initial: 250 mg once a day; maintenance: 100–250 mg/day (max. 750 mg/day) *Elderly:* begin 100–125 mg/day (avoid in elderly due to increased risk of prolonged reactions; use shorter-acting agent)	Nausea, vomiting, anorexia, hypoglycemia, liver function elevations, jaundice, blood dyscrasias, rash, urticaria, SIADH	*Interactions:* alcohol—flushing, headache, "Antabuse reaction"; → metabolism with chloramphenicol; ↑ response with salicylates or sulfonamides; ↓ response with rifampin, β-blockers, thiazides; numerous other interactions *Contraindications:* infection, ketosis prone, juvenile onset; also severe hepatic, renal, or endocrine dysfunction, pregnancy

Drug	Dosage	Side Effects	Notes
Chlorthalidone (Hygroton, various) Tabs.: 25, 50, 100 mg	Initial: 12.5–25 mg once daily; increase to 50 mg; maintenance: use lowest effective dose	Hypokalemia, hyponatremia, hyperuricemia, hyperglycemia, GI disturbances, rash, photosensitivity, muscle cramps, weakness, blood dyscrasias, hepatitis	Doses above 25 mg may not produce greater reductions in BP. No clinical advantage over hydrochlorothiazide; see Hctz
Cholestyramine (Questran) (Questran) Contains 4 gm of drug per 9 gm of powder Packets: 4 gm Can: 378 gm (Questran Light) contains 4 gm of drug per 5 gm powder Can: 210 gm	Initial: 1 scoop BID; increase slowly up to 3 scoops BID; See Table 16–4 for comparison	Bloating, gas, constipation, vitamin deficiencies (A, D, K) rare	Mix each scoop in 4 oz of fruit juice (noncarbonated). Bulk is less expensive than packets. There are numerous drug interactions when taken together, e.g., digoxin, thyroid, warfarin, antibiotics. Give other drugs 1 hr before or 4–6 hr after Questran
Cimetidine (Tagamet) Tabs.: 200, 300, 400, 800 mg Liq.: 300 mg/5 cc Inj.: 300 mg/2 cc	*Adults:* active benign gastric or duodenal ulcer: 300 mg 4 × daily for 6 weeks; or 400 mg BID, or 800 mg hs; prophylaxis: 400 mg hs; severe renal impairment: 300 mg q12h; Zollinger-Ellison: max. dose 2,400 mg/day. *Children* < 16 yr (limited experience): 20–40 mg/kg/day in 4 doses	Dizziness, somnolence, diarrhea, hallucinations, bradycardia, neutropenia, agranulocytosis; confusion in elderly or with renal dysfunction; impotence and gynecomastia seen, especially with high doses	Take with meals and h.s. Use liberal antacids for pain relief. *Interactions:* ↑ response to warfarin, phenytoin, β-blockers, lidocaine, theophylline, benzodiazepines, carbamazepine (due to ↓ metabolism); ↑ absorption of ketoconazole. Single 800 mg hs dose more effective for acute disease

Continued.

TABLE 16–11.—Continued

DRUG	DOSAGE	ADVERSE REACTIONS	COMMENTS
Ciprofloxacin (Cipro) Tabs.: 250, 500, 750 mg	250–500 mg q12h, 750 mg q12h for more severe infections Adjust dose with CrCl <50 cc/min.	GI, CNS seizures have been reported, crystalluria	The most useful quinolone Do not give with antacids May increse theophylline serum levels 25% Contraindicated in pregnancy or in children
Clonidine (Catapres) Tabs.: 0.1, 0.2, 0.3 mg Topical patch: 0.1, 0.2, 0.3 mg	Initial: 0.1 mg b.i.d.; increase by 0.1 mg/day to max. of 2.4 mg/day (usual, 0.2–0.8 mg/day) Topical patch: apply once weekly	Dry mouth, sedation, drowsiness, impotence, rebound hypertension on abrupt withdrawal, orthostatic dizziness, high incidence of rash with topical	Tricyclic antidepressants may block antihypertensive effect Avoid abrupt discontinuation Avoid in noncompliant patients
Clotrimazole Topical (Lotrimin, Mycelex) Cr.: 1%—15, 30, 45, 90 gm Soln.: 1%—10, 30 ml Vaginal (Gyne-Lotrimin, Mycelex G): Tabs.: 100 mg Cr.: 1%—45 gm, 90 gm	Topical: Apply twice a day Vaginal tab.: 1 h.s. × 7 days Vaginal Cr.: applicatorful h.s. × 7–14 days	Erythema, irritation, pruritis, urticaria	Discontinue if irritation or sensitivity develops Vaginal—14 days may produce greater cures than 7 days 1st trimester—insufficient safety data
Cloxacillin (Cloxapen, Tegopen, various) Caps.: 250, 500 mg Soln.: 125 mg/5 cc	*Adults:* 250–500 mg q6h *Children:* 50–100 mg/kg/day in 4 doses	Rash, urticaria, anaphylaxis, GI disturbances	Indicated for staph. infection but will also inhibit streptococci (*S. pyogenes*, *S. pneumoniae*)

Cromolyn (Intal) Inhalar spray Soln.: 20 mg/2 cc Nasal spray (Nasalcrom) Ophth (Opticrom)	*Adults, Children* > 5 yr: 2 puffs inhaled 4 × daily Nasal (allergic rhinitis): 1 spray each nostril 3–4 × daily Ophth: 1–2 drops each eye 4–6 × daily	Rash, urticaria, wheezing, sneezing, nasal itching, cough, stinging	Inhalation of gelatin capsules, mouthpiece, or propeller have occurred with Spinhaler; use inhaled spray instead. Inhaler not effective for acute asthma Improvement may require days or weeks
Desipramine (Norpramine, Pertofrane) Tabs.: 25, 50, 75, 100, 150 mg Caps.: 25, 50 mg	Initial: 50–75 mg h.s.; increase every 2–3 days by 25 mg/day; max. 200 mg/day outpatient, 300 mg/day inpatient *Elderly:* Use ½ the above doses See Table 16–8 for comparison	Dry mouth, sedation, urinary retention, constipation, orthostatic dizziness, tachycardia, rash, photosensitivity, overdose	Long duration allows once-daily administration Titration minimizes adverse reactions Less sedation and anticholinergic than imipramine or amytriptyline Avoid other CNS depressants and MAO inhibitors Interferes with action of methyldopa, clonidine, guanethidine

Continued.

TABLE 16–11.—Continued

DRUG	DOSAGE	ADVERSE REACTIONS	COMMENTS
Diazepam (Valium, various) Tabs.: 2, 5, 10 mg Inj.: 5 mg/ml Sustained release (Valrelease): 15 mg	*Adults:* Oral: 2–10 mg 2–4 × daily; parenteral: 2–20 mg q3–4h if necessary *Children:* Oral: 1–2.5 mg 3–4 × daily; do not use in children < 6 mo; parenteral: do not exceed 0.25 mg/kg; may repeat in 15–30 min *Geriatrics:* 2–2.5 mg, 1–2 × daily *Status epilepticus:* 5–10 mg at 10–15-min intervals; max. adults 30 mg, children 10 mg, infants 5 mg	Sedation, drowsiness, ataxia, bradycardia, hypotension, skin rash, respiratory depression, paradoxical excitement	Half-life 20–50 hr sustained release is generally unnecessary Inject IV at 1 ml/min or slower in large vein Cautions: may cause dependence, do not give during shock or depressed vitals; associated with ↑ risk of congenital malformations Avoid other CNS depressants *Interactions:* ↑ diazepam levels with cimetidine, disulfiram, isoniazid; → diazepam levels with rifampin
Dicloxacillin, (various) Caps.: 125, 250, 500 mg Susp.: 62.5 mg/5 cc	*Adults:* 125–250 mg q6h *Children:* 12.5–25 mg/kg/day in 4 doses	Rash, hypersensitivity, urticaria, anaphylaxis, GI disturbances	High blood levels achieved compared to other oral penicillins. (Note lower dosage range.) Indicated for staph. infections but will inhibit streptococci (*S.pyogenes, S. pneumoniae*)

Drug	Dosage	Side Effects	Comments
Dicyclomine (Bentyl, various) Caps.: 10, 20 mg Tabs.: 20 mg Syrup: 10 mg/5 cc Inj.: 10 mg/ml	*Adults*: 10–20 mg, 3–4 × daily PO; IM: 20 mg q4–6h *Children*: 10 mg, 3–4 × daily *Infants*: 0.5–1.0 mg/kg day in 3–4 doses	Drowsiness, dry mouth, blurred vision, urinary hesitancy, constipation, tachycardia, lightheadedness with injection	Do not administer IV Usually take 30 min before meals *Contraindications*: narrow-angle glaucoma, unstable cardiac status, GI or GU obstruction, and infants <6 mo.
Digoxin (Lanoxin, various) Tabs.: 0.125, 0.25, 0.5 mg Caps.: 0.05, 0.1, 0.2 mg Elix.: 0.05 mg/ml Inj.: 0.1, 0.25 mg/ml	See chapter 7 for dosage calculations	GI: nausea, vomiting, diarrhea CNS: weakness, disorientation, hallucinations Cardiac: dysrhythmias-bradycardia, PVCs, heart block most common	Lanoxin brand tablets are recommended due to bioavailability differences Many patients (up to 50%) have dysrhythmias before GI signs of toxicity Serum levels should be drawn at least 6–8 hr after dosing Digoxin levels ↑ by quinidine, verapamil, nifedipine, erythromycin, tetracycline
Diltiazem (Cardizem) Tabs.: 30, 60, 90, 120 mg Sustained release: 90 mg, 120 mg	Initial: 30 mg, 3–4 × daily; Sustained release: 60–120 mg twice daily; increase gradually to max. of 360 mg/day See Table 16–3 for comparison	Headache, flushing, dizziness, rash, urticaria, bradycardia, heart block edema	Additive prolongation of AV conduction with digoxin or β-blockers. Contraindicated in nodal dysfunction, heart block, hypotension *Interactions*: Carbamazepine, cimetidine, digoxin, cyclosporine

Continued.

477

TABLE 16–11.—Continued

DRUG	DOSAGE	ADVERSE REACTIONS	COMMENTS
Diphenhydramine (Benadryl, various) Caps.: 25, 50 mg Inj.: 10, 50 mg/ml	*Adults:* 25–50 mg, 3–4 × daily PO; injection: 10–100 mg, max. 400 mg/day *Children:* (>10 kg): 5 mg/kg/ day in 4 doses; max. 300 mg/day	Drowsiness, dizziness, sedation, GI distress, dry mouth, constipation, urinary retention, hypotension, rash, urticaria, photosensitivity, blurred vision	Highly sedating *Contraindications:* newborns, MAO inhibitors, narrow-angle glaucoma, acute asthma, stenosing peptic ulcer, duodenal obstruction, symptomatic prostatic hypertrophy Avoid other CNS depressants
Disopyramide (see Table 16–1)			
Disulfiram (Antabuse, various) Tabs.: 250, 500 mg	Initial: 250–500 mg once daily for 1–2 weeks; maintenance: 125–500 mg/ day	Drowsiness, fatigue, skin eruptions, dermatitis, hepatotoxicity, blood dyscrasias Monitor LFTs 2 weeks after starting and monitor CBC and LFTs every 6 mo.	Do not give until patient is free of alcohol for >12 hr Avoid all alcohol including vinegars, cooking wine, cough syrups, aftershave lotions *Contraindications:* severe myocardial disease, coronary occlusion, psychoses Skin rash often controlled by antihistamines or lower dose *Interactions:* ↑ blood levels or response to warfarin, phenytoin, diazepam, chlordiazepoxide

Drug	Dosage	Adverse Effects	Comments
			Acute psychosis reported with disulfiram and metronidazole
Doxycycline (Vibramycin, various) Caps.: 50, 100 mg Tabs.: 100 mg Susp.: 25 mg/5 ml Syrup: 50 mg/5 ml Inj.: 100 mg, 200 mg/vial	*Adults:* 100 mg, 1–2 × daily *Children:* (>8 yr): 1–2 mg/lb once daily; chlamydia: 100 mg b.i.d. × 7–10 days	Nausea, vomiting, diarrhea, skin rash, photosensitivity, suprainfections; rare: hepatic toxicity, blood dyscrasias	Administer infusion over 1–4 hr ↑ Doxycycline metabolism with barbiturates, phenytoin, carbamazepine Should not be used in pregnancy, lactation, or children <8 yr Caution: hepatic and renal disease
Enalapril (Vasotec) Tabs.: 2.5, 5.0, 10, 20 mg	Initial: 2.5–5 mg once daily; increase to 10–40 mg daily given in 1–2 doses. Reduce dose with renal impairment	Hypotension, dizziness, headache, rash, altered taste, and cough Hypotension and elevated BUN more common with volume depletion or renal artery stenosis	Discontinue other BP drugs before starting if possible. Caution with renal impairment or renal artery stenosis Avoid using potassium or potassium-sparing diuretics
Encainide (see Table 16–1) Erythromycin Base (E-mycin, various) Tabs./caps. (enteric): 250, 333 mg; tabs.: 250, 500 mg	*Adults:* 250 (400 ethylsuccinate) q6h, up to 500 q6h *Children:* 30–50 mg/kg/day in 3–4 doses; IV infusion: 15–	Nausea, vomiting, cramping, diarrhea, allergy, rash, hepatotoxicity	Spectrum: *S. pyogenes, S. pneumoniae,* most *S. aureus, Mycoplasma, Chlamydia, Treponema, Legionnella*

Continued.

TABLE 16–11.—Continued

DRUG	DOSAGE	ADVERSE REACTIONS	COMMENTS
Estolate (Ilosone) Tabs. (chewable): 125, 250 mg Caps.: 125, 250 Liq.: 125, 250/5 cc Stearate (Erythrocin, various) Tabs.: 125, 250, 500 mg Ethylsuccinate (EES, various) Tabs.: 200, 400 mg Susp.: 200, 400 mg/5 cc	20 mg/kg/day (4 gm max.) (continuous infusion is preferable to prevent irritation)		400 mg ethylsuccinate = 250 mg base Avoid estolate due to age-related hepatitis. ↑ serum levels of theophylline (30% increase), carbamazepine, cyclosporine, warfarin, digoxin (10% of patients)
Famotidine (Pepcid) Tabs.: 20, 40 mg Susp.: 40 mg/5 cc Inj: 10 mg/cc	Acute: 40 mg h.s. × 4–8 weeks Maint.: 20 mg h.s. IV: 20 mg q12h	Headache, diarrhea, dizziness, constipation	Reduce dose with severe renal impairment No significant drug interactions yet reported
Flecainide (see Table 16–1)			
Fluoxetine (Prozac) Caps.: 20 mg	Initial: 20 mg q A.M. increase to 20 mg b.i.d. if needed (max. 80 mg daily) See Table 16–8 for comparison	High incidence of headache, nervousness, insomnia, tremor, nausea, diarrhea, anorexia, anxiety, rash, and weight loss	Anticholinergic and cardiac side effects are rare May take up to 4 weeks for antidepressant effects. Selective serotonin uptake inhibitor

Drug	Dosage	Adverse Effects	Comments
Flurazepam (Dalmane) Caps.: 15, 30 mg	*Adults:* 15–30 mg h.s. *Elderly:* 15 mg h.s. Not recommended in children < 15 yr	Drowsiness, sedation, ataxia, disorientation, GI disturbances	*Contraindicated* in pregnancy Avoid other CNS depressants; see also diazepam
Furosemide (Lasix, various) Tabs.: 20, 40, 80 mg Soln.: 10 mg/ml Inj.: 10 mg/ml	*Adults:* Hypertension: 20–40 mg b.i.d.; edema: 20–80 mg/day (increase no sooner than q8h by 20–40 mg, max. 600 mg/day); parenteral: 20–40 mg IM or IV slowly, increase as needed *Children:* 1–2 mg/kg; doses > 6 mg/kg not recommended	Anorexia, nausea, vomiting, hypokalemia, hyperglycemia, hyperuricemia, hyponatremia, volume depletion, hypotension, rash, blood dyscrasias, ototoxicity	*Contraindications:* anuria, hepatic coma, severe electrolyte disturbances ↑ Lithium levels; ↑ ototoxicity with aminoglycosides; indomethacin and other anti-inflammatories may → diuresis
Gentamicin (Garamycin, various) Inj., ophthalmic oint., soln., topical	Dosage must be individualized based on age and CrCl. See Table 16–2.	Nephrotoxicity, ototoxicity, rash, urticaria, numbness, tingling, ↑ liver function tests	Monitor serum creatinine, and serum levels, keep peaks < 10 μg/ml and troughs < 2.0 μg/ml ↑ Ototoxicity with furosemide Synergistic with β-lactam agents
Glipizide (Glucotrol) Tabs.: 5, 10 mg	Initial: 5 mg (2.5 mg in elderly) 30 min before breakfast; increase by 2.5–5 mg up to 20 mg b.i.d.	Uncommon: GI, hypoglycemia, diarrhea	Fewer drug interactions than with 1st-generation agents
Glyburide (Micronase, Diabeta) Tabs.: 1.25, 2.5, 5 mg	Initial: 1.25–2.5 mg with breakfast; increase by no more than 2.5 mg/week up to 20 mg daily	See glipizide	See glipizide. Equivalent dose of glyburide is less than glipizide.

Continued.

TABLE 16–11.—Continued

DRUG	DOSAGE	ADVERSE REACTIONS	COMMENTS
Griseofulvin (various) Micro-Caps: 125, 250 mg Tabs.: 125, 250, 500 mg Susp.: 125 mg/5 cc Ultramicro tabs.: 125, 250, 330 mg (equivalent to 250 and 500 mg microsize)	*Adults:* 500 mg (250 ultramicro) to 1,000 mg daily. *Children:* 10 mg/kg/day of microsize	Skin rash, urticaria, nausea, vomiting Rare: proteinuria, leukopenia	Take with a fatty meal to increase absorption *Contraindicated* in hepatocellular failure, porphyria Duration: tinea corporis, 2–4 weeks; capitis, 4–6 weeks; peditis, 4–8 weeks; fingernails, > 4 mo.; toenails, > 6 mo.
Haloperidol (Haldol) Tabs.: 0.5, 1, 2, 5, 10, 20 mg Liq.: 2 mg/ml Inj.: 5 mg/ml	Initial: 0.5–5 mg, 2–3 × daily; gradually increase to 100 mg/day if necessary *Geriatrics:* 0.5–2 mg 2–3 × daily *Children* (3–12 yr): Initial, 0.5 mg/day; if necessary, increase weekly by 0.5 mg/day up to 0.05–0.15 mg/kg/day	Drowsiness, sedation, dry mouth, constipation, blurred vision, urinary retention, dizziness, tachycardia, ECG changes, pseudoparkinsonism, dystonia, akathesia, tardive dyskinesia, photosensitivity, rash, jaundice, heat stroke, hyperpyrexia, blood dyscrasia, lowered seizure threshold	High extrapyramidal symptoms; low sedative and anticholinergic effects Once daily dosing often sufficient for chronic dosing Periodically evaluate long-term therapy to limit adverse effects See Table 16–9 for comparison of antipsychotics

Drug	Dosage	Side effects	Comments
Heparin Inj.: various	*Prophylaxis:* 5,000 units q8–12h SC *Continuous infusion:* load 50–100 units/kg then infuse 15–25 units/kg/hr (20,000–40,000 units/day); adjust to PTT *Intermittent IV:* 10,000 units as bolus, then 5,000–10,000 q4–6h (PTT will change during dosing interval)	Hemorrhage, fever, chills, urticaria, increased platelet aggregation with thrombocytopenia, osteoporosis with long-term use, alopecia	Avoid IM injection; less bleeding and better control with infusion compared to intermittent IV Monitor PTT, platelets; maintain PTT at 1.5–2.0 × control (minidose does not markedly ↑ PTT) Overdose: Protamine sulfate 1 mg neutralizes 100 units of heparin; inject slowly (50 mg over 10 min)
Hydralazine (Apresoline, various) Tabs.: 10, 25, 50, 100 mg Inj.: 20 mg/ml	Initial: 10 mg, 4 × daily, slowly increase to 50 mg 4 × daily (can be given 2 × daily); parenteral: 20–40 mg IM or IV, repeat as necessary	Headache, palpitations, flushing, dizziness, tachycardia, angina, rash, urticaria, lupus (dose related), peripheral neuropathy	Absorption ↑ with food. *Contraindications:* coronary artery disease, mitral valve disease Monitor ANA or LE if arthralgias develop Minimize tachycardia with β-blockers
Hydrochlorothiazide (Hydrodiuril, various) Tabs.: 25, 50, 100 mg	*Adults:* 12.5–50 mg once daily *Children:* < 2 yr, 12.5–37.5 mg/day in 2 doses; 2–12 yr, 37.5–50 mg/day in 2 doses	Hypokalemia, hyperlipidemia, hyperglycemia, hyperuricemia, hyponatremia, ectopy, GI disturbances, rash, photosensitivity, muscle cramps, weakness, blood dyscrasias, hepatitis	Can give once daily Will ↑ lithium levels; ↓ Diuresis, natriuresis with anti-inflammatory drugs Not effective with renal impairment (CrCl < 30 ml/min); *contraindicated* in renal decompensation

Continued.

483

TABLE 16–11.—Continued

DRUG	DOSAGE	ADVERSE REACTIONS	COMMENTS
Hydroxyzine (Atarax, various) Tabs.: 10, 25, 50, 100 mg Caps.: 25, 50 mg Liq.: 10 mg/5 cc, 25 mg/5 cc Inj.: 50, 75, 100 mg/dose	*Adults:* 25–100 mg 3–4 × daily *Children:* >6 yr, 50–100 mg/day in 3 doses; <6 yr, 50 mg/day in 3 doses IM: *adults:* 25–100 mg, *children:* 1.1 mg/kg	Drowsiness, dry mouth, sedation, dizziness, GI disturbances, constipation, urinary retention, hypotension, rash, urticaria, photosensitivity, blurred vision	For allergic rhinitis, titrate upward to limit side effects Avoid other CNS depressants
Ibuprofen (Motrin, various) Tabs.: 200, 300, 400, 600, 800 mg	RA: 300–600 mg, 3–4 × daily, max. 3.2 gm Pain, dysmenorrhea: 400 mg q4–6h	Nausea, vomiting, abdominal pain, GI bleeding, heartburn, ulcer, elevated BUN or creatinine, rash, urticaria, visual disturbances, ocular reactions	Take with meals Avoid aspirin *Contraindicated* in patients with aspirin allergy (angioedema and bronchospasm) Caution with impaired renal function or CHF Interactions: ↓ effect of BP meds, diuretics, ↑ effects or toxicity with phenytoin, oral hypoglycemics, lithium, methotrexate, warfarin
Imipenem-Cilastatin (Primaxin) Injection	Dose is based on imipenem Usual: 250–500 mg q6h Severe infections: 1 gm q6–8h; reduce dose if CrCl is <70 cc/min	Similar to penicillins and, there may be cross-reactivity in penicillin allergic patients Seizures (1.5%)	The broadest spectrum agent currently available Not reliably active against methicillin-resistant *Staph.*, enterococci, *Chlamydia.* Should not be used alone against *Pseudomonas.*

Drug	Dosage	Adverse Effects	Comments
Imipramine (Tofranil, various) Tabs.: 10, 25, 50	Initial: 50–75 mg h.s.; increase every 2–3 days by 25 mg/day; max.: 200 mg/day outpatient, 300 mg/day inpatient. *Elderly:* ½ the above doses. *Enuresis* (children >6 yr): 25 mg/day, increase to 50 mg/day (6–12 yr) or 75 mg/day (>12 yr) if necessary	Dry mouth, sedation, urinary retention, constipation, orthostatic dizziness, tachycardia, rash, photosensitivity.	Long duration allows once-daily use—sustained release is unnecessary; usually can be given once daily. Titration minimizes adverse effects. Avoid other CNS depressants and MAO inhibitors. Interferes with action of methyldopa, clonidine, guanethidine. See Table 16–8 for comparison of antidepressants
Indomethacin (Indocin, various) Caps.: 25, 50 mg Caps. (sustained release): 75 mg	25–50 mg, 3 × daily; sustained release: 75 mg 1–2 × daily; not recommended in children <14 yr; patent ductus: 0.1 mg/kg × 1–3 doses via orogastric tube	Nausea, vomiting, abdominal pain, headache, dizziness, GI bleeding, sodium and fluid retention, increased BUN and creatinine, blood dyscrasias.	Take with meals. Adverse effects increase with dose, use lowest dose. *Contraindications:* hypersensitivity, aspirin allergy. Caution in impaired renal function, elderly with CHF. *Interactions:* see ibuprofen for similar interactions

Continued.

TABLE 16–11.—Continued

DRUG	DOSAGE			ADVERSE REACTIONS	COMMENTS
	Onset (hr)	Peak (hr)	Duration (hr)		
Insulin					
Rapid					
Regular insulin	0.5–1	2–4	5–7		Only regular insulin can be given IV
Insulin zinc, prompt (semilente, semitard)	1–2	4–6	12–16		Pure pork less antigenic than beef; most insulins available in beef plus pork, purified pork, or purified beef or human form
Intermediate					Patient should not change order of mixing or change brands without careful monitoring
Isophane (NPH)	1–1.5	6–14	24+		When mixing insulin, regular insulin should be drawn up first; once mixed, these are stable for 30 days (90 days if refrigerated)
Insulin zinc (Lente, Lentard)	1–2.5	6–14	24+		Complete mixing of regular and NPH insulin takes 15 min and regular with Lente takes 15 min to 24 hr
Long-Acting					
Protamine zinc (PZI)	4–8	14–24	36+		
Ultralente	4–8	18–24	36+		
Isoniazid (various) Tabs.: 50, 100, 300 mg Inj.: 100 mg/ml	Prevention: *adults,* 300 mg/day; *children,* 10 mg/kg/day up to 300 mg Treatment: *adults,* 5 mg/kg/day, up to 300 mg; *children,* 10–20 mg/kg/day up to 300 mg			Peripheral neuropathy, GI disturbances, elevated liver function, hepatitis, blood dyscrasias	Hepatitis incidence is age-related Supplemental B6 (10–50 mg) recommended in adolescents and malnourished *Contraindicated* in acute or chronic liver disease INH ↑ blood levels of phenytoin, carbamazepine, benzodiazepines, and ↑ CNS toxicity with cyclosporine

Drug	Dosage	Side Effects	Comments
Isosorbide dinitrate (Isordil, Sorbitrate, various) SL: 2.5, 5, 10 mg Chew: 5, 10 mg Tab.: 5, 10, 20, 30 mg Sustained: 40 mg	Initial: 5–10 mg b.i.d., increase gradually, much higher doses than recommended may be necessary (up to 120 mg t.i.d.)	Headache, flushing, dizziness (↑ with alcohol)	SL and chewable provide no major advantage over SL NTG See nitrate comparison in chapter 7 Tolerance is reduced with 2 or 3 daily doses instead of 4
Ketoconazole (Nizoral) Tab.: 200 mg Suspension: 100 mg/5 cc Cream	*Adults:* 200 mg/day; serious infections; 400 mg/day *Children* >2 yr: 3.3–6.6 mg/kg; <2 yr: not established Topical: once daily	Nausea, vomiting, abdominal pain, gynecomastia, hepatic toxicity	Monitor liver function tests Antacids, cimetidine, ranitidine, and anticholinergics inhibit absorption ↑ cyclosporine serum levels, may interact with phenytoin
Labetalol (Normodyne, Trandate) Tabs: 100, 200, 300 mg Inj.: 5 mg/cc	Usual dosage: 200 mg, 2–3 × daily PO; max. dose approximately 2,400 mg/day IV: 20 mg over 2 min, then 40–80 mg q-10 min up to 300 mg	Drowsiness, fatigue, dizziness, orthostasis, dry mouth, headache, impotence, CHF, bronchospasm, scalp tingling, goose flesh, cold extremities, rash, GI distress, positive ANA See Table 16–2	Blocks β- and α-receptors, causing vasodilation; probably more side effects than β-blockers Reserve for patients who require β-blockade and vasodilation or urgencies Avoid in CHF, asthma, diabetes

Continued.

TABLE 16–11.—Continued

DRUG	DOSAGE	ADVERSE REACTIONS	COMMENTS
Levodopa/Carbidopa (Sinemet) Tabs.: 10/100 (100 mg levo); 25/100; 25/250	Initial: 25/100 3 × daily; increase every other day by one tab. daily to 6 tabs./day; if more levodopa is needed, change to 25/250 3 × daily and continue titration if needed; tablets are scored	Dystonia, chorea, anorexia, nausea, vomiting, dry mouth, dysphagia, ataxia, dizziness, weakness, cardiac irregularities, hypotension, mental changes, GI bleeding, agranulocytosis, elevations in renal and hepatic function tests	Max. carbidopa needed to inhibit dopa decarboxylase is 70–100 mg Stop levodopa for at least 8 hr before starting Sinemet Monitor glucose in diabetics *Contraindicated* in malignant melanoma; caution with cardiac, pulmonary, renal, hepatic, endocrine disease or psychosis *Interactions:* ↑ BP with MAO inhibitors; ↓ effect with phenothiazines, haloperidol, phenytoin, pryidoxine (B6); ↑ levodopa levels with metoclopramide (Reglan)
Lisinopril (Prinivil, Zestril) Tabs.: 5, 10, 20 mg	Initial: 5 mg once daily; increase gradually to 20–40 mg daily	See enalapril	See enalapril or captopril
Lithium (various) Caps., tabs.: 300 mg Tabs. (slow release): 300, 450 mg Syrup: 300 mg/5 cc	Acute mania: 1,200–3,000 mg/day in 2–3 doses; can be given as single h.s. dose if ≤ 1,200 mg/day, or q12h if ≤ 2,400 mg/day (see serum levels)	*Serum level related:* nausea, vomiting, diarrhea, polyuria, thirst, lethargy, tremor, ECG changes, ataxia, seizures, arrhythmia, hypothyroidism *Others:* weight gain;	Combine neuroleptic (e.g., haloperidol) in highly active manics for a short time Serum levels 0.9–1.4 mEq/L for acute mania, 0.6–1.0 for prophylaxis; draw 12 hr

Drug	Dose		
		glomerular and interstitial fibrosis; increased neurotoxic effects with haloperidol, phenytoin, carbamazepine, phenothiazines	after last dose New steady state reached in 5–7 days Nausea ↑ with high peak serum levels Monitor thyroid, CBC, SCr, UA Teratogenic ↑ Serum levels occur with diuretics, salt restriction, indomethacin, ibuprofen other nonsteroidals
Lorazepam (Ativan) Tabs.: 0.5, 1.0, 2.0 mg Inj.: 2 mg/ml, 4 mg/ml	*Adults:* 1–10 mg/day PO; IM (preop.): 0.05 mg/kg, up to 4 mg; IV (sedation): 0.04 mg/kg or 2 mg, whichever is smaller No data in children < 18 yr	Sedation, drowsiness, ataxia, bradycardia, hypotension, skin rash, paradoxical excitement	Half-life 10–15 hr Cautions: may cause dependence; do not give during shock or depressed vitals; avoid other CNS depressants Dilute before IV and inject slower than 2 mg/min
Lovastatin (Mevacor) Tab: 20 mg	Initial: 20 mg with evening meal; increase to 80 mg daily (1 or 2 daily doses) if needed See Table 16–4 for a comparison	Constipation, diarrhea, flatus, headache, elevations in LFTs, myalgia or rhabdomyolysis more common when given with niacin or clofibrate or gemfibrozil or cyclosporine	Monitor LFTs q4–6 weeks for the first 15 mo.; slit-lamp exam should be performed at baseline, then q12 mo. *Contraindicated* in pregnancy

Continued.

TABLE 16–11.—Continued

DRUG	DOSAGE	ADVERSE REACTIONS	COMMENTS
Mebendazole (Vermox) Tabs.: 100 mg	Pinworm: 100 mg × 1 dose; trichuriasis, hookworm, ascariasis: 100 mg b.i.d. × 3 days	Abdominal pain, diarrhea, fever	Adult and children's dose is the same Tablets may be chewed or crushed and mixed with food 5%–10% absorbed; *contraindicated* in pregnancy; caution in children < 2 yr
Medroxyprogesterone (Provera, various) Tabs.: 2.5, 10 mg	Secondary amenorrhea: 5–10 mg × 5–10 days; abnormal uterine bleeding: 5–10 mg × 5–10 days on days 16 or 21.	Edema, menstrual irregularities, cervical erosion, jaundice, rash, acne, depression, breast changes, alopecia, hirsutism	*Contraindications:* thrombophebitis (or history), cerebral apoplexy, liver impairment, carcinoma of breast or genital organs, undiagnosed vaginal bleeding, missed abortion, pregnancy diagnosis Discontinue with visual disturbances or thrombosis

Drug	Dosage	Side Effects	Comments
Meperidine (Demerol, various) Tabs.: 50, 100 mg Syrup: 50 mg/5 cc Inj.: 25, 50, 75, 100 mg/dose	*Adults:* 50–150 mg IM, SC, or PO, q3–4h PRN *Children:* 1–2 mg/kg IM, SC, or PO, q3–4h (do not exceed adult dose) Anesthesia support: dilute to 10 mg/ml and give by slow injection or 1 mg/ml infusion	Lightheadedness, sedation, dizziness, nausea, vomiting, euphoria, constipation, hypotension, syncope, tachycardia, rash, urticaria, respiratory depression, apnea, shock, arrest	Less effective orally Reduce dose 25%–50% with phenothiazines *Contraindicated* with MAO inhibitors, ↑ intracranial pressure, respiratory depression, asthma, COPD, corpulmonale, emphysema, hyposcoliosis May cause dependence; avoid other CNS depressants
Metaproterenol (Alupent, Metaprel) Tabs.: 10, 20 mg Syrup: 10 mg/5 cc Aerosol	Inhaler: 2 inhalations 3–4 × daily, do not exceed 12 inhalations; oral: *adults,* 20 mg 3–4 × daily; *children* (> 9 yr, > 60 lb), 20 mg 3–4 × daily; 6–9 yr (< 60 lbs), 10 mg 3–4 × daily; < 6 yr, not recommended, but 1.3–2.6 mg/kg/day has been used	Restlessness, nervousness, headache, tachycardia, palpitations, tremor	Approx. 300 doses in aerosol Duration 3–5 hr Less cardiac stimulation than isoproterenol Warnings: diabetes, hyperthyroid, heart disease, MAO inhibitors Excess inhaler use may signal onset of severe asthma Inhaled is more effective than oral.

Continued.

TABLE 16–11.—Continued

DRUG	DOSAGE	ADVERSE REACTIONS	COMMENTS
Methyldopa (Aldomet, various) Tabs.: 125, 250, 500 mg Susp.: 250 mg/5 cc Inj.: 250 mg/5 ml	*Adults:* Initial 250 mg, 2–3 × daily, PO; usual maintenance is 500–3,000 mg daily in 2–3 doses; IV: (dilute in 100 ml D5W), 250–500 mg q6h if needed; max. 1 gm q6h *Children:* 10 mg/kg/day in 2–3 doses; max. is 65 mg/kg/day	Sedation, drowsiness, dizziness, orthostasis, edema, bradycardia, impotence, rash, Coombs-positive hemolytic anemia, elevated liver function tests, hepatitis	*Contraindications:* active hepatitis or previous liver disease with methyldopa Monitor Hgb, Hct, RBC, hepatic function May ↑ lithium levels Reduce dose in elderly or those with impaired renal or hepatic function
Methylphenidate (Ritalin, various) Tabs.: 5, 10, 20 mg SR tabs.: 20 mg	Initial: 0.3 mg/kg A.M.; may increase to A.M. and noon (max. 60 mg/day)	Nervousness, insomnia, headache, hypertension, anorexia	May lower seizure threshold, Monitor CBC and platelets
Metoclopramide (Reglan) Tabs.: 10 mg Syrup: 5 mg/5 ml Inj.: 5 mg/ml	Gastroparesis secondary to diabetes or malignancy: 10 mg 30 min before meals and h.s for 2–8 wk; IV (inject over 1–2 min), single dose: *adults:* 10 mg; *children:* 2.5–5.0 mg; *children* < 6 yr: 0.1 mg/kg Cisplatin emesis: Initial 2 mg/kg 30 min before then 2 hr after, followed by 1–2 mg/kg q3h × 3 doses	Drowsiness, dizziness, pseudo-Parkinson's, dystonic reactions, nausea, diarrhea	Administer diphenhydramine (Benadryl), 50 mg, if extrapyramidal or dystonic reactions occur Avoid CNS depressants Antagonized by anticholinergics ↑ Absorption of levodopa, → ↑ absorption of digoxin, cimetidine, antibiotics

Drug	Dosage	Side Effects	Comments
Metolazone (Diulo, Zaroxolyn) Tabs.: 0.5, 2.5, 5.0, 10.0 mg	Hypertension: 0.5–5.0 mg once daily; edema (cardiac): 5–10 mg/day; edema (renal): 5–20 mg/day	Hypokalemia, hyperlipidemia, hyperglycemia, hyperuricemia, hyponatremia, ectopy, GI disturbances, rash, photosensitivity, muscle cramps, weakness, blood dyscrasias, hepatitis	May have additive effects with furosemide (Lasix) in renal dysfunction. Only thiazide with activity in renal impairment *Contraindications:* hypersensitivity, anuria, hepatic coma. Will ↑ lithium levels. ↓ Diuresis with anti-inflammatory drugs
Metoprolol (Lopressor) Tabs.: 50, 100 mg Inj.: 1 mg/ml	Initial: 100 mg/day in 1–2 doses; increase to 450 mg/day if necessary; dose > 150 mg will block β_2-receptors	See Table 16–2	See Table 16–2
Metronidazole (Flagyl, various) Tabs.: 250, 500 mg Inj.: 500 mg	Trichomoniasis: 2 gm single dose, or 250 mg 3 × daily for 7 days; treat partner *Gardnerella vaginitis* (not approved): 500 mg 2 × daily for 7–10 days. Amebiasis: Adults, 750 mg 3 × daily × 5–10 days; children: 35–50 mg/kg/day in 3 doses × 10 days. Anaerobic infections: Load: 15 mg/kg infused over 1 hr; maintenance: 7.5 mg/kg q6h; max., 4 gm/24 hr	Nausea, vomiting, headache, metallic taste, rash, candidiasis, seizures, neuropathy, dizziness, ataxia, encephalopathy	Do not inject via aluminum needles or equipment. Infuse IV over 1 hr; do not give bolus injection. Mix IV according to package insert. Contraindicated in first trimester of pregnancy. Avoid alcohol; may darken urine. Carcinogenic in rodents. May ↑ effects of warfarin; Causes psychotic reaction with disulfiram

Continued.

493

TABLE 16–11.—Continued

DRUG	DOSAGE	ADVERSE REACTIONS	COMMENTS
Miconazole Vaginal cream and suppository (Monistat) Topical cream, lotion, powder (Monistat-Derm, Micatin) Inj.: Monistat-IV	Vaginal: 1 applicatorful h.s. × 7 days Topical: Apply b.i.d. × 2 wk (4 wk for tinea pedis) IV, see labeled indications	Burning, itching, irritation, rash, hives	Discontinue if irritation occurs Three-day suppository may not be as effective as 7-day cream
Minocycline (Minocin) Caps., tabs.: 50, 100 mg Susp.: 50 mg/5 cc Inj.: 100 mg	*Adults:* Initial, 200 mg followed by 100 mg q12h *Children* (> 8 yr): 4 mg/kg, followed by 2 mg/kg q12h	Anorexia, nausea, vomiting, ataxia, vertigo, rash, photosensitivity, suprainfections Rare: hepatic toxicity, blood dyscrasias	Avoid using this drug due to frequent vestibular toxicity *Contraindications:* pregnancy, children < 8 yr, lactation Caution: hepatic and renal disease
Morphine Tab.: 10, 15, 30 mg Sustained release tab (MS Contin): 30 mg Soln.: 10 mg/5 cc, 20 mg/5 cc Inj.: multiple	SC or IM: *adults,* 5–20 mg q4–6h; *children,* 0.1–0.2 mg/kg/dose IV (*adults*): 4–10 mg *very slowly* Oral: 10–30 mg q4h	Sedation, dizziness, drowsiness, euphoria, constipation, flushing, tachycardia, bradycardia, hypotension, syncope, rash, urticaria	*Contraindications:* hypersensitivity, increased intracranial pressure, respiratory depression, COPD, asthma, emphysema, cor pulmonale, kyphoscoliosis May cause dependence ↑ Confusion and apnea with cimetidine Avoid other CNS depressants

Nadolol (Corgard) Tabs.: 40, 80, 120, 160 mg	Initial: 40 mg once daily; gradually increase by 40 mg/day weekly if necessary (usual, 80–320 mg/day) Renal dysfunction: lower dosage and increase interval	See Table 16–2	See Table 16–2
Nafcillin (Nafcill, Unipen) Caps.: 250 mg Tabs.: 500 mg Soln.: 250 mg/5cc Inj.: Multiple	Oral not recommended due to low serum levels *Adults:* 250–500 mg q4–6h IM or IV *Children:* 25–50 mg/kg/day in 4 doses *Neonates:* 10 mg/kg 2–4 × daily	Rash, hypersensitivity, urticaria, anaphylaxis, GI disturbances, bleeding abnormalities, IV—phebitis, tissue necrosis with extravasation	Indicated for *S. aureus* but will inhibit *S. pyogenes, S. pneumoniae* Use dicloxacillin for oral anti-*Staph.* penicillin
Naproxen Tabs. (Naprosyn): 250, 375, 500 mg Tabs. (Anaprox): 275 mg as sodium salt (= 250 mg Naprosyn), 550 mg Susp. (Naprosyn): 125 mg/5 cc	Arthritis and gout: 250–375 mg b.i.d., increase to 500 mg b.i.d. Dysmenorrhea, tendonitis: 500 mg, followed by 250 mg q6–8h	Nausea, abdominal pain, heartburn, drowsiness, pruritis, fluid retention, tinnitus, asthma, anaphylaxis, GI bleeding	No clear therapeutic difference between Anaprox and Naprosyn Take with meals *Contraindications:* hypersensitivity, aspirin allergy Cautions: impaired renal function and elderly, CHF Interactions: see ibuprofen

Continued.

TABLE 16–11.—Continued

DRUG	DOSAGE	ADVERSE REACTIONS	COMMENTS
Netilmicin (Netromycin) Inj.: 10 mg/ml, 25 mg/ml, 100 mg/ml	Dosage must be individualized based on CrCl See Table 16–12	Nephrotoxicity, ototoxicity, purpura, drug fever, rash, neuromuscular blockade	Maintain peak serum levels <16 and trough levels <4 Monitor serum creatinine Inactivated by penicillins when combined in IV solution Synergistic with β-lactam agents
Niacin (Various) Tabs.: 25, 50, 100, 250, 500 mg No advantage for sustained release	For lipids: Initial: 50 mg TID with meals. Increase very slowly to 3–12 Gm daily.	Flushing, pruritis, GI, peptic ulcer, hepatotoxicity. See Table 16–4 for comparison	Take 1 aspirin daily to diminish flushing Monitor LFTs, uric acid, glucose *Contraindicated* in liver disease or peptic ulcer.
Nifedipine (Procardia, Adalat) Caps.: 10, 20 mg Sustained release tablets: 30, 60, 90 mg	Initial: 10 mg 3–4 × daily; Sustained release, 30–60 mg once daily increase slowly if needed; max. 180 mg/day See Table 16–3 for comparison	Headache, flushing, reflex tachycardia, dizziness, edema (due to vasodilation), syncope, angina pain, myocardial ischemia	For SL absorption, bite capsules Caution with β-blockers, but can be used together ↑ Side effects with other *vasodilators*
Nitrofurantoin (Furadantin, Macrodantin, various) Tabs., caps.: 50, 100 mg Susp.: 25 mg/5 cc	*Adults*: 50–100 mg 4 × daily × 10–14 days; suppression: 25 –50 mg 4 × daily	Anorexia, nausea, emesis, rashes, urticaria, pulmonary reactions (dyspnea, cough, fever, chills, interstitial	Macrocrystals recommended—less nausea and vomiting Take with food or milk

Inj.: 180 mg Macrocrystals (Macrodantin): 25, 50, 100 mg	Children: 5–7 mg/kg/day in 4 doses; suppression: 1 mg/kg/day IV (diluted): >55 kg: 180 mg 2 × daily; <55 kg: 6.6 mg/kg/day in 2 doses	pneumonitis), peripheral neuropathy, hepatitis, anemia (G-6-PD deficiency)	*Contraindications:* infants <1 month, impaired renal function (<40 cc/min), term pregnancy, G-6-PD deficiency
Nitroglycerin SL tab.: 0.15, 0.3, 0.4, 0.6 mg Spray (sublingual)	Initial: 0.3–0.4 mg SL PRN; may repeat q5min; may take 5–10 min before precipitating activities	Headache, flushing, dizziness, palpitation, syncope for all nitrate products	Compare with nitrates in chapter 7 Refill SL tabs. 6–8 mo. after opening; keep in original container, tightly sealed
Sustained release (Nitro-BID, various): 2.5, 6.5, 9 mg	Initial: 2.5–6.5 mg q8h; increase as necessary; much higher doses may be required due to extensive first-pass metabolism		Compare with nitrates in Chapter 7
Ointment (Nitro BID, Nitrol, various): 2%	Initial: ½ inch, q8h increase by ½ inch; apply thin layer over 6 × 6 inches	Topical allergic reactions to ointment	Do not rub or massage Wash hands after application Contains about 60 1-inch applications
Transdermal (Nitrodisc, NitroDur, Transderm-Nitro): 2.5, 5, 7.5, 10, 15 mg/24 hr	Initial: 2.5–5.0 mg patch once daily; increase slowly as needed	Irritation at site of patch	Compare with transdermal in chapter 7 Recent data shows that duration is *not* 24 hours Patch should be removed at bedtime to diminish tolerance

Continued.

TABLE 16–11.—Continued

DRUG	DOSAGE	ADVERSE REACTIONS	COMMENTS
IV 0.8, 5 mg/ml	Initial: 5 μg/min; increase at 5 μg/min increments q3–5 min if necessary; use infusion pump		*Contraindications* to IV: hypotension, hypovolemia, constrictive pericarditis, tamponade, poor cerebral circulation See product literature to avoid absorption to plastic materials
Nitroprusside (Nipride, various) Inj.: 50 mg	0.5–10 μg/kg/min; use lower doses with concomitant antihypertensives; dilute in D5W and wrap in aluminum foil to protect from light	Nausea, vomiting, headache, diaphoresis, palpitations, dizziness, methemoglobinemia *Long-term therapy:* hypothyroidism; thiocyanate toxicity—blurred vision, tinnitus, confusion, delirium, convulsions, cyanide toxicity	Administer by IV infusion only *Contraindications:* compensatory hypertension, poor cerebral circulation Cautions: hepatic or renal impairment Long-term use: monitor serum thiocyanate, acid-base; discontinue if metabolic acidosis occurs
Norfloxacin (Noroxin) Tabs.: 400 mg	400 mg b.i.d.; for CrCl <30 cc, then 400 mg daily	Nausea, headache, dizziness, crystalluria	Useful only for UTI's resistent to other agents Does not achieve adequate serum levels Do not give with antacids May ↑ theophylline levels

Drug	Dosage	Adverse Effects	Comments
Nortriptyline (Aventyl, Pamelor) Caps.: 10, 25, 75 mg Soln.: 10 mg/5cc	Initial: 25–50 mg h.s.; increase by 25 mg/day at 3-day intervals; max., 100 mg/day Elderly: use ½ above doses	Sedation, dry mouth, blurred vision, urinary hesitancy, constipation, orthostatic hypotension, tachycardia, rash; poisoning See Table 16–8	Due to long duration, can be given once daily Adequate trial—3–4 weeks Contraindications: recent MI, seizure disorders, MAO inhibitors
PENICILLINS			
Aqueous penicillin G (crystalline)	Adults: 5–30 million units/day in 4–6 doses, depending on severity Children: 25,000–300,000 units/kg/day Newborns: 50–200,000 units/kg/day in 2–3 doses	Rash, hypersensitivity, urticaria, anaphylaxis, electrolyte imbalance; neurotoxicity with high doses, especially with renal failure	Sodium salt contains 2.0 mEq per million units K salt contains 1.7 mEq K and 0.3 mEq Na per million units
Aqueous procaine penicillin G (APPG) (Wycillin, various)	Adults: 0.6–1.2 million once daily Children: 0.3–1.2 million once daily	Same as penicillin, plus procaine allergy, mental disturbances from procaine	
Benzathine penicillin G (Bicillin LA)	Adults: 1.2 million units Children (< 60 lb): 0.3–0.6 million units Rheumatic fever prophylaxis: 1.2 million units once a month		Failures reported with benzathine used for neurosyphilis in recommended doses
Penicillin V Tabs.: 125, 250, 500 mg Susp.: 125, 250 mg/5 cc	Adults: 250–500 mg q.i.d. Children: 15–50 mg/kg day in 4 doses Rheumatic fever prophylaxis: 125–250 mg 2 × day		Strep. pharyngitis should be treated for 10 days; 500 mg b.i.d. as effective as 250 q.i.d. for Strep. pharyngitis

Continued.

TABLE 16–11.—Continued

DRUG	DOSAGE	ADVERSE REACTIONS	COMMENTS
Phenobarbital (various) Tabs.: 8, 15, 30, 65, 100 mg Liq.: 15, 20 mg/ml Inj.: 30, 60, 130 mg/ml	*Adults*: 30–100 mg, 2–3 × daily; parenteral: 100–300 mg IM or IV *Children*: 4–15 mg/kg/day	Sedation, somnolence, ataxia, hypoventilation, respiratory depression, hypotension, rash, paradoxical excitement in children and elderly	Therapeutic levels 15–40 μg/ml (anticonvulsant) *Contraindications*: porphyria, severe cardiovascular disease, shock Associated with congenital malformations Interactions: ↑ phenobarbital effect with valproic acid, chloramphenicol, MAO inhibitors, CNS depressants; phenobarbital may ↓ effects of warfarin, oral contraceptions, quinidine, phenytoin
Phenytoin (Dilantin, various) Chew tabs.: 50 mg Susp.: 30, 125 mg/5 ml Caps.: (phenytoin sodium, 92% phenytoin) 30, 100 mg	*Adults*: Initial, 100 mg 3 × daily; adjust by small doses (30–50 mg) every 2 weeks and individualize *Children*: 5 mg/kg/day in 2–3 doses; usual maintenance	Nausea, vomiting Dose-related (levels > 20): nystagmus, ataxia, slurred speech, somnolence Rapid IV: hypotension, cardiovascular collapse,	Only Dilantin Kapseals can be given once a day Bioavailability differences exist—avoid interchanging brands or dosage forms NOTE: tabs. and susp. are

Inj.: (phenytoin sodium, 92% phenytoin): 50 mg/ml

4–8 mg/kg/day
IM: Avoid—erratic absorption
IV: Do not exceed 50 mg/min; 150–250 mg IV, then 100 mg 30 min later if needed; max., 1 gm load

dysrhythmias
Other: rash, urticaria, toxic epidermal necrolysis, blood dyscrasias, lymphadenopathy (mimicking Hodgkin's), gingival hyperplasia, hepatitis, folate deficiency (therapy controversial since folate may lower phenytoin levels)

100% phenytoin, caps. and inj. are only 92%
Dose-dependent elimination—large increases in serum levels may occur with small dosage increase
Monitor serum levels (10–20 µg/ml)
Contraindications: hypersensitivity; IV—sinus bradycardia heart block, Stokes-Adams
↑ Incidence of birth defects associated
Interactions: ↑ phenytoin effect or levels with cimetidine, warfarin, disulfiram, INH, chloramphenicol, sulfas, salicylates
→ Phenytoin effect with barbiturates, folic acid, calcium, antacids
Phenytoin may ↓ effect of oral contraceptives, corticosteroids, quinidine, disopyramide
← Effect of warfarin
↑→ Phenytoin protein binding with valproic acid—monitor free phenytoin levels

Continued.

TABLE 16–11.—Continued

DRUG	DOSAGE	ADVERSE REACTIONS	COMMENTS
Pindolol (Visken) Tabs.: 5, 10 mg	Initial: 10 mg 2 × daily; increase q2–4 weeks by 10 mg/day to max. 60 mg/day	See Table 16–2	Less bradycardia than other β-blockers See Table 16–2
Piperacillin (Pipracil) Inj.: multiple	Serious infection: 12–18 gm/day in 4–6 doses Other infection: 6–16 gm/day in 3–4 doses Dosages not established in children < 12 yr *Renal impairment:* CrCl (ml/min) Dose 20–40 9–12 gm/day < 20 6–8 gm/day	Hypersensitivity, rash, anaphylaxis, fever High doses (especially with renal dysfunction): neurotoxicity, edema, platelet dysfunction with bleeding abnormalities	1.85 mEq sodium per gm (0.4–0.9 gm daily) Inactivates aminoglycosides when combined in IV solution Reserve for serious infection and usually combined with an aminoglycoside
Piroxicam (Feldene) Caps.: 10, 20 mg	20 mg once daily	Nausea, vomiting, abdominal pain, GI bleeding, heartburn, ulcer, elevated BUN or creatinine, rash, urticaria	Take with meals Avoid aspirin May reduce efficacy of BP medications, ↑ lithium levels, interact with warfarin *Contraindicated* in patients with aspirin allergy (angioedema and bronchospasm)

Drug	Dose	Adverse Effects	Comments
Potassium chloride Liq.: 10% = 20 mEq/15 cc 20% = 40 mEq/15 cc Powders: 15, 20, 25, 50 mEq Tabs., Caps.: 7, 8, 10 mEq Slow K, Micro K = 8 mEq Kaon Cl-10 Klotrix, K-Tab = 10 mEq Inj.: multiple	Individualize: Oral: for depletion, 40–100 mEq/day; for maintenance, 16–24 mEq/day IV: 10–40 mEq/hr, max. = 200–400 mEq/24 hr; max. concentration, 40–80 mEq/L	Bitter salty taste (liquids), nausea, vomiting, abdominal discomfort, gastric erosion, hyperkalemia	Dilute liquid KCl, take with meals; do not crush or chew tabs.; wax matrix may be found in stool *Contraindications:* severe renal impairment, hyperkalemia, untreated Addison's, K-sparing diuretics; wax-matrix tabs. contraindicated in esophageal compression or delayed GI transit
Prazosin (Minipress) Caps.: 1, 2, 5 mg	Initial: 1 mg h.s., then 1 mg 2 × daily; increase initially the h.s. dose to max. of 20 mg/day	Dizziness, headache, drowsiness, weakness, palpitations, nausea, tachycardia, first dose syncope	Syncope may occur on dosage increases
Primidone (Mysoline, various) Tabs.: 50, 250 mg Susp.: 250 mg/5 cc	Initial: 100–125 mg/day; increase q3–7 days by 100–125 mg/day, up to 250 mg 3 × daily; max. 2,000 mg *Children* <8 yr, ½ above doses; usual maintenance dose is 10–25 mg/kg/day in 3 doses	Drowsiness, dizziness, ataxia, vertigo, nausea, nystagmus, rash, folate deficiency, rare blood dyscrasias	Converted to phenobarbital; monitor primidone and phenobarbital serum levels (see phenobarbital)
Probucol (Lorelco) Tabs.: 250 mg	500 mg b.i.d. with meals	QT prolongation, headaches, dizziness, GI	See Table 16–4 for comparison

Continued.

503

TABLE 16–11.—Continued

DRUG	DOSAGE	ADVERSE REACTIONS	COMMENTS
Procainamide (see Table 16–1)			
Prochlorperazine (Compazine, various) Tabs.: 10, 25 mg Liq.: 1, 10 mg/ml Sustained release: 10, 15, 30, 75 mg Inj.: 5 mg/ml Supp.: 2.5, 5, 25 mg	*Adults:* for nausea, 5–10 mg 3–4 × daily orally; rectally, 25 mg 2 × daily; IM, 5–10 mg 3–4 × daily; max. dose for psychosis, 100–150 mg/day orally or 50–100 mg IM *Children* (>2 yr): Oral or rectal, 9–13 kg—2.5 mg 1–3 × daily; 14–18 kg—2.5 mg 2–4 × daily; 18–39 kg—2.5–5 mg 2–3 × daily; IM: 0.1 mg/kg, then use oral	Dry mouth, sedation, blurred vision, constipation, tachycardia, ECG changes, pseudoparkinsonism, dystonia, tardive dyskinesia, akathesia, photosensitivity, rash, jaundice, heat stroke, hyperpyrexia, blood dyscrasias, lowered seizure threshold	*Contraindications:* pediatric surgery, coma, CNS depression, bone marrow depression, liver disease, Parkinson's, severe hypertension or hypotension. See Table 16–9 for comparison of antipsychotics
Promethazine (Phenergan, various) Tabs.: 12.5, 25, 50 mg Syrup: 6.25 mg, 25 mg/5 cc supp.: 12.5, 25, 50 mg Inj.: 25, 50 mg/ml	Motion sickness or nausea: 12.5–25 mg 2 × daily PO, supp, or IM Sedation: 25–50 mg *Children:* 12.5–25 mg	Drowsiness, sedation, dry mouth, dizziness, paradoxical excitement, dystonia, photosensitivity, rash	*Contraindications:* newborn or premature infants, narrow angle glaucoma, asthmatic attack, stenosing peptic ulcer, prostatic hypertrophy See Table 16–9 for comparison
Propranolol (Inderal) Tabs.: 10, 20, 40, 80 mg Long-acting.: 80, 160 mg Inj.: 1 mg/ml	Initial: 20–40 mg 2 × daily; increase gradually to max. of 480 mg/day; 3–4 daily doses may be needed for dysrhythmias, migraine, IHSS	See Table 16–2	Long-acting may not be equivalent dose for dose; monitor control There may not be a significant advantage for long-acting See Table 16–2

Drug	Dosage	Adverse Effects	Comments
Protriptyline (Vivactil) Tabs.: 5, 10 mg	*Adults:* 15–60 mg in 1–2 doses *Adolescents and elderly:* 5–20 mg in 1–2 doses	Dry mouth, urinary retention, blurred vision, constipation, excitement, insomnia, tachycardia, orthostatic hypotension See Table 16–8 for comparison of tricyclics	Little or no sedation—may be stimulatory; given in A.M. 3–4 wk is adequate trial *Contraindications:* recent MI, MAO inhibitors, seizure disorders
Pseudoephedrine (Sudafed, various) Tabs.: 30, 60 mg Caps. (timed-release): 120 mg Liq.: 30 mg/5 cc	*Adults:* 60 mg q6–8h or 120 mg timed-release q12h *Children* (6–12 yr): 30 mg q6h, max. 120 mg/day; 2–5 yr: 15 mg q6h; max. 60 mg/day *Infants:* 7.5–15 mg q6h; max. 60 mg/day	Nervousness, tremor, restlessness, insomnia, palpitations, tachycardia, hypertension, urinary retention	*Contraindications:* MAO inhibitors, hypertension, coronary artery disease *Caution:* hyperthyroid, diabetes, prostatic hypertrophy *Interactions:* ↑ BP with β-blockers, MAO inhibitors, reserpine, methyldopa, nonsteroidals
Pyrantel pamoate (Antiminth) Susp.: 50 mg/ml	Ascariasis, enterobiasis: 11 mg/kg in single dose, up to 1 gm	Anorexia, nausea, vomiting, diarrhea, drowsiness, rash	Caution: pre-existing liver disease
Quinidine (see Table 16–1)			
Ranitidine (Zantac) Tabs.: 150, 300 mg Inj.: 25 mg/cc	150 mg 2 × daily or 300 mg h.s.; renal impairment: 150 mg 1–2 × daily Maintenance: 150 mg h.s.	Headache, nausea, dizziness, constipation, abdominal pain, rash, hepatic enzyme elevations	Drug interactions ↑ effect of warfarin, procainamide, glipizide.

Continued.

TABLE 16–11.—Continued

DRUG	DOSAGE	ADVERSE REACTIONS	COMMENTS
Reserpine (various) Tabs.: 0.1, 0.2, 0.5, 1.0 mg Inj.: 2.5 mg	Initial: 0.1 mg once daily; increase to 0.25 mg/day if necessary; higher doses not recommended	Nausea, vomiting, GI distress, peptic ulcer, orthostatic hypotension, drowsiness, sedation, depression, rash, asthma, nasal congestion	Association with depression is controversial *Contraindications:* acute asthma, acute depression, peptic ulcer, ulcerative colitis, pheochromocytoma, ECT
Rifampin (Rifadin, Rimactane) Caps.: 150, 300 mg	TB-*Adults:* 600 mg once daily. *Children:* 10–20 mg/kg day up to 600 mg *Meningococcal carriers:* above dose × 4 days Give on an empty stomach	Flu-like symptoms, heartburn, GI distress, rash, urticaria, elevations in hepatic functions, hepatitis, blood dyscrasias	Suspension can be compounded with simple syrup May discolor urine, stools, saliva, etc. a reddish orange. *Interactions:* rifampin ↑ metabolism of warfarin, β-blockers, oral contraceptives, quinidine, corticosteroids
Spironolactone (Aldactone, various) Tabs.: 25 mg	Hypertension: 25–50 mg 2 × daily; edema (hyperaldosteronism): 25–200 mg/day *Children:* 1.7–3.3 mg/kg/day in 2–3 doses	Diarrhea, abdominal pain, drowsiness, headache, impotence, irregular menses, hirsutism, gynecomastia, rash	Weak diuretic—add to a thiazide for hypertension *Contraindications:* anuria, renal insufficiency, hyperkalemia Avoid with potassium supplements or captopril

Drug	Dosage	Side Effects	Comments
Sucralfate (Carafate) Tabs.: 1 gm	1 gm 4 × daily on an empty stomach × 4–8 wk; can give 2 gm b.i.d.	Constipation, nausea, diarrhea, indigestion	Avoid giving with food or antacids May reduce absorption of tetracycline; digoxin, phenytoin, cimetidine
Sulfamethoxazole (Gantanol, various) Tabs.: 500, 1000 mg Susp.: 500 mg/5 ml	*Adults:* 1 gm b.i.d. *Children:* (>2 mo.): 25–50 mg/kg b.i.d.	GI disturbances, rash, urticaria, blood dyscrasias, hepatitis, cystalluria, fever, photosensitivity	*Contraindications:* term pregnancy, lactation, infants < 2 mo., porphyria Take with full glass of water
Sulfasalazine (Azulfidine, various) Tabs.: 500 mg Enteric-coated: 500 mg Susp.: 250 mg/5 cc	Initial: *Adults,* 3–8 gm/day in divided doses; *children,* 40–60 mg/kg/day in 3–4 doses Maintenance: *Adults,* 500 mg 4 × daily; *children,* 30 mg/kg/day in 4 doses	GI disturbances, rash, urticaria, blood dyscrasias, hepatitis, fever, folate deficiency, oligospermia	GI irritation may be ↓ by more frequent dosing or enteric tabs May discolor urine orange-yellow *Contraindications:* Infants < 2 mo., term pregnancy, lactation, porphyria, salicylate allergy, sulfa allergy, GI obstruction *Interactions:* see sulfonamides
Sulfisoxazole (Gantrisin, various) Tabs.: 500 mg Liq.: 500, 1,000 mg/5 ml Inj.: 400 mg/ml	*Adults:* 1–2 gm 4 × daily *Children* (>2 mo.): 150 mg/kg/day in 4 doses; max. 6 gm/day	See sulfamethoxazole	See sulfamethoxazole

Continued.

TABLE 16–11.—Continued

DRUG	DOSAGE	ADVERSE REACTIONS	COMMENTS
Sulindac (Clinoril) Tabs.: 150, 200 mg	150–200 mg 2 × daily	Nausea, vomiting, abdominal pain, GI bleeding, ulcer, elevated BUN or creatinine, rash, urticaria	Take with meals; avoid aspirin *Contraindications:* aspirin allergy (angioedema, bronchospasm) *Interactions:* see ibuprofen
Temazepam (Restoril, various) Caps.: 15, 30 mg	*Adults:* 15–30 mg h.s. *Elderly:* 15 mg h.s.	Drowsiness, sedation, ataxia, disorientation, GI disturbances, paradoxical stimulation	*Contraindication:* pregnancy Avoid other CNS depressants
Terazosin Hytrin) Tabs.: 1, 2, 5 mg	Initial: 1 mg h.s., then 1 mg once daily (max. 20 mg/day in 1–2 doses)	Headache, weakness, fatigue, hypotension, dizziness, palpitations	Same mechanism as prazosin. May cause 1st dose effect
Terbutaline (Brethine, Bricanyl) Tabs.: 2.5, 5.0 mg Inj.: 1 mg/ml Inhaler (Brethaire)	*Adults:* 2.5–5 mg 3 × daily *Children* (12–15 yr): 2.5 mg 3 × daily; not recommended in children <12 yr Parenteral: 0.25 mg SC; may repeat in 15–30 min Inhaled: 2 puffs 4 × daily	Restlessness, nervousness, insomnia, tremor, palpitations, tachycardia	*Contraindications:* cardiac dysrhythmias with tachycardia Inhaled is more effective than oral
Terfenadine (Seldane) Tabs.: 60 mg	*Adults:* 60 mg b.i.d., then titrate, 6–12 yr: 30–60 mg b.i.d. 3–5 yr: 15 mg b.i.d.	Alopecia, angioedema, rash itching, cough, drowsiness	May cause less drowsiness than chlorpheniramine. Therapeutic doses may be cost prohibitive

Drug (preparations)	Dosing	Side effects	Comments
Tetracycline (various) Caps, tabs.: 250, 500 mg Susp.: 125 mg/5 cc Inj.: Ophth. drops and oint. Topical	*Adults:* 1–2 gm/day in 3–4 doses *Children* (>8 yr): 25–50 mg/kg/day in 3–4 doses Acne maintenance: 125–500 mg/day Chlamydia: 500 mg 4 × daily × 7 days	Anorexia, nausea, vomiting, esophageal ulceration, rash, photosensitivity, increased BUN, blood dyscrasia, superinfection	Take on empty stomach; avoid dairy products, antacids, or iron Outdated product may cause a Fanconi-like syndrome Warnings: do not use in children, pregnancy, lactation, renal impairment Topical may color skin yellow
Theophylline (various) Numerous liquids, tabs., caps., and IV	For outpatients: attempt to use a slow-release product—Theodur and Slobid have the least peak-trough fluctuations in serum levels (see *N. Engl. J. Med.* 1983; 308:760–4) See chapter 8 for dosing	Nausea, vomiting, headache, insomnia, restlessness, tremor, tachycardia, dysrhythmias, seizures	Monitor serum levels 10–20 μg/ml, measure 4–6 hr after dose with sustained release or 1–2 hr after rapid release. ↑ Theophylline serum levels with cimetidine, ciprofloxacin, norfloxacin, erythromycin, flu vaccine, term pregnancy ↓ Theophylline levels with smoking, phenobarbital 24-hr theophylline products require further study; will not be acceptable with rapid eliminators (children, smokers), avoid using these

Continued.

TABLE 16–11.—Continued

DRUG	DOSAGE	ADVERSE REACTIONS	COMMENTS
Thioridazine (Mellaril, various) Tabs.: 10, 15, 25, 50, 100 150, 200 mg Susp.: 25, 100 mg/5 ml Concentrate: 30, 100 mg/ml	Initial: 10–25 mg 3 × daily; increase to max of 200–800 mg/day Children (>2 yr): 0.5–3 mg/ kg/day See Table 16–9 for comparison of antipsychotics	Dry mouth, sedation, blurred vision, constipation, urinary retention, orthostatic dizziness, tachycardia, ECG changes, pseudoparkinsonism, dystonia, tardive dyskinesia, akathesia, photosensitivity, rash, jaundice, heat stroke, blood dyscrasia, lowered seizure threshold	High: sedation, orthostasis, anticholinergic; low: extrapyramidal symptoms Periodically evaluate long- term therapy to limit adverse effects Contraindications: coma, marrow depression, blood dyscrasias, Parkinson's, liver damage, coronary disease, severe hypertension or hypotension
Ticarcillin (Ticar) Inj.: multiple	Adults: 150–300 mg/kg/day in 4–6 doses Children (<40 kg): 50–200 mg/kg/day in 3–4 doses Neonates mg/kg/day <2 kg, 0–7 days 150 <2 kg, 7 days 225 >2 kg, 0–7 days 225 >2 kg, > 7 days 300 Renal Dysfunction: Reduce dosage	Hypersensitivity, rash, anaphylaxis, fever, hypokalemia, sodium retention, edema High dose (especially with renal dysfunction): neurotoxicity, edema, platelet dysfunction with bleeding abnormality	Contains 5.2 mEq sodium/gm (2–4 gm/day) Inactivates aminoglycosides when mixed in IV solution Usually combined with aminoglycosides for severe infections (e.g., Pseudomonas)

Drug	Dose	Side effects	Comments
Timolol (Blocadren) Tabs.: 10, 20 mg Ophth. (Timoptic drops): 0.25%, 0.5%	Initial: 10 mg 2 × daily Glaucoma: 0.25%, 1 drop 2 × daily; increase to 0.5%, 1 drop 2 × daily if needed	See Table 16–2	See Table 16–2
Tobramycin (Nebcin) Inj.: various Ophth. drops	See aminoglycoside dosing, Table 16–12	Nephrotoxicity, ototoxicity, purpura, drug fever, rash, neuromuscular blockade	Monitor serum creatinine, keep peak serum levels <10 and troughs <2 Inactivated by penicillins when combined in IV soln. Synergistic with β-lactam agents
Tolbutamide (Orinase, various) Tabs.: 250, 500 mg	Initial: 0.5–1 gm 2 × daily; maintenance: 0.25–3 gm/day	Nausea, vomiting, anorexia, hypoglycemia, liver function elevations, jaundice, blood dyscrasias, rash, urticaria	*Contraindications:* infections, ketosis prone juvenile onset, severe hepatic or renal disease, endocrine dysfunction, pregnancy *Interactions:* with alcohol flushing, headache, "Antabuse reaction" → Metabolism with chloramphenicol ↑ Response with salicylates, sulfonamides → Response with rifampin, β-blockers, thiazides

Continued.

TABLE 16-11.—Continued

DRUG	DOSAGE	ADVERSE REACTIONS	COMMENTS
Tolmetin (Tolectin) Tabs.: 200 mg Caps.: 400 mg	Initial: 400 mg 3 × daily; increase to 1,600–2,000 mg/day *Children* (>2 yr): initial, 20 mg/kg/day; maintenance, 15–30 mg/kg/day	Nausea, vomiting, abdominal pain, GI bleeding, heartburn, ulcer, elevated BUN or creatinine, rash, urticaria	Take with meals; avoid aspirin *Contraindicated* in patients with aspirin allergy (bronchospasm and angioedema) Caution in renal impairment, elderly, CHF *Interactions:* see ibuprofen
Trazadone (Desyrel) Tabs.: 50, 100, 150 mg	Initial: 100–150 mg h.s.; Increase q3 days by 50 mg until max of 400 mg/day (600 mg for inpatients) (Note: higher doses are required than with other antidepressants)	Drowsiness, sedation, dizziness, hypertension, hypotension, tachycardia, congestion, rash, impotence, dysrhythmias, priapism	Enhanced absorption with food Administer h.s. to take advantage of sedation Avoid with cardiac disease, particularly dysrhythmias See Table 16–8 for comparison with antidepressants
Trimethoprim-sulfamethoxazole (Bactrim, Septra, various) Tabs.: 80 mg T, 400 mg S DS Tabs.: 160 mg T, 800 mg S Susp.: 40 mg T, 200 mg S/ 5 cc	*Adults:* 160 mg T, 400 mg S 2 × daily; IV: 8–10 mg/kg/ day (of T) *Children:* 8 mg/kg/day T and 40 mg/kg/day S e.g., 10 kg 5 cc b.i.d. 15 kg 7.5 cc b.i.d. 20 kg 10 cc b.i.d.	GI disturbances, rash, blood dyscrasias, photosensitivity, fever, purpura, Stevens-Johnson Side effects are greatly increased in AIDS patients	Renal dysfunction: (CrCl 15–30 ml/min) cut dose 50%; not recommended if CrCl < 15 Avoid rapid IV injection *Contraindications:* hypersensitivity to sulfa or trimethoprim, folate

Inj.: 80 mg T, 400 mg S/5 cc	Pneumocystis: Adults, 20 mg/kg/day (T) in 4 doses; children, 160 mg T/800 mg S q6h		deficiency anemia, term pregnancy, lactation, children < 2 mo. Interactions: ↑ response to warfarin, oral hypoglycemics, methotrexate, phenytoin, ↓ response to cyclosporine and ↑ nephrotoxicity Do not use for Strep. pharyngitis
Valproic acid (Depakene, Depakote) Caps.: 250 mg Syrup: 250 mg/5 cc Enteric tabs.: 125, 250, 500 mg	Initial: 15 mg/kg/day in 2 doses; increase weekly by 5–10 mg/kg/day until seizures controlled; max. 60 mg/kg/day	Nausea, indigestion, abdominal cramps, sedation, decreased platelet aggregation, bruising, hepatotoxicity	Monitor levels and liver function Contraindications: hepatic disease May be ↑ risk of neural tube defects when given in pregnancy Interactions: ↑ bleeding tendency with warfarin, salicyclates; Valproic may ↓ phenytoin levels, but free phenytoin unchanged—monitor levels and control

Continued.

TABLE 16–11.—Continued

DRUG	DOSAGE	ADVERSE REACTIONS	COMMENTS
Verapamil (Calan, Isoptin) Tabs.: 40, 80, 120 Sustained release: 240 mg Inj.: 5 mg/2 ml	Initial: 40–80 mg b.i.d.; (max. dose 480 mg/day) Parenteral (for SVT): 5–10 mg (0.075–0.15 mg/kg) by slow IV injection over 2 min; repeat in 30 min if not effective Children 0–1 yr: 0.1–0.2 mg/kg IV (2–5 mg); do not exceed 5 mg; 1–15 yr: 0.1–0.3 mg/kg IV; repeat in 30 min if necessary	Headache, flushing, hypotension, peripheral edema, bradycardia, heart block, constipation, hepatotoxicity, CHF See Table 16–3 for comparison	Half-life increases after 48 hours of treatment Contraindications: severe hypotension, AV block, SSS, cardiogenic shock, severe CHF unless due to tachycardia responsive to verapamil, patients receiving IV β-blockers Interactions: ↑ cardiac depression with β-blockers or disopyramide; verapamil ↑ digoxin and carbamazepine levels

Continued.

TABLE 16–12.—AMINOGLYCOSIDE DOSING

DOSE	AMIKACIN*	GENTAMICIN*	TOBRAMYCIN*
Dose with Normal Renal Function	5–7.5 (mg/kg/dose)	1–2 (mg/kg/dose)	1–1.7 (mg/kg/dose)
Dose with CrCl† of (cc/min):	(the following are based on dosing q8h)**		
75	4.0–6.0	0.80–1.6	0.80–1.4
60	3.5–5.3	0.70–1.4	0.70–1.2
50	3.3–4.9	0.65–1.3	0.65–1.1
40	2.8–4.1	0.55–1.1	0.55–0.90
	(the following are based on dosing q12h)**		
30	3.2–4.7	0.65–1.3	0.65–1.10
20	2.5–3.7	0.50–1.0	0.50–0.90
15	2.1–3.1	0.40–0.8	0.40–0.70
10	1.7–2.6	0.33–0.66	0.33–0.58
5	1.2–1.7	0.23–0.46	0.23–0.39
0	0.55–0.80	0.11–0.22	0.11–0.19
Keep peak	<30	<10	<10
Keep trough	<5	<2	<2

*These are the actual mg/kg dosages *(based on lean weight)* that should be given q8h *(or 12h for moderate to severe impairment)*. **These are approximate dosages that should be adjusted based on pharmacokinetic analysis. These are not accurate predictions for neonates, patients with burns, pregnancy, postpartum, or morbid obesity.
†To estimate CrCl from serum creatinine, see appendix.

17 *Poisoning*

Barry L. Carter, Pharm.D.

TABLE 17–1.—GENERAL MANAGEMENT FOR POISONING

General measures include emesis, gastric lavage, activated charcoal, and cathartics. The comparative efficacy of emesis and gastric lavage is currently controversial.

Emesis

Recent evidence suggests gastric lavage may be more effective. However, syrup of ipecac (not the fluid extract) is useful for moderately severe ingestions and for prehospital administration.

Contraindications

Decreased level of consciousness

Caustic ingestions

Ingested material that leads to rapid, significant neurologic symptoms

Relative contraindications

Age <6 mo.

Most hydrocarbons

Late-stage pregnancy

Severe hypertension, cardiac or respiratory disease

Syrup of ipecac dose

6–12 mo.	5–10 ml	(A second dose of equal amount can be given in
1–12 yr	15 ml	20–30 min. if emesis did not occur.)
> 12 yr	30 ml	

Follow ipecac with fluids (not milk, which delays emesis): 2–4 oz in young children and 8–16 oz in older children and adults.

Do not give activated charcoal with ipecac because the ipecac is inactivated.

Save vomitus for inspection and/or analysis.

Gastric lavage

When indicated, lavage should be performed even if 3–4 hr has elapsed. Lavage may even be beneficial after 8–10 hr for drugs that delay gastric emptying (e.g., salicylates, tricyclics, anticholinergics).

Contraindications

Caustic ingestions

Most hydrocarbon ingestions

Seizures or coma

Methods

To prevent aspiration in an unconscious patient, insert and inflate a cuffed endotracheal tube before performing gastric lavage.

Place patient on left side in the Trendelenburg position.

Use the largest diameter tube possible (gastric hose or Ewald tube). Use 36–40F in adults or 32–36F in children.

Lavage with normal saline (0.9%) at 15 ml/kg/cycle in children and up to 200–400 ml/cycle in adults. Lavage until several passes are clear (5–20 L total).

Save first pass for toxicology analysis.

516

Activated charcoal:
  Activated charcoal effective for adsorption of most toxins *except* boric acid, acids, alkali, hydrocarbons, alcohols, cyanide, iron, and lithium.
  Do not give before ipecac (inactivates ipecac) or *N*-acetylcysteine (unless co-ingestion of other poison).
Availability:
  Powder or liquid suspensions in sorbitol in bottles containing 25, 30, 50 gm (Charcoaid, Liqui-Char, Superchar). Superchar may adsorb 3 times as much as other preparations due to greater surface area.
Acute dose (in 70% sorbitol)
  Small children: 15–30 gm
  > 12 yr: 50–100 gm
Multiple doses (intestinal dialysis)
  Is effective long after the drug is absorbed and has increased the systemic removal of theophylline, digoxin, digitoxin, barbiturates, tricyclic antidepressants, carbamazepine and cyclosporine.
  Small children: 5–10 gm q4–8h × 24–48h
  > 12 yr 20–60 gm q4–12h × 24–48h
Carthartics
  Particularly useful following charcoal to move contents through the GI tract.
Contraindications
  Caustic ingestions
  CHF (sodium containing agents)
  Renal impairment (magnesium containing agents)
  Recent bowel surgery
  Absence of bowel sounds
Dose
  Sorbitol: 70% (with charcoal)
  Magnesium or sodium sulfate: 250 mg/kg
  Magnesium citrate: 4 ml/kg (up to 200 ml)
Dialysis
  Most effective for small nonpolar molecules such as barbiturates, boric acid, meprobamate, quinidine, salicylates, strychnine, methanol, or ethylene glycol.

*Adapted from Rodgers GC, Matyunas NJ: *Pediatr Clin North Am* 1986; 33:261–285, Park GD, et al: *Arch Intern Med* 1986; 146:969–973; Jones J, et al: *Am J Emerg Med* 1987; 5:305–310, Watson WA: *Drug Intell Clin Pharm* 1987; 21:160–166, and Yarbrough BE: *South Med J* 1988; 81:892–901.

TABLE 17–2.—ACETAMINOPHEN INGESTION*

Symptoms
  Within minutes to a few hours after ingestion, anorexia, nausea, vomiting, and diaphoresis occur.
  Symptoms continue to improve over 48 hours, but bilirubin, hepatic enzymes and PT levels rise.
  After 3–5 days with large ingestion, jaundice, coagulation defects, encephalopathy, and renal failure may occur due to hepatic necrosis.

Continued.

TABLE 17–2.—Continued

Estimating risk of hepatotoxicity

Hr After Ingestion	No Risk (μg/ml)	Probable Risk (μg/ml)	High Risk (μg/ml)
4	<200	200–300	>300
6	<150	150–200	>200
8	<100	100–150	>150
10	<75	75–120	>120
12	<50	50–75	>75
14	<35	35–60	>60
16	<25	25–40	>40
18	<20	20–28	>28
20	<12	12–20	>20
22	<9	9–12	>12
24	<7	7–10	>10

To use the table: Acetaminophen serum levels should be drawn 4 hr, or later, following ingestion. Serum levels drawn before 4 hr are not reliable when estimating risk. Based on the time the serum level is drawn, estimate the risk of hepatotoxicity. Patients with serum levels in the Probable or High Risk category should receive therapy with acetylcysteine.

For laboratories that report in mmol/L: 20 μg/ml = 0.13 mmol/L; 60 μg/ml = 0.4 mmol/L; 100 μg/ml = 0.62 mmol/L; 200 μg/ml = 1.32 mmol/L.

Emergency treatment

Empty stomach by emesis (within 1 hr of ingestion) and/or lavage with a large-bore tube (see Table 17–1).

Activated charcoal should not be given if acetylcysteine will be given unless there is co-ingestion of other poison. Lavage charcoal from stomach before giving acetylcysteine.

With unknown or large ingestions, begin acetylcysteine before serum level results are known (see later).

After 4 hr of ingestion, measure acetaminophen serum level and calculate risk using the values listed in the earlier section for estimating risk.

If serum level is in the safe range and acetylcysteine has been started, discontinue acetylcysteine.

If serum level is in the probable or high-risk category, continue acetylcysteine.

Acetylcysteine should be given as soon as possible. It is most effective if given within 10–16 hr, but it may be effective even up to 24 hr after ingestion. *Free consultation: 1-800-525-6115, 24 hr daily.*

Oral acetylcysteine (Mucomyst) 20%. Mix to prepare a 5% solution in carbonated beverage or fruit drink.

Loading dose: 140 mg/kg PO or NG

Maintenance: 70 mg/kg q4h for a total of 18 doses

If vomiting occurs within 1 hr of a dose, repeat that dose. Cold solutions and a straw may increase palatability. Severe vomiting can be treated with metoclopramide (Reglan) at 1 mg/kg IV or IM.

Intravenous acetylcysteine is used in Canada and Europe (the sterile injectable form is not available in the United States except through an investigational protocol with the National Capital Poison Center or the Rocky Mountain Poison Center):

150 mg/kg in 200 ml NS or D5W over 15 min, then 50 mg/kg in 500 ml NS or D5W in the next 4 hr, then 100 mg/kg in 1,000 ml NS or D5W in the next 16 hr (total dose 300 mg/kg over 20 hr).

Monitor liver function tests, electrolytes, and CBC.

Charcoal hemoperfusion may be beneficial but has not been adequately evaluated. This might supplement the previous measures in very large ingestions or with late presentations.

*Adapted from Rumack BH, et al: *Arch Intern Med* 1981; 141:380–385; Smilkstein MJ, et al: *N Engl J Med* 1988; 319:1557–1562, Meredith TJ, Vale JA: *Drugs* 1986; 32 (suppl 4):177–205, Rumack BH, Matthews H: *Pediatrics* 1975; 55:871–876, Rumack BH: *Pediatr Clin North Am* 1986; 33:691–701, and Mann KV: *Clin Pharm* 1988; 7:563–564.

TABLE 17–3.—POISONING BY ASPIRIN AND OTHER SALICYLATES*

Signs and symptoms
Nausea, vomiting, tinnitus, fever, dehydration, lethargy, excitability, disorientation, convulsions, coma, hyperpnea, respiratory alkalosis, metabolic acidosis.

Severity
Ingestions of >150 mg/kg are expected to cause toxicity. Ingestions of 300–500 mg/kg are serious, and ingestions >500 mg/kg are potentially lethal.

Chronic ingestion of much lower doses may be toxic.

Estimating risk
Measure serum levels 6 hr or later after acute ingestion. Compare the level with the following estimation of severity. Make serial determinations to examine elimination. Levels measured before 6 hr may indicate toxicity but may not reflect severity.

Hr After Ingestion	Potential Severity (mg/dl)		
	Mild	Moderate	Severe
6	45–65	65–90	>90
12	38–55	55–80	>80
24	22–36	36–50	>50
30	20–30	30–40	>40
36	13–22	22–32	>32
42	12–20	20–28	>28
48	10–13	13–21	>21
60	—	10–13	>13

Therapy (begin before serum level is known)
Emesis or gastric lavage with large-bore tube followed by charcoal and cathartics.

Fluid management
Initially: Ringer's lactate in D5W at 10–15 ml/kg/hr for 1–2 hr to achieve a urine flow of 3–6 cc/kg/hr.

Continued.

TABLE 17–3.—Continued

Then: Continue D5W containing bicarbonate 20–35 mEq/L (depending on the degree of acidosis), 20–40 mEq/L KCl, 40–50 mEq/L of sodium, and 50 mEq/L of chloride at a rate of 4–8 ml/kg/hr until salicylate level is therapeutic. Attempt to maintain urinary pH >7–8. Maintenance fluids can then be administered at 2–3 ml/kg/hr.

Monitor blood gas, blood glucose, serum electrolyte, and calcium values, coagulation status, urine pH, and specific gravity, I/O, and salicylate levels.

Both hemodialysis and hemoperfusion remove salicylate. These procedures are indicated when (1) salicylate level > 130 mg/dl 6 hr after ingestion; (2) severe, unresponsive acidosis (pH <7.1); (3) renal failure; (4) unresponsive seizures; or (5) progressive deterioration despite other measures (see earlier).

*Adapted from Temple AR: *Arch Intern Med* 1981; 141:364–369, and Snodgrass WR: *Pediatr Clin North Am* 1986; 33:381–391.

TABLE 17–4.—Overdose With Anticholinergic Drugs (Atropine, Belladonna, Antihistamines, Tricyclics)

Signs and symptoms

Dry mouth, mydriasis, flushing, urinary retention, decreased bowel sounds, fever, tachycardia, hypertension, AV dissociation, restlessness, irritability, delirium, hallucinations, coma (drowsiness and ataxia with antihistamines).

Therapy

Emesis (unless contraindicated), lavage, activated charcoal, cathartics. These drugs slow GI motility and lavage may be effective long after ingestion.

Lavage may be more effective for antihistamines due to their *antiemetic* properties.

Tachycardia may respond to propranolol.

Physostigmine:

Indications:

1. To establish the diagnosis of anticholinergic poisoning. Most signs and symptoms will disappear in minutes if diagnosis is correct.

2. To treat convulsions, hallucinations, hypertension or arrythmias.

Contraindications: Gangrene, asthma, GI or GU obstruction.

Dose: Adults, 2 mg IM or *slow* IV repeat 1–2 mg in 20 min if no reversal. Repeat 1–4 mg (lowest effective dose) every 60 minutes.

Children and elderly: 0.5 mg IM or *slow* IV. Give at 5-minute interval up to 2 mg.

Neostigmine and pyridostigmine do not enter brain and do *not* correct CNS toxicity.

TABLE 17–5.—INGESTION OF CAUSTIC SUBSTANCES*

Signs and Symptoms
 Vomiting, drooling, dysphagia, refusal to drink, and edema or ulceration of pal-
 ate and pharynx.
Treatment
 Do *not* attempt to chemically neutralize. Do *not* induce emesis or give charcoal.
 Immediately dilute with water, 15 ml/kg, up to a maximum of 250 ml. Antacids
 or MOM can be used for strong acids.
 All patients should be admitted. Make NPO, begin IV fluid, and observe for 12
 to 24 hr. Treatment should be initiated before endoscopy unless it can be
 performed immediately.
 Endoscopy should be performed within 24 to 48 hr using a small, flexible fiberoptic endoscope.
 Steroid use is controversial but may reduce stricture formation for 2nd-degree
 burns. Use IV methylprednisolone 2 mg/kg/day or equivalent. Discontinue
 steroids if endoscopy shows 1st degree burn. Continue steroids for all 2nd-
 or 3rd-degree burns for 2 to 3 wk (e.g., prednisone 1 mg/kg/day) or until reepithelialization has occurred.
 If steroids are used, there is increased infection risk, so use antibiotic such as
 IV ampicillin. Discontinue if endoscopy shows 1st-degree burn.
 Use H_2 blocker such as IV cimetidine or antacid to suppress gastric acid formation (continue oral form for 6–8 wk for 2nd- or 3rd-degree burns).
Additional follow-up
 Close follow-up will be necessary to detect stricture formation and to perform
 dilation or surgery as necessary.
 These patients may be at high risk for the development of esophageal carci-
 noma (as early as 13 yr and a mean of 40 yr later), and they should be
 followed for this disease.

*Adapted from Rothstein FC: *Pediatr Clin North Am* 1986; 33:665–674, and Knopp R:
JACEP 1979; 8:329–336.

TABLE 17–6.—POISONING FROM DIGITALIS GLYCOSIDES (DIGOXIN, DIGITOXIN)*

Signs and Symptoms
  Acute ingestion
    Nausea, vomiting, hyperkalemia (with large ingestions), bradycardia, supra-
    ventricular arrhythmias, 1st- or 2nd-degree heart block. With large inges-
    tions PAT with block, ventricular ectopy with block, 3rd-degree block.
  Chronic toxicity
    Nausea, vomiting, CNS disturbances, arrhythmias (see earlier), abnormal
    vision, usually hypokalemia
Assessment
  Potential toxicity is increased by hypokalemia, hypomagnesemia, or hypercal-
    cemia.
  Digoxin levels drawn within 6 hr are still in distributive phase. These may not
    reliably correlate with the "therapeutic range" and should be repeated later.
  Serum digoxin level does not predict toxicity, and treatment should be based
    on clinical assessment. Healthy children often tolerate high digoxin levels
    with little toxicity (e.g., levels of < 10 ng/ml).
Therapy
  Emesis (unless contraindicated), lavage, activated charcoal, saline cathartics.
  Begin continuous ECG monitoring and monitoring serial electrolyte values, di-
    goxin level, and magnesium and calcium concentrations.
  Multiple-dose charcoal (see Table 17–1) can markedly increase digoxin elimi-
    nation long after ingestion or even with chronic toxicity.
  Symptomatic bradycardia and heart block
    Atropine
      Adults: 0.5 mg IV
      Children: 0.01 mg/kg/ IV
      May repeat in 5 min × 2–4 doses
  Ventricular arrhythmias
    Lidocaine:
      1–1.5 mg/kg load, then infusion of 1–4 mg/min; can repeat bolus of 0.5–
        1.0 mg/kg every 8–10 min × 3 more doses *or*
    Phenytoin:
      1–2 mg/kg IV (do not give faster than 50 mg/min); repeat every 5 min up
        to 10 doses (1.0 gm max).
  Do not give potassium until electrolytes status is known.
  For severe hyperkalemia (uncommon) or life-threatening arrhythmias, give di-
    goxin specific antibodies (Digibind). It is also indicated when >10 mg of
    digoxin is ingested by an adult or >4 mg by a healthy child.

$$\text{Digibind Dose (in \# of vials)} = \frac{\text{Body load (mg)}}{0.6 \text{ (mg/vial)}}$$

$$\text{Body load in mg} = \frac{\text{Dig level} \times 0.56 \times \text{Weight (kg)}}{1,000}$$

  Each vial of Digibind will bind about 0.6 mg of digoxin or digitoxin.

*Adapted from Lalonde RL, et al: *Clin Pharmacol Ther* 1985; 37:367–371, Lake KD, et al: *Pharmacotherapy* 1984; 4:161–163, Bigger JT: *J Clin Pharmacol* 1985; 25:514–521, Cole PL, Smith TW: *Drug Intell Clin Pharm* 1986; 20:267–269, and Lewander WJ, et al: *Am J Dis Child* 1986; 140:770–773.

TABLE 17-7.—HYDROCARBON INGESTIONS*

Signs and Symptoms
Most morbidity and mortality are from aspiration pneumonitis. Symptoms include choking, coughing, tachypnea, respiratory effort, retractions, fever, irritability, drowsiness, lethargy, seizures, and coma.

Therapy
Gastric emptying increases the risk of aspiration. Emesis and lavage are generally *contraindicated* unless the substance contained pesticides, benzene, toluene, heavy metals, or other systemic toxins. Some recommend gastric emptying when the estimated ingested volume is >1-2 ml/kg, but this is controversial. If emesis is indicated, it should be performed only in an alert patient. If mental status is deteriorating, intubation with a cuffed endotracheal tube should be performed before lavage.

Examine and observe for at least 6-8 hr; obtain chest x-ray film and blood gas values.

Monitor BP, heart rate and rhythm, and respiratory rate, and begin oxygen. Intubate and ventilate if necessary.

All patients who become symptomatic during observation should be admitted.

Asymptomatic patients with x-ray abnormalities should be admitted and observed unless close follow-up can be ensured.

Do not use steroids or epinephrine.

Prophylactic antibiotics should not be used unless the patient is debilitated or has preexisting respiratory disease. Infectious pneumonia can be difficult to distinguish due to fever and other signs of aspiration, and Gram stains and cultures should be performed.

*Adapted from Anas N, et al: *JAMA* 1981; 246:840-843, Klein BL, Simon JE: *Pediatr Clin North Am* 1986; 33:411-419, and Truemper E, et al: *Pediatr Emerg Care* 1987; 3:187-193.

TABLE 17-8.—INSECTICIDES (CARBAMATES AND ORGANOPHOSPHATES)*

Signs and symptoms
Rapidly absorbed through skin and mucous membranes. Symptoms progress rapidly and occur within minutes and almost always before 12 hr of exposure.

Salivation, Lacrimation, Urination, Defecation, vomiting, miosis, sweating, fasciculations, tremors, convulsions, coma, and respiratory arrest. CNS signs are uncommon with carbamates. Pneumonitis may occur with liquid insecticides that are in a petroleum base.

Therapy
Establish airway and ventilate if necessary. Obtain RBC cholinesterase if possible (for organophosphates and this must be obtained prior to the use of 2-PAM to follow progress). Serum cholinesterase levels: 20%-50% of normal = mild poisoning; 10%-20% of normal = moderate poisoning; <10% of nomal = severe poisoning.

Continued.

TABLE 17–8.—Continued

Atropine (will not treat muscle weakness due to stimulation of nicotine receptors and patients can still develop respiratory depression):
Adult: 1–2 mg q 10–30 min
Child (<12 yr): 0.05 mg/kg q 10–30 min
Very large doses may be necessary (40–50 mg daily are common, and much higher doses may be needed). Do not underdose. The endpoint should be drying of secretions and elevation of heart rate (if the patient had bradycardia). It will be necessary to continue atropine for 24 hr (up to 5–10 days for lypophillic poisons) and then to slowly taper atropine.
Pralidoxime (2-PAM) is the specific antidote and should be used as soon as possible. It is effective for organophosphates, but it may not be effective for carbamates. Some authors consider it contraindicated in carbamate poisoning.
Adult: 0.5–1.0 gm in 100–200 ml D5W infused over 15–30 min; Can be repeated in 1–2 hr and then every 8–12 hr
Child: 25–50 mg/kg given in the same intervals as in the adults
Do not give morphine, theophylline, physostigmine, phenothiazines, ethacrynic acid, or furosemide. These are contraindicated.
Once stabilized, decontaminate by removing clothing and washing all contaminated areas with soap and copious amounts of water. For oral ingestions, induce emesis (unless contraindicated) or lavage. Give activated charcoal and cathartics (see Table 17–1).

*Adapted from Mortensen ML: *Pediatr Clin North Am* 1986; 33:421–445; and Tafuri J, Roberts J: *Ann Emerg Med* 1987; 16:193–202.

TABLE 17–9.—Iron Ingestion*

Signs and Symptoms
Phase I (within 12 hr of ingestion):
abdominal pain, vomiting, diarrhea, hemorrhagic gastritis. Rarely seizures, shock, coma.
Phase II (stability—4–48 hours): improvement of symptoms but the existance of this phase is disputed.
Phase III (shock—12–48 hours): hypoperfusion and shock, hepatic necrosis or failure, hypoglycemia, metabolic acidosis, bleeding abnormalities, coma, seizures.
Phase IV (2–8 weeks): pyloric or antral stenosis, CNS damage, cirrhosis.
Estimating severity (for children < 5 yr)
Care should be taken to make an accurate assessment of the ingestion or the most that could have been ingested. If < 20 mg/kg, no therapy is needed. For 20–60 mg/kg, patients can be treated with syrup of ipecac and followed closely at home. For > 60 mg/kg, or symptomatic, patients should be evaluated by a physician.
Deferoxamine challenge: Give 1 gm of deferoxamine IM. A pink-orange (vin rose) color indicates iron complex in urine and a significant ingestion.

Serum iron: Should be obtained within 2–4 hr after ingestion because this provides the best correlation with severity of poisoning. Serum iron 300–500 μg/dl with symptoms or serum level exceeding iron-binding capacity should receive chelation therapy. All patients with levels >500 μg/dl should receive chelation therapy.

Therapy

Emesis unless contraindicated (see Table 17–1). Charcoal does not absorb iron.

Lavage with 5% sodium bicarbonate solution. Oral deferoxamine is controversial and discouraged.

Obtain abdominal x-ray film after lavage to identify remaining iron.

Correct shock, electrolyte imbalance, or hypoglycemia. Large IV volumes may be necessary, and urine output should be maintained at least 1–2 ml/kg/hr.

Deferoxamine (if the previous criteria are met): Give IV at 15 mg/kg/hr until serum iron is <300 μg/dl (can reduce to 6 mg/kg/hr after stabilization). For less severe ingestions, give 40–90 mg/kg q4–8h IM (but not to exceed 1 gm per dose). Not all patients will have vin rose–colored urine. For those who do, the chelation therapy should continue for 24 hr after the urine color returns to normal.

*Adapted from Banner W, Tong TG: *Pediatr Clin North Am* 1986; 33:393–409, and Mann KV, et al: *Clin Pharm* 1989; 8:428–440.

TABLE 17–10.—Lead Poisoning*

Signs and Symptoms

Anorexia, weight loss, irritability, fatigue, headache, lead lines, and anemia. Severe cases may signal impending encephalopathy and include ataxia, persistent vomiting, irritability, paralysis, severe anemia or frank papilledema, seizures, and coma.

Screening and Diagnosis

Lead poisoning is suggested by a low hemoglobin level and basophilic stippling on a peripheral smear and by x-ray evidence of lead lines at ends of growing bones. Width of lead lines indicates duration of exposure, not extent. X-ray film of abdomen may show radiopaque particles if ingestion was recent.

Diagnosis is established by elevated blood lead and erythrocyte protoporphyrin (EP) levels.

Risk classification of asymptomatic children[†]

Risk is more urgent than indicated for symptomatic children, children < 3 yr, children in the upper part of the following categories, and in children whose siblings are in a higher category.

Blood Lead (μg/dl)	EP Levels by Extraction Method (μg dl)			
	<35 (<35)	35–109 (35–74)	110–249 (75–174)	>250 (>175)
<24	I	Ia	Ia	EP
25–49	Ib	II	II	III
50–69	—	III	III	IV
>70	—	—	IV	IV

Continued.

TABLE 17–10.—Continued

Values in parentheses indicate values for zinc protoporphyrin by hematofluore-meter.

EP is erythropoietic protoporphyria (rarely, iron deficiency may elevate EP lev-els up to 300 μg/dl).

I and Ib are low risk, Ia is low risk (may be iron deficiency), II is moderate risk, III is high risk, and IV is urgent risk. However, recent evidence suggests possible long-term impairment with levels much lower than 24 μg/dl.

The dash indicates not observed clinically.

Therapy

For acute ingestion, use emesis, charcoal, and cathartics unless contraindi-cated. If lead is detected on abdominal x-ray films, use enema (see chelator therapy).

For all levels of blood lead, the patient should be removed from all lead sources, and iron deficiency should be treated. For patients with moderate or high risk, prescribe a low-fat diet with sufficient minerals, especially cal-cium and iron.

Asyptomatic patients

Blood lead level 25–55 μg/ml: Perform CaEDTA provocation test, 500 mg/m^2 in 5% D5W IV over 1 hr. Collect all urine and calculate the ratio of lead excreted:

$$(\mu g)/Ca\ EDTA\ given\ (mg)$$

If the ratio is <0.6, do not treat but repeat lead level and provocation test periodically. If ratio is 0.6–0.69 in children >3 yr, do not treat but follow as above. If ratio is 0.6–0.69 and the patient is <3 yr, treat with Ca EDTA for 3 days IV or IM (see later). If the ratio is >0.7 treat with Ca EDTA for 5 days IV or IM (see later).

Blood lead level 56–69 μg/ml: Treat with Ca EDTA for 5 days.

Blood lead >70 μg/ml: Use BAL 50 mg/m^2 IM q4h, and after 4 hr start Ca EDTA and give for 5 days. BAL can be discontinued after 3 days if lead level is < 50 μg/ml. BAL is contraindicated with hepatic insufficiency and should be used with caution in patients with G-6-PD deficiency.

Ca EDTA regimen is 1,000 mg/m^2/day by continuous IV infusion (inpatient), or with a 1-hr infusion (outpatient), or mixed with procaine and given IM. Ca EDTA is contraindicated with renal insufficiency. (An alternative to Ca EDTA is D-penicillamine, 25–40 mg/kg/day PO on an empty stomach. Cannot be given to penicillin allergic patients and may cause rash, neutro-penia, proteinuria. Monitor for these and discontinue therapy if adverse effects occur.

Symptomatic patients

Provide adequate fluid replacement for chelator therapy. Establish urine flow with D5W 10–20 ml/kg and then provide maintenance with careful avoid-ance of excessive fluids.

Without encephalopathy: Treat with BAL 50–60 mg/m^2 IM q4h. Then after the first 4 hr add Ca EDTA 1,000 mg/m^2/day for 5 days (see earlier). BAL can be stopped after 3 days if lead level is < 50 μg/ml.

Acute encephalopathy: Treat with BAL 75–85 mg/m^2 IM q4h. After the first 4 hr add Ca EDTA 1,500 mg/m^2/day for 5–7 days (see earlier). If encephalopathy continues after 4 days, the usual 5-day regimen can be cautiously lengthened to 7 days.

D-Penicillamine can be given for 1–2 mo., which may reduce the chances of rebound of lead levels.

Monitor serial lead levels and EP on day 3–5, 1 wk, 2 wk, and then every 2–4 wk for 6 mo.

*Adapted from Piomelli S, et al: *J Pediatr* 1984; 105:523–532, Shannon M, et al: *J Pediatr* 1988; 112:799–804; American Academy of Pediatrics: *Pediatrics* 1987; 79:457–465, and Ibels LS, Pollock CA: *Med Toxicol* 1986; 1:387–410.
†Information from Centers for Disease Control: *MMWR* 1985; 34:67–68.

TABLE 17–11.—Poisoning With Narcotics and Their Analogues

Signs and Symptoms
Stupor, coma, slow respirations, cyanosis, hypotension, shock, constricted pupils (dilated with anoxia), flaccid musculature.

Therapy
Maintain airway; intubate and ventilate if necessary.

Immediately give naloxone (Narcan) to any patient with depressed mental status of unknown cause. Narcan dosages are:

Adults: 0.4–0.8 mg IV bolus

Children: 0.01 mg/kg IV bolus

Emesis only if the patient is fully conscious. Gastric lavage after tracheal intubation.

Give activated charcoal and cathartics every 3–4 hr until charcoal appears in stool.

If response does not occur in minutes, repeat the Narcan. For large ingestions, much higher doses may be necessary, e.g., 2–4 mg IV for both children and adults. Narcan has a short duration, so repeat injections every 20–60 min.

For large ingestions or long-acting narcotics, consider a Narcan infusion. Mix Narcan in normal saline or D5W and infuse at 2.5–5.0 μg/kg/hr. Continue infusion for 24 hr or 48 hr for large ingestions or long-acting agents (methadone). Attempt to discontinue the infusion every 12 hr, but the patient's vital signs and respiratory rate should be monitored closely for at least 2 hr after discontinuation.

For all patients, monitor vital signs, respiratory rate, and sensorium frequently, and periodically monitor blood gas and electrolyte values.

TABLE 17–12.—Poisoning With Tricyclic Antidepressants*

Signs and Symptoms
 Hypotension, shock, arrhythmias, tachycardia, AV block, mydriasis, urinary re-
  tention, decreased bowel sounds, fever, restlessness, irritability, delirium,
  and seizures.
Assessment
 Tricyclic serum levels do not predict toxicity. These agents prolong the QRS
  on ECG, and this is a better guide to toxicity. Doses >10 mg/kg are potentially toxic.
Therapy
 Provide cardiovascular and respiratory support. If the patient has CNS depres-
  sion or seizures, give Narcan (see Table 17–10).
 Induce emesis (unless contraindicated or gastric lavage; see Table 17–1). Tri-
  cyclics slow GI emptying, and these measures may be effective even 18 hr
  after ingestion.
 Give repeated doses of charcoal (intestinal dialysis; see Table 17–1).
 Begin IV and continuous ECG monitoring (measure QRS and QT intervals). If
  hypotension occurs, increase IV flow to expand plasma volume.
 If hypotension, acidosis, ventricular arrhythmias, or widened QRS occurs, give
  sodium bicarbonate (keep blood pH 7.5–7.55).
 Seizures should be treated with IV diazepam. Arrhythmias should be treated
  with volume and bicarbonate. Ventricular arrhythmias can be treated with
  lidocaine or phenytoin (see Table 17–5 for regimen). Supraventricular arrhythmias can be treated with propranolol. Physostigmine might be considered if other measures fail *except* for bradycardia. Quinidine, procainamide,
  and disopyramide are contraindicated (similar cardiac effects).
 If patient is asymptomatic, monitor at least 6–12 hrs due to possible delayed
  absorption.
 If patient is symptomatic, do not discharge unless patient is asymptomatic and
  without arrhythmias for at least 24 hr.

*Adapted from Braden NJ, et al: *Pediatr Clin North Am* 1986; 33:287–297, Boehnert
MT, Lovejoy FH: *N Engl J Med* 1985; 313:474–479, and Ware MR: *South Med J* 1987;
80:1410–1415.

TABLE 17–13.—Carbon Monoxide Poisoning*

Signs and Symptoms
 Carboxyhemoglobin (COHb) of:
  20%–30%: headache
  30%–40%: headache, nausea, fatigue, dizziness, weakness
  40%–50%: headache, syncope, confusion
  50%–60%: seizures
  60%–70%: seizures, coma, death with prolonged exposure
     80%: death
 Complications
  Arrhythmias, pulmonary edema, myoglobinuria and renal failure, seizures,
   cerebral edema, visual defects, or temporary blindness.

Late complications (1–2 wk after exposure)
    Personality changes, decreased mentation, visual impairment, agnosia, and movement disorders.
Therapy
Immediately remove patient from the source of carbon monoxide.
Provide 100% oxygen until COHb levels are <10%. (CO half-life at room air is 5 hr, at 100% oxygen it is 90 min, and with hyperbaric oxygen it is < 30 min.)
If available and as soon as possible, provide hyperbaric oxygen at 2–2.5 atm for COHb >20%, if there is mental impairment, if there are cardiac abnormalities, or if the patient is pregnant. Give for 30–60 min and then provide 100% oxygen until COHb is <20%.

*Adapted from Norkool DM, Kirkpatrick, JN: *Ann Emerg Med* 1985; 14:1168–1171, and Zimmerman SS, Truxal B: *Pediatrics* 1981; 68:215–224.

TABLE 17–14.—THEOPHYLLINE AND AMINOPHYLLINE TOXICITY AND POISONING*

Signs and Symptoms
    Levels > 20–25 μg/ml
        Nausea, vomiting, diarrhea, insomnia, tremor, irritability, headache (seizures and death rarely at 25 μg/ml)
    Levels > 30–35 μg/ml
        Tachycardia, arrhythmias, seizures, hypotension, cardiac arrest
Therapy
Obtain serial theophylline levels but begin therapy before the results are known.
Support cardiac and respiratory status, establish airway, start IV, and administer oxygen.
If seizures occur, treat with diazepam.
If serious ventricular arrhythmias occur, treat with lidocaine or procainamide (see Table 17–5 for lidocaine). Verapamil or propranolol can be used to slow ventricular rate for atrial arrhythmias.
Induce emesis for acute ingestion unless contraindicated. If contraindicated, perform gastric lavage.
For both acute ingestions and serious chronic toxicity (levels >30–40 μg/ml), give multiple doses of charcoal at 20–50 gm q4h PO or NG until level is <20 μg/ml to increase systemic elimination (see intestinal dialysis in Table 17–1). This method should be performed even in the absence of symptoms, and it may be preferred even to charcoal hemoperfusion. Give cathartics to allow evacuation of the charcoal.
For serious, life-threatening toxicity, charcoal hemoperfusion will rapidly remove theophylline. Indicated if patient has cardiorespiratory failure, hepatic dysfunction, recurrent seizures, or serum level >60 μg/ml.

*Adapted from Park GD, et al: *Arch Intern Med* 1986; 146:969–973, Gal P, et al: *JAMA* 1984; 251:3130–3131, and Albert S: *Pediatr Clin North Am* 1987; 34:61–73.

TABLE 17–15.—Poisoning With Methanol or Ethylene Glycol*

Sources
  Methanol
    Carburetor fluid, gas antifreeze, model engine fuel, windshield washer fluid, and bootleg whiskey
  Ethylene glycol
    Auto radiator antifreeze or coolant and brake fluid
Lethal dose
  Methanol
    30 ml of 100% methanol (but death has occurred with 15 ml of 40%)
  Ethylene glycol
    100 ml of 100% ethylene glycol
Signs and Symptoms
  Methanol
    Cloudy, blurred vision, yellow spots, central scotoma, reversible or irreversible blindness, anion gap metabolic acidosis, confusion, slurred speech, CNS depression, and seizures.
  Ethylene glycol
    Nausea, vomiting, ataxia, nystagmus, seizures, hypothermia, myoclonic jerks, fever, coma with metabolic acidosis and anion gap (may be up to 12 hr after ingestion); calcium oxalate crystals in urine (within 4–8 hr) may lead to renal failure.
Therapy
  Provide cardiopulmonary support, induce emesis (unless contraindicated), and give charcoal (see Table 17–1).
  Correct acidosis promptly with sodium bicarbonate and provide forced diuresis for ethylene glycol poisoning.
  Administer ethanol (which has higher affinity for alcohol dehydrogenase). Give IV or PO loading dose of 7.6–10 ml/kg of 10% ethanol in D5W (or 1 ml/kg of 95% ethanol in fruit juice), then a maintenance dose of 1.4 ml/kg/hr (continuous infusion) of 10% ethanol in D5W IV or 0.15 ml/kg/hr of 95% ethanol in fruit juice PO.
  Continuously monitor blood ethanol levels and adjust ethanol dose to maintain blood level of 100 mg/dl. Dose will need to be increased if hemodialysis is performed.
  Hemodialysis is indicated along with ethanol therapy for serum methanol or ethylene glycol >50 mg/dl or with renal failure from ethylene glycol.
  For methanol, administer folate 1 mg/kg (up to 50 mg/dose) IV q4h × 6 doses.
  For ethylene glycol, give thiamine 100 mg IM and pyridoxine 100 mg IM or IV.

*Adapted from Litovitz T: *Pediatr Clin North Am* 1986; 33:311–323.

18 *Hematology-Oncology*

Charles E. Driscoll, M.D.

HEMOSTASIS

TABLE 18–1.—Pathologic Bleeding

Pathologic bleeding may be secondary to vascular fragility, platelet factors (cellular), or plasma coagulation factors.

Localize the defect by history:

History	Vascular	Cellular	Plasma
Bleeding from multiple sites		+	+
Hemarthrosis; large ecchymoses			+
Petechiae, purpura, mucosal bleeding	+	+	
Bleeding after trauma		Immediate	Delayed
Congenital disorders; prior bleeding episodes			+

Order selective screening tests to complete the diagnosis.

TABLE 18–2.—PRESUMPTIVE DIAGNOSIS OF COMMON BLEEDING DISORDERS BASED ON ROUTINE SCREENING TESTS*

PRESUMPTIVE PROBLEM	PLATELET COUNT	BLEEDING TIME	PROTHROMBIN TIME (PT)	PARTIAL THROMBOPLASTIN TIME (PTT)	THROMBIN TIME (TT)	MISCELLANEOUS
Thrombocytopenia	↓	N, ↑	N	N	N	
Platelet function defect or vascular defect	N	↑	N	N	N	
Von Willebrand's disease	N	↑	N	↑	N	↓ VIIIcr, ↓ VIIIag, ↓ VIIIvwf
Extrinsic pathway defect (VII)	N	N	↑	N	N	
intrinsic pathway defect (VIII, IX, XI, XII, prekallikrein, high-molecular-weight kininogen, inhibitor)	N	N	N	↑	N	
Common pathway or multiple pathway defects, excluding fibrinogen	N	N	↑	↑	N	
Fibrinogen deficiency or dysfunction, vitamin K deficiency, liver disease, primary fibrinolysis	N	N	↑	↑	↑	High levels of fibrin(ogen) degradation products (FDP)
Disseminated intravascular coagulation	↓	N, ↑	↑	↑	↑	High levels of FDP
Factor XIII deficiency	N	N	N	N	N	Positive clot solubility

*Adapted from Blacklow RS (ed): *MacBryde's Signs and Symptoms: Applied Pathologic Physiology and Clinical Interpretation*, ed 6. Philadelphia, JB Lippincott Co, 1983, p 551.
N = normal; ↓ = decreased; ↑ = increased.

TABLE 18–3.—CHARACTERISTICS OF COAGULATION FACTORS*

FACTOR	DESCRIPTIVE NAME	SOURCE	APPROXIMATE HALF-LIFE (hr)	FUNCTION‡
I	Fibrinogen	Liver	120	Substrate for fibrin clot (CP)
II	Prothrombin	Liver VKD†	60	Serine protease (CP)
V	Proaccelerin, labile factor	Liver	12–36	Cofactor (CP)
VII	Serum prothrombin conversion accelerator, proconvertin	Liver VKD	6	? Serine protease (EP)
VIII	Antihemophilic factor or globin	Endothelial cells and ? elsewhere	12	Cofactor (IP)
IX	Plasma thromboplastin component, Christmas factor	Liver VKD	24	Serine protease (IP)
X	Stuart-Prower factor	Liver VKD	36	Serine protease (CP)
XI	Plasma thromboplastin antecedent	? Liver	40–84	Serine protease (IP)
XII	Hageman factor	? Liver	50	Serine protease, contact activation (IP)
XIII	Fibrin stabilizing factor	? Liver	96–180	Transglutaminase (CP)
Prekallikrein	Fletcher factor	? Liver	?	Serine protease, contact activation (IP)
High-molecular-weight kininogen	Fitzgerald factor Flaujeac or Williams factor	? Liver	?	Cofactor, contact activation (IP)

*From Blacklow RS (ed): *MacBryde's Signs and Symptoms: Applied Pathologic Physiology and Clinical Interpretation*, ed 6. Philadelphia, JB Lippincott Co, 1983, p 539. Reproduced by permission.
†Vitamin K–dependent (VKD).
‡Common pathway (CP), extrinsic pathway (EP), intrinsic pathway (IP).

DISSEMINATED INTRAVASCULAR COAGULOPATHY

TABLE 18–4.—COMPARISON OF SCREENING AND SPECIFIC TESTS BETWEEN DIC
AND ENTITIES CONFUSED WITH DIC*

Consumptive coagulopathy may need to be differentiated from other coagulation disorders. Causes of DIC include septic shock, severe RDS in newborns, malignancies, rickettsial diseases, head trauma, obstetric hemorrhage, and postoperatively (lung and prostate).

ASPECT	DIC	LIVER DISEASE	VITAMIN K DEFICIENCY	DILUTIONAL	SEPSIS WITHOUT SHOCK
Partial thromboplastin time	P	P	P	P	P
Prothrombin time	P	P	P	P	P
Fibrinogen	R	R	N	R	E
Factor II	R	R	R	R	R
Factor V	R	R	N	R	E
Factor VIII	R	N-E	N	R	E
Platelets	R	N-R	N	R	N-R
FSPs	+	+/−	O	O	O
"Soluble fibrin"	+	O	O	O	O

*From Corrigan JD: *Pediatr Rev* 1979; 1:37–45. Reproduced by permission.
Abbreviations used: P, prolonged; N, normal; R, reduced; +, present; O, absent; E, elevated; FSPs, fibrinolytic split products.

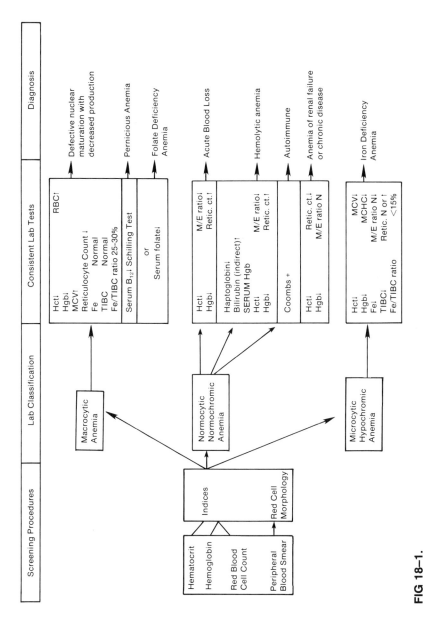

FIG 18–1.

Laboratory diagnosis of anemia. (From Bolinger AM, Korman NR: Anemias, in Young LY, Koda-Kimble MA [eds]: *Applied Therapeutics: The Clinical Use of Drugs,* ed 4. Vancouver, Wash, Applied Therapeutics, 1988, p 1053. Reproduced by permission.)

TABLE 18–5.—Differential Diagnosis of the Hypochromic-Microcytic States*

	DEFICIENCY	TRANSFERRIN DEFECT	DEFECT IN IRON UTILIZATION	DEFECT IN IRON RE-UTILIZATION
Peripheral blood				
Microcytosis (*M*) vs. hypochromia (*H*)	M > H	M > H	M > H	M < H
Polychromatophilic targeted cells	Absent	Absent	Present	Absent
Stippled red cells	Absent	Absent	Present	Absent
RDW[†]	Increased	Increased	Increased	Normal
Serum iron				
Iron-binding capacity	↓ : ↑	↓ : ↓	↑ : Normal	↓ : ↓
% saturation of transferrin	<10%	0	>50%	>10%
Serum ferritin (normal 30–300 ng/mL)	<12	(No data available)	>400	30–400
Bone marrow				
Erythrocyte-granulocyte ratio (normal 1:3 to 1:5)	1:1—1:2	1:1—1:2	1:1—5:1	1:1—1:2
Marrow iron	Absent	Present	Increased	Present
Ringed sideroblasts	Absent	Absent	Present	Absent

*From Berkow R, Fletcher AJ (eds): Hematology and oncology, in *The Merck Manual*, ed 15. Rahway, NJ, Merck & Co., 1987, p 1102. Adapted from Frenkel EP: *Houston Med* 1976: June, vol 11. Reproduced by permission.
[†]RDW = Red blood cell volume distribution width expressing the degree of anisocytosis (i.e., variation in cell size).

TABLE 18–6.—Characteristics of the Thalassemias*

CATEGORY	ANEMIA	MCV	% Hb A$_2$	% Hb F
β Thalassemia				
Heterozygous	Mild	↓	↑	Variable
Homozygous	Severe	↓	Variable	↑ up to 90%
β-δ Thalassemia				
Heterozygous	Mild	↓	N or ↓	> 5%
Homozygous	Moderate-severe	↓	Absent	100%
α Thalassemia				
Single gene defect	None	N— ↓	N	N
Double gene defect	Mild	↓	N— ↓	< 5%
Triple gene defect	Moderate	↓	N— ↓ (Hb H or Bart's present)	Variable

*From Berkow R, Fletcher AJ (eds): Hematology and oncology, in *The Merck Manual*, ed 15. Rahway, NJ, Merck & Co, 1987, p 1123. Reproduced by permission.

TABLE 18–7.—Normal Microhematocrit Values*

AGE	AVERAGE NORMAL	MINIMAL NORMAL
Children—Both Sexes		
At birth	56.6	51.0
First day	56.1	50.5
End of 1st wk	52.7	47.5
End of 2d wk	49.6	44.7
End of 3d wk	46.6	42.0
End of 4th wk	44.6	40.0
End of 2d mo.	38.9	35.1
End of 4th mo.	36.5	32.9
End of 6th mo.	36.2	32.6
End of 8th mo.	35.8	32.3
End of 10th mo.	35.5	32.0
End of 1st yr	35.2	31.7
End of 2d yr	35.5	32.0
End of 4th yr	37.1	33.4
End of 6th yr	37.9	34.2
End of 8th yr	38.9	35.1
End of 12th yr	39.6	35.7
Men		
End of 14th yr	44	39.6
End of 18th yr	47	42.3
18–50 yr	47	42.3
50–60 yr	45	40.5
60–70 yr	43	38.7
70–80 yr	40	36.0
Nonpregnant Women		
14–50 yr	42	36
50–80 yr	40	36
Pregnant Women		
End of 4th mo.	42	30
End of 5th mo.	40	30
End of 6th mo.	37	30
End of 7th mo.	37	30
End of 8th mo.	39	30
End of 9th mo.	40	30

*Courtesy of Dr M Strumia.

TABLE 18–8.—NORMAL LEUKOCYTE
COUNT IN PERIPHERAL BLOOD*

	LEUKOCYTE COUNT (CELLS/CU MM)	
AGE	Average	95% Range[†]
Birth	18,100	9,000–30,000
12 hr	22,800	13,000–38,000
24 hr	18,900	9,400–34,000
1 wk	12,200	5,000–21,000
2 wk	11,400	5,000–20,000
4 wk	10,800	5,000–19,500
2 mo.	11,000	5,500–18,000
4 mo.	11,500	6,000–17,500
6 mo.	11,900	6,000–17,500
8 mo.	12,200	6,000–17,500
10 mo.	12,000	6,000–17,500
12 mo.	11,400	6,000–17,500
2 yr	10,600	6,000–17,000
4 yr	9,100	5,500–15,500
6 yr	8,500	5,000–14,500
8 yr	8,300	4,500–13,500
10 yr	8,100	4,500–13,500
12 yr	8,000	4,500–13,500
14 yr	7,900	4,500–13,000
16 yr	7,800	4,500–13,000
18 yr	7,700	4,500–12,500
20 yr	7,500	4,500–11,500
21 yr	7,400	4,500–11,000

*Adapted from Albritton EC: *Standard Values in Blood.* Philadelphia, WB Saunders Co, 1952, pp 50–51.
[†]Average value ± 2 SD.

TABLE 18–9.—Normal Leukocyte Differential Count in Peripheral Blood[*][†]

AGE	SEGMENTED NEUTROPHILS		BAND NEUTROPHILS		EOSINOPHILS		BASOPHILS		LYMPHOCYTES		MONOCYTES	
	%	No./mm³	%	No./mm³	%	No./mm³	%	No./mm³	%	No./mm³	%	No./mm³
At birth	52	9,400	9.1	1,650	2.2	400	0.6	100	31 ± 5	5,500	5.8	1,050
12 hr	58	13,200	10.2	2,330	2.0	450	0.4	100	24	5,500	5.3	1,200
24 hr	52	9,800	9.2	1,750	2.4	450	0.5	100	31	5,800	5.8	1,100
1 wk	39	4,700	6.8	830	4.1	500	0.4	50	41	5,000	9.1	1,100
2 wk	34	3,900	5.5	630	3.1	350	0.4	50	48	5,500	8.8	1,000
4 wk	30	3,300	4.5	490	2.8	300	0.5	50	56 + 15	6,000	6.5	700
2 mo.	30	3,300	4.4	490	2.7	300	0.5	50	57	6,300	5.9	650
4 mo.	29	3,300	3.9	450	2.6	300	0.4	50	59	6,800	5.2	600
6 mo.	28	3,300	3.8	450	2.5	300	0.4	50	61	7,300	4.8	580
8 mo.	27	3,300	3.3	410	2.5	300	0.4	50	62	7,600	4.7	580
10 mo.	27	3,200	3.3	400	2.5	300	0.4	50	63	7,500	4.6	550
12 mo.	28	3,200	3.1	350	2.6	300	0.4	50	61	7,000	4.8	550
2 yr	30	3,200	3.0	320	2.6	280	0.5	50	59	6,300	5.0	530
4 yr	39	3,500	3.0	270	2.8	250	0.6	50	50 ± 15	4,500	5.0	450
6 yr	48	4,000	3.0	250	2.7	230	0.6	50	42	3,500	4.7	400
8 yr	50	4,100	3.0	250	2.4	200	0.6	50	39	3,300	4.2	350
10 yr	51	4,200	3.0	240	2.4	200	0.5	40	38 ± 10	3,100	4.3	350
12 yr	52	4,200	3.0	240	2.5	200	0.5	40	38	3,000	4.4	350
14 yr	53	4,200	3.0	240	2.5	200	0.5	40	37	2,900	4.7	380
16 yr	54	4,200	3.0	230	2.6	200	0.5	40	35 ± 10	2,800	5.1	400
18 yr	54	4,200	3.0	230	2.6	200	0.5	40	35	2,700	5.2	400
20 yr	56	4,200	3.0	230	2.7	200	0.5	40	33	2,500	5.0	380
21 yr	56	4,200	3.0	220	2.7	200	0.5	40	34 ± 10	2,500	4.0	300

*Adapted from Albritton EC: Standard Values in Blood. Philadelphia, WB Saunders Co, 1952, pp 50–51.
†Average values based on the average normal leukocyte counts in Table 18–6.

539

IMMUNE FACTORS

T cells (thymus-dependent) and B cells (lymphocytes from bursa of Fabricius) cannot be separated morphologically, but a functional assessment is possible. T cells are screened by a white cell count with differential; B cells are evaluated by means of immunoglobulin assay.

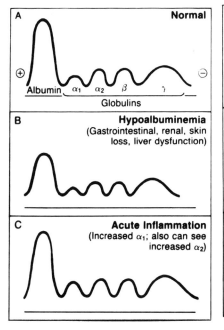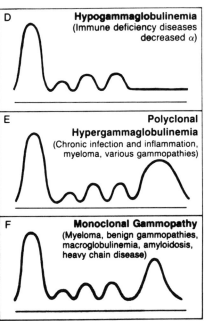

FIG 18–2.
Serum immunoelectrophoretic patterns. (From Goodwin JS: Clinical assessment of the immune system: Which tests? When? in Goodwin JS [ed]: *Mediguide to Inflammatory Diseases.* New York, Dellacorte Publications, 1983, vol 1, no 2, p 2. Reproduced by permission.)

TABLE 18–10.—Clinical and Laboratory Features of Various Forms of Chronic Leukemia Commonly Seen at Diagnosis*

SYMPTOMS	PHYSICAL FINDINGS	LABORATORY FINDINGS
Chronic myelogenous leukemia (CML)		
Abdominal discomfort, fullness	Slight hepatomegaly	Blood
Fatigue	Mild to moderate splenomegaly	Philadelphia chromosome (Ph¹)
Malaise		Granulocytic leukocytosis
Night sweats		Mild normochromic normocytic anemia
Weight loss		Thrombocytosis (platelet count >450,000/mm³)
		Increase in vitamin B12 serum level and binding activity
		Decrease in leukocyte alkaline phosphatase (LAP) activity
		Bone marrow
		Basophilia
		Eosinophilia
		Hypercellularity with elevated myeloid-erythroid ratio
Chronic lymphocytic leukemia (CLL)		
Same as in CML	Anemia	Blood
	Lymphadenopathy	Lymphocytosis
	Hepatomegaly	Positive Coombs test
	Splenomegaly	Hypogammaglobulinemia
	Thrombocytopenia (degree of all depending on disease stage)	Neutropenia
		Bone marrow
		Lymphocytosis

Continued.

TABLE 18–10.—Continued

SYMPTOMS	PHYSICAL FINDINGS	LABORATORY FINDINGS

Hairy cell leukemia (HCL)
Same as in CML
	Moderate to massive splenomegaly
	Mild hepatomegaly
	Minimal lymphadenopathy
		Blood
		  Pancytopenia
		  Mononuclear cells with cytoplasmic
		    extensions (hairy cells)
		  Leukocyte count $<3,000/mm^3$
		  Granulocytopenia
		  Moderate thrombocytopenia
		  Normochromic normocytic anemia

Prolymphocytic leukemia (PLL)
Same as in CML
	Massive splenomegaly
	Moderate hepatomegaly
	No significant lymphadenopathy
		Blood
		  Extreme leukocytosis (leukocyte count
		    $>100,000/mm^3$)
		  Mild anemia
		  Thrombocytopenia

*From Hurd DD: *Postgrad Med* 1983; 73(5):217–231. Reproduced by permission.

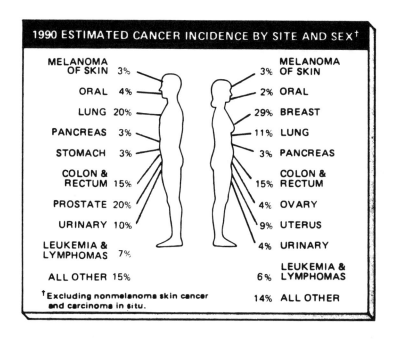

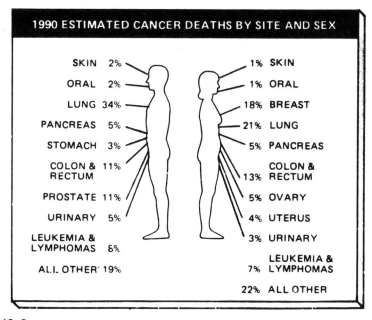

FIG 18–3.
1990 estimated cancer incidence and deaths by site and sex (excluding nonmelanoma skin cancer and carcinoma in situ). (From Silverberg E, Boring CC, Squires TS: CA 1990; 40(1):9–26. Reproduced by permission.)

CANCER DETECTION

TABLE 18–11.—Risk Assessment*

FACTOR	INCREASED RISK FOR CANCER
Carcinogenic factor	
Alcohol	Head and neck, esophagus
Alkylating agents	Leukemia, bladder
Aromatic amines	Bladder
Asbestos	Lung, mesothelioma
Estrogen	Uterus
Other chemicals	
Radiation (especially thyroid, spine, skin, breast)	Leukemia, sarcoma thyroid
Tobacco	Lung, head and neck, larynx
Cigarettes	
Cigar	
Pipe	
Chew	
NOTE: Some combinations are *very* dangerous	
Alcohol and tobacco	Head and neck, esophagus
Asbestos and tobacco	Very high incidence of lung cancer
Genetic predisposition	
Dysplastic nevus syndrome	Melanoma
Familial cancers of breast, ovary, uterus, colon	Breast, ovary, uterus, colon
Multiple endocrine neoplastic syndrome	Neuroendocrine
Polyposis coli	Colon
von Recklinghausen's neurofibromatosis	CNS
Personal history of cancer	
Breast	Breast, colon, uterus, ovary
Cervix	Rectum
Colon	Colon, prostate, ovary
Lung	Lung, larynx, oral cavity, bladder
Lymphoma	Leukemia (especially if heavily treated with chemotherapy or radiotherapy)
Oral cavity	Oral cavity (particularly if patient continues to smoke), lung, larynx, bladder
Ovary	Leukemia (if treated with alkylating chemotherapy)
Uterus	Rectum
Family history of cancer	
Breast, colon, lung, melanoma, prostate, stomach	Breast, colon, lung, melanoma prostate, stomach

Certain associated diseases

Cirrhosis of liver	Liver
Colonic polyps, ulcerative colitis	Colon
Dermatomyositis	Viscera
Molar pregnancy	Choriocarcinoma
Paget's disease	Osteogenic sarcoma
Pernicious anemia, achlorhydria	Stomach
Scleroderma	Bronchiolar carcinoma
Sjögren's syndrome	Lymphoma
Undescended testes	Testes

Other

Early or multiple coital partners	Cervix
Nulliparity, late parity	Breast
Obesity, nulliparity	Uterus

*Adapted from Costanza ME, Li FP, Greene HL, et al: Cancer prevention and detection: Strategy for the office practice, in American Cancer Society: *Cancer: A Manual for Practitioners,* ed 6. Boston, American Cancer Society, Massachusetts Division, 1982, pp 6–7.

TABLE 18–12.—AMERICAN CANCER SOCIETY GUIDELINES FOR EARLY DETECTION OF CANCER IN ASYMPTOMATIC PATIENTS*

	POPULATION		
TEST OR PROCEDURE	SEX	AGE	FREQUENCY
Sigmoidoscopy	M/F	50 and over	Every 3 to 5 years, based on advice of physician.
Stool Guaiac Slide Test	M/F	Over 50	Every year
Digital Rectal Examination	M/F	Over 40	Every year
Pap Test	F	All women who are, or who have been, sexually active, or have reached age 18, should have an annual Pap test and pelvic examination. After a woman has had three or more consecutive satisfactory normal annual examinations, the Pap test may be performed less frequently at the discretion of her physician.	
Pelvic Examination	F		
Endometrial Tissue Sample	F	At menopause, women at high risk†	At menopause

Continued.

TABLE 18–12.—Continued

TEST OR PROCEDURE	SEX	AGE	FREQUENCY
		POPULATION	
Breast Self-examination	F	20 and over	Every month
Breast Physical	F	20–40	Every 3 years
Examination		Over 40	Every year
Mammography	F	35–39	Baseline
		40–49	Every 1–2 years
		50 and over	Every year
Chest X-ray			Not recommended
Sputum Cytology			Not recommended
Health Counseling and	M/F	Over 20	Every 3 years
Cancer Checkup[‡]	M/F	Over 40	Every year

*From Summary of Current Guidelines for the Cancer-Related Checkup: Recommendations. Atlanta, American Cancer Society, 1988. Reproduced by permission.
[†]History of infertility, obesity, failure to ovulate, abnormal uterine bleeding, or estrogen therapy.
[‡]To include examination for cancers of the thyroid, testicles, prostate, ovaries, lymph nodes, oral region, and skin.

TABLE 18–13.—SYMPTOMATIC METASTASES IN PATIENTS WITH CANCER*

GENERAL AREA OF METASTASES	COMMON SYMPTOMS	POSSIBLE PHYSICAL FINDINGS	INITIAL DIAGNOSTIC TESTS	POSSIBLE SPECIFIC FINDINGS
Lung and mediastinum	Hemoptysis,[†] dyspnea, dry cough, pleuritic pain, hoarseness	Bronchospasm, stridor, rhonchi, distended neck veins, pulsus paradoxus, Horner's syndrome, cord paralysis	Chest radiography	Intrapulmonary metastases, tracheal or caval compression by tumor masses,[‡] pleural effusion,[†] pericardial effusion,[†] rib fracture
CNS	Headaches, mental confusion, extremity weakness,[‡] visual difficulty, leg pain, bowel or bladder control loss[‡]	Papilledema, deficits of cranial nerves, muscle strength, tendon reflexes, sensation, cranial function, sphincter tone	*Not* lumbar puncture; brain scan, spine radiographs, serum calcium, ? bone scan, ? myelogram, ? CT scan	Intracranial metastases,[†] spinal cord compression (either epidural or vertebral body metastases)[‡]

Continued.

TABLE 18–13.—Continued

GENERAL AREA OF METASTASES	COMMON SYMPTOMS	POSSIBLE PHYSICAL FINDINGS	INITIAL DIAGNOSTIC TESTS	POSSIBLE SPECIFIC FINDINGS
Bone metastases	Pain with weight-bearing, radiating pain, pleuritic pain, nighttime pain, obtundation	Point tenderness to percussion, decreased tendon reflexes	Radiography, bone scan, serum calcium	Large lytic metastases[†] with impending vertebral body collapse or pathologic fracture, diffuse metastases with hypercalcemia[†]
Abdomen and pelvis	Pain, vomiting, GI bleeding, obstipation, fatigue	Tenderness, distention, abnormal or absent bowel sounds, ascites, hepatomegaly, palpable masses, blood in stool	Radiography, hematocrit, leukocyte count, blood urea nitrogen	Bowel obstruction,[‡] bowel perforation,[‡] diffuse metastases, liver metastases, urinary obstruction[†]

*From Osteen RT, McDonough EF, Harris JR: The history and physical examination for cancer detection, in American Cancer Society: *Cancer: A Manual for Practitioners*, ed. 6. Boston, American Society, Massachusetts Division, 1982, p 27. Reproduced by permission.
[†]Urgent treatment sometimes indicated.
[‡]Emergency treatment usually necessary for good palliation.

TABLE 18–14.—THE PARANEOPLASTIC SYNDROMES

ENDOCRINE SUBSTANCE	DIAGNOSIS	TUMOR
Inappropriate ADH	Low serum osmolality and Na^+, high urinary sodium	Oat cell lung, thymoma, pancreas, lymphoma
ACTH	Excess adrenocortical hormones, abnormal GII	Oat cell, bronchial carcinoid, islet cell of pancreas, pheochromocytoma, ovary
Parathormone	Hypercalcemia, low serum phosphorus, high urinary calcium, no boney metastases, metabolic alkalosis	Lung squamous cell, head and neck, kidney, ovary, cervix, hepatoma, pancreas
Insulin	Hypoglycemia	Pancreatic insulinoma, hepatoma, mesothelioma, fibrosarcoma
HCG	Elevated serum HCG	Hepatoblastoma, stomach, lung, melanoma, ovary, carcinoid
Erythropoietin	Hematocrit >54% in men, 47% in women; normal leukocyte alkaline phosphatase	Renal cell, Wilms's, sarcoma, hepatoma, cerebellum, uterus, ovary, pheochromocytoma
Thyroid-stimulating substance	Elevated serum T_3 and T_4; thyroid scan diffusely active	Trophoblastic tumors of testes, choriocarcinoma, moles
Gastrin	High serum gastrin, diarrhea, steatorrhea, GI ulcerations (Zollinger-Ellison syndrome)	Pancreatic islet cell, pheochromocytoma, lung cancer
Vasoactive intestinal peptide	Hypokalemia, hypochlorhydria, hypercalcemia, severe watery diarrhea (Verner-Morrison syndrome)	
Serotonin, kinins, histamine, prostaglandins	Elevated serum 5-HIAA	Carcinoid with hepatic metastases
Prolactin	Hyperprolactinemia	Renal
Placental alkaline phosphatase	Elevated serum alkaline phosphatase	Lung, breast, colon, ovary, pancreas, stomach, cervix, lymphoma
Growth hormone	Elevated serum GH	Lung, endometrium

TABLE 18–15.—Skin and Connective Tissue and Other Changes

CONDITION	DIAGNOSIS	TUMOR
Acanthosis nigricans	Pigmented hyperkeratosis in skin flexures of axillae and perineum; pruritus	Stomach and other visceral adenocarcinomas
Icthyosis	Generalized drying and scaling	Lung, Hodgkin's disease
Dermatomyositis	Violaceous malar and extremity skin rash; proximal muscle weakness and pain; elevated serum CPK, aldolases, and transaminases	Stomach, breast, lung
Hypertrophic pulmonary osteoarthropathy	Clubbing of fingers and toes, polyarticular arthritis, periosteal proliferation	Lung
Reverse myasthenia gravis	Eaton-Lambert syndrome: males over 40 with proximal muscle weakness, facilitation after repeated stimuli	Oat cell lung (true myasthenia-thymoma)
Carcinomatous neuropathy	Symmetric motor, sensory, or mixed peripheral neuropathy	All types of malignancy
Proteinuria	Bence Jones proteinuria and renal amyloidosis	Multiple myeloma
	Extensive proteinuria with nephrotic syndrome	Breast, colon, lung, Hodgkin's disease

TABLE 18–16.—Common Oncologic Emergencies*

EMERGENCY	IMPLICATION	TREATMENT OPTIONS
Ascites	Portal hypertension Tumor extension	Spironolactone, paracentesis Tumor control
Bilateral ureteral obstruction	Tumor extension	Ureteral catheters, or percutaneous nephrostomies, hemodialysis
Bowel obstruction	Primary tumor or peritoneal metastases	Decompression by tube, surgery, or radiation
Bowel perforation	Rupture secondary to chemotherapy, radiation, or unattended obstruction	Fluids, antibiotics, surgical exploration
Disseminated infections: viral, fungal, parasitic	Immunocompromise	Organism specific, supportive
Disseminated intravascular coagulation	Seen in initial therapy of AML and prostate cancer	Fresh frozen plasma, heparin
Esophageal obstruction and perforation	Esophageal or gastric tumor extension	Nutritional support, tumor reduction

Hypercalcemia	Bone metastases, ectopic parathormone	Vigorous hydration, furosemide, mithramycin
Hypoglycemia	Insulinoma	50% glucose, tumor reduction
Hyperuricemia	Result of treatment of leukemias and lymphomas	Diuresis, alkalinization of urine, dialysis, allopurinol
Increased intracranial pressure	CNS tumor	Corticosteroids, surgery, radiation, chemotherapy
Lactic acidosis	Rapidly growing tumors, e.g., lymphoma	Sodium bicarbonate
Leukostasis	Leukemia (blastic crisis)	Chemotherapy (hydroxyurea 5,000–6,000 mg as single dose)
Pathologic fractures	Lytic bone metastases	Orthopedic surgery, radiation
Pericardial tamponade	Metastatic tumor to pericardium, radiation pericarditis	Pericardiocentesis, surgery
Pleural effusion	Pleural metastases, ascites, CHF, tumor obstructing lymph system	Treat cause, thoracentesis
Pneumothorax and tension pneumothorax	Misadventure, tumor extension	Chest tube
Sepsis	Leukopenia	Antibiotics, cultures, supportive
Spinal cord compression	Tumor extension	Corticosteroids, radiation, surgery, chemotherapy
Superior vena cava syndrome	Tumor extension	Radiation, chemotherapy
Thrombocytopenic hemorrhage	Myelosuppression	Platelets
Tumor lysis syndrome	Rapid necrosis of tumor secondary to chemotherapy	Diuresis, electrolyte management, dialysis
Upper airway obstruction	Tumor extension	Radiation, tracheostomy, chemotherapy
Visual changes	Ocular primary or metastasis	Radiation, chemotherapy

*From Bope ET: Follow-up of the cancer patient: Surveillance for metastases, in Driscoll CE (ed): *Primary Care: The Management of the Cancer Patient.* Philadelphia, WB Saunders Co, 1987, pp 391–401. As adapted from Rubin P, Arsenlau JC: *Clinical Oncology, A Multidisciplinary Approach,* ed 6. New York, American Cancer Society, 1983, pp 516–525. Reproduced by permission.

CANCER THERAPIES

TABLE 18–17.—Common Combination Chemotherapy Regimens*

CANCER	NAME	DRUGS AND DOSAGES
A. Breast	1. ACe (breast cancer, metastatic or recurrent)	Cyclophosphamide 200 mg/m^2/day, PO, days 3–6 Doxorubicin (Adriamycin) 40 mg/m^2/, IV, day 1 Repeat every 21–28 days
	2. CAF (breast cancer, metastatic disease)	Cyclophosphamide 100 mg/m^2/day, PO, days 1–14 Doxorubicin 30 mg/m^2/day, IV days 1 and 8 Fluorouracil 500 mg/m^2/days, IV, days 1 and 8 Repeat every 4 weeks until a total cumulative dose of 450 mg/m^2 of doxorubicin is given, then discontinue doxorubicin and substitute methotrexate 40 mg/m^2, IV, and increase fluorouracil to 600 mg/m^2, IV
	3. CMF (breast cancer, metastatic or recurrent disease and various adjuvant regimens)	Cyclophosphamide 100 mg/m^2/day, PO, days 1–14 Methotrexate 40–60 mg/m^2/day, IV, days 1 and 8 Fluorouracil 600 mg/m^2/day, IV, days 1 and 8 Repeat every 28 days
	4. CMFP (breast cancer, metastatic disease)	Same as CMF but fluorouracil is 700 mg/m^2/day days 1 and 8 plus Prednisone 40 mg/m^2/day, PO, days 1–14

		Repeat every 28 days
	5. FAC	Fluorouracil 500 mg/m^2/day, IV, days 1 and 8
		Doxorubicin 50 mg/m^2, IV, day 1
		Cyclophosphamide 500 mg/m^2, IV, day 1
		Repeat every 3 weeks
B. Hodgkin's	1. ABVD (Hodgkin's induction resistant to MOPP)	Doxorubicin 25 mg/m^2/day, IV, days 1 and 14
		Bleomycin 10 units/m^2/day, IV, days 1 and 14
		Vinblastine 6 mg/m^2/day, IV, days 1 and 14
		Dacarbazine 375 mg/m^2/day, IV, days 1 and 14
		Repeat every 38 days for 6 cycles
	2. A-COPP Hodgkin's induction (children only)	Doxorubicin 60 mg/m^2, IV, day 1
		Cyclophosphamide 300 mg/m^2/day, IV, days 14 and 20
		Vincristine 1.5 mg/m^2/day, IV, days 14 and 20 (Max 2 mg)
		Procarbazine 100 mg/m^2/day, PO, days 14–28
		Prednisone 40 mg/m^2/day, PO, days 1–27 (1st and 4th cycles; then days 14–27 durin 2nd, 3rd, 5th, and 6th cycles)
		Repeat every 42 days for 6 cycles
	3. MOPP	Mechlorethamine 6 mg/m^2/day, IV, days 1 and 8
		Vincristine 2 mg/m^2/day, IV, days 1 and 8 (max 2 mg)

Continued.

TABLE 18–17.—Continued

CANCER	NAME	DRUGS AND DOSAGES
		Procarbazine 100 mg/m^2/day, PO days 1–14
		Prednisone 40 mg/m^2/day, PO, days 1–14
		Repeat every 28 days for 6 cycles
C. Non-Hodgkin's lymphoma	1. CHOP (Non-Hodgkin's lymphoma with unfavorable histology)	Cyclophosphamide 750 mg/m^2, IV, day 1
		Doxorubicin 50 mg/m^2, IV, day 1
		Vincristine 1.4 mg/m^2, IV, day 1 (max 2 mg)
		Prednisone 60 mg/day, PO, days 1–5
		Repeat every 21–28 days for 6 cycles
	2. COP (Non-Hodgkin's lymphoma with unfavorable histology)	Cyclophosphamide 800–1,000 mg/m^2, IV, day 1
		Vincristine 1.4 mg/m^2, IV, day 1 (max 2 mg)
		Prednisone 60 mg/m^2/day, PO, days 1–5
		Repeat every 21 days for 6 cycles
	3. C-MOPP (or COPP) (Hodgkin's or non-Hodgkin's lymphoma with unfavorable histology)	Cyclophosphamide 650 mg/m^2/day, IV, days 1 and 8
		Vincristine 1.4 mg/m^2/day, IV, days 1 and 8 (max 2 mg)
		Procarbazine 100 mg/m^2/day, PO, days 1–14
		Prednisone 40 mg/m^2/day, PO, days 1–14
		Repeat every 28 days for 6 cycles
D. Leukemia (ALL)	1. MTX + MP + CTX	Methotrexate 20 mg/m^2/week, IV
		Mercaptopurine 50 mg/m^2/day, PO

		Cyclophosphamide 200 mg/m^2/week, IV Continue until relapse or after 3 years of remission
	2. VP	Vincristine 2 mg/m^2/week, IV, for 4–6 weeks (max dose 2 mg) Prednisone 60 mg/m^2/day, PO, in divided doses for 4 weeks Taper weeks 5–7
E. Leukemia (AML)	1. AraC ADR	Cytarabine 100 mg/m^2/day, continuous 24 hour infusion, for 7–10 days Doxorubicin 30 mg/m^2/day, IV, for 3 days
	2. AraC + DNR + Pred + MP	Daunorubicin 25 mg/m^2, IV, for 1 day Cytarabine 80 mg/m^2/day, IV, for 3 days Prednisolone 40 mg/m^2/, PO, daily Mercaptopurine 100 mg/m^2, PO, daily Repeat weekly until remission, then repeat every month
F. Leukemia (CLL)	1. CHL + Pred	Chlorambucil 0.4 mg/kg/day, PO, for 1 day every other week Prednisone 100 mg/day, PO, for 2 days every other week Adjust CHL according to blood counts and increase every 2 weeks by 0.1 mg/kg until toxicity or disease control
	2. M-2 (also used for multiple myeloma)	Vincristine 0.03 mg/kg, IV, day 1 (max 2 mg) Carmustine 0.5 mg/kg, IV, day 1

Continued.

TABLE 18–17.—Continued

CANCER	NAME	DRUGS AND DOSAGES
		Cyclophosphamide 10 mg/kg, IV, day 1
		Melphalan 0.25 mg/kg/day, PO, days 1–4
		Prednisone 1.0 mg/kg/day, PO, days 1–7, then taper to day 21
		Continue treatment cycle throughout remission period until progression of disease
G. Lung	1. CAMP (non-oat cell)	Cyclophosphamide 300 mg/m^2/day, IV, days 1 and 8
		Doxorubicin 20 mg/m^2/day, IV, days 1 and 8
		Methotrexate 15 mg/m^2/day, IV, days 1 and 8
		Procarbazine 100 mg/m^2/day, PO, days 1–10
		Repeat every 28 days
	2. CAV (small-cell)	Cyclophosphamide 750 mg/m^2, IV, every 3 weeks
		Doxorubicin 50 mg/m^2, IV, every 3 weeks
		Vincristine 2 mg, IV, every 3 weeks
	3. CHOR (small-cell)	Cyclophosphamide and doxorubicin doses same as CAV but give both drugs on days 1 and 22
		Vincristine 1 mg, IV, days 1, 8, 15, 22
		Radiation total dose, 3,000 rad, 10 daily fractions over a 2-week period beginning with day 36

	4. FAM (non-oat cell, also used for gastric and pancreatic but daily schedule differs)	Fluorouracil 600 mg/ m^2/day, IV, days 1, 8, 28 36 Doxorubicin 30 mg/m^2/ day, IV, days 1 and 28 Mitomycin 10 mg/m^2, IV, day 1 Repeat every 8 weeks
	5. MACC (non-oat cell)	Methotrexate 40 mg/ m^2, IV, day 1 Doxorubicin 40 mg/m^2, IV, day 1 Cyclophosphamide 400 mg/m^2, IV, day 1 Lomustine 30 mg/m^2, PO, day 1 Repeat every 21 days
H. Soft tissue sarcomas	1. CY-VA-DIC	Cyclophosphamide 500 mg/m, IV, day 1 Vincristine 1.4 mg/m^2, IV, days 1 and 5 (max 2 mg) Doxorubicin 50 mg/m^2, IV, day 1 Dacarbazine 250 mg/ m^2/day, IV, days 1– 5 Repeat every 21 days
	2. VAC standard	Vincristine 2 mg/m^2/ week, IV, weeks 1– 12 (max 2 mg) Dactinomycin 0.015 mg/kg/day, IV, for 5 days, every 3 months for 5–6 courses (max 0.5 mg/day) Cyclophosphamide 2.5 mg/kg/day, PO, continue for 2 years
I. Testicular (disseminated)	1. VBP	Vinblastine 0.2 mg/kg/ day, IV, days 1 and 2 (every 3 weeks for 5 courses)

Continued.

TABLE 18–17.—Continued

CANCER	NAME	DRUGS AND DOSAGES
		Cisplatin 20 mg/m²/ day, IV infusion over 15 minutes, 6 hours after vinblastine, days 1–5; Repeat every 3 weeks for 3 courses
		Bleomycin 30 units/ week, IV, 6 hours after vinblastine on the 2nd day of each week for 12 weeks to a total cumulative dose of 360 units

*Adapted from Carter BL: Common chemotherapeutic agents, in Driscoll CE (ed): *Primary Care: Management of the Cancer Patient.* Philadelphia, WB Saunders Co, 1987; pp 293–315; and Olin BR (ed): Antineoplastics, in *Facts and Comparisons.* St Louis, CV Mosby Co, 1990, pp 643–643h.

TABLE 18–18.—IMMEDIATE TOXICITIES OF COMMONLY USED CHEMOTHERAPEUTIC AGENTS*

AGENT	TRADE OR OTHER NAME	LOCAL IRRITANT	ANAPHYLAXIS	FACIAL FLUSHING	FEVER	NAUSEA AND VOMITING	MUCOSITIS	ALOPECIA	SKIN REACTIONS	MISCELLANEOUS
Alkylating agents										
Chlorambucil	Leukeran					+			Rash, dermatitis	
Cyclophosphamide	Cytoxan		+	+	+	++	+	++	↑ PIG†	Hemorrhage, cystitis, SIADH
Melphalan	Alkeran		+			+			Dermatitis	
Nitrogen mustard	Mustargen	+++	+		+	+++			PIG, dermatitis	
Antimetabolites										
Cytarabine (ARA-C)	Cytosar	+			+	+	+			
5-Fluorouracil (5FU)	Adrucil				+	++	++	+	↑ PIG, rash, photosens.	Ataxia, cerebellar syndrome
Mercaptopurine (6-MP)	Purinethol	+			+	+/−	++	+++	↑PIG, dermatitis	Headache, weakness
Methotrexate	Methotrexate		+		+‡		++		Dermatitis	Renal toxicity
Thioguanine (6-TG)	Tabloid					+/−	++§	+	Rash	
Vinca alkaloids										
Vinblastine	Velban	++			+	+	+	+	Dermatitis, rash, pruritis	Constipation, SIADH
Vincristine	Oncovin	++			+	+	+	+	Dermatitis, pruritis, rash	Constipation, SIADH
Antibiotics										
Actinomycin-D	Cosmegen	++	+			+++	+++	+/−	↑ PIG, folliculitis	Acneiform lesions
Bleomycin	Blenoxane		+	+	+++	+	++	++	↑PIG, urticaria, dermatitis	Pneumonitis
Daunomycin	Cerubidine	+				++	++	+++	Rash, urticaria	
Doxorubicin	Adriamycin	+++		++	+	++	+++	+++	↑PIG, rash, urticaria	Drowsiness, cardiotoxicity
Mitomycin	Mutamycin	++	+		+		+		Dermatitis	Lethargy, weakness

Continued.

559

TABLE 18–18.—Continued

AGENT	TRADE OR OTHER NAME	LOCAL IRRITANT	ANAPHYLAXIS	FACIAL FLUSHING	FEVER	NAUSEA AND VOMITING	MUCOSITIS	ALOPECIA	SKIN REACTIONS	MISCELLANEOUS
Nitrosoureas										
BCNU	Carmustine			+		+				
CCNU	Lamustine					+				
Miscellaneous agents										
L-Asparaginase	Elspar		+ +		+ +	+			Urticaria	Pancreatis, lethargy
5-Azacytidine						+ +			Rash	
Busulfan	Myleran					+			↑ PIG, rare urticaria	
Cisplatinn	Platinol		+			+ + +				Renal toxicity
Imidazole carboxamide (DTIC)	Dacarbazine	+		+	+	+ + +				Flu-like syndrome
Prednisone		+		+		+			↑ PIG, photosens.	
Procarbazine	Matulane			+∥	+/−	;			Rash (10%), dermatitis	Constipation

*Adapted from Spiegel RJ: *Cancer Treat Rev* 1981; 8:197–207.
†PIG indicates increased pigmentation.
‡A 10% incidence after intrathecal administration.
§Increased incidence with high dose infusions.
∥Increased with concomitant alcohol use.

560

TABLE 18–19.—CURATIVE DOSES OF RADIATION FOR SPECIFIC TUMORS*

2,000–3,000 rad	*6,000–6,500 rad*
Acute lymphocytic leukemia	Larynx (<1 cm)
Central nervous system	Breast cancer (lumpectomy)
	Pancreas
3,000–4,000 rad	
Neuroblastoma	*7,000–7,500 rad*
Seminoma	Bladder cancers
Wilms' tumor	Cervical cancer
	Lung cancer (<3 cm)
4,000–4,500 rad	Lymph nodes, metastatic (1–3 cm)
Hodgkin's disease	Oral cavity (2–4 cm)
Lymphosarcoma	Oro-naso-laryngo-pharyngeal cancer
Seminoma	Ovarian cancer
Skin cancer (basal and squamous)	Uterine fundal cancer
5,000–6,000 rad	*≥8,000 rad*
Breast cancer	Breast cancer (>5 cm)
Ewing's tumor	Glioblastoma
Embryonal cancer	Head and neck cancer (>4 cm)
Lymph nodes, metastatic	Lymph nodes, metastatic (>6 cm)
Ovarian cancer	Melanomas
Medulloblastoma	Soft tissue sarcoma (>5 cm)
Retinoblastoma	Thyroid cancer

*From Carter BL: Commonly used chemotherapeutic agents, in Driscoll CE (ed): *Primary Care: Management of the Cancer Patient.* Philadelphia, WB Saunders Co, 1987, pp 293–315. As adapted from Rubin P, Siemann D: Principles of radiation oncology and cancer radiotherapy, in Rubin P (ed): *Clinical Oncology,* ed 6. American Cancer Society, Rochester, Minn, 1983, pp 58–71.

TABLE 18–20.—REPORTING RESULTS OF CANCER THERAPY: RECOMMENDATIONS FOR GRADING OF ACUTE AND SUBACUTE TOXICITY*

	GRADE 0	GRADE 1	GRADE 2	GRADE 3	GRADE 4
Hematologic (adults)					
Hemoglobin (gm/dl)	≥11.0	9.5–10.9	8.0–9.4	6.5–7.9	<6.5
Leukocytes (1,000/mm³)	≥4.0	3.0–3.9	2.0–2.9	1.0–1.9	<1.0
Granulocytes (1,000/mm³)	≥2.0	1.5–1.9	1.0–1.4	0.5–0.9	<0.5
Platelets (1,000/mm³)	≥100	75–99	50–74	25–49	<25
Hemorrhage	None	Petechiae	Mild blood loss	Gross blood loss	Debilitating blood loss
Gastrointestinal					
Bilirubin	≤1.25 × N†	1.26–2.5 × N	2.6–5 × N	5.1–10 × N	>10 × N
SGOT/SGPT	≤1.25 × N	1.26–2.5 × N	2.6–5 × N	5.1–10 × N	>10 × N
Alkaline phosphatase	≤1.25 × N	1.26–2.5 × N	2.6–5 × N	5.1–10 × N	>10 × N
Oral	None	Soreness/erythema	Erythema, ulcers, can eat solids	Ulcers, requires liquid diet only	Alimentation not possible
Nausea/vomiting	None	Nausea	Transient vomiting	Vomiting requiring therapy	Intractable vomiting
Diarrhea	None	Transient, <2 days	Tolerable but >2 days	Intolerable, requiring therapy	Hemorrhagic dehydration
Renal, bladder					
BUN or blood urea	≤1.25 × N	1.26–2.5 × N	2.6–5 × N	5–10 × N	>10 × N
Creatinine	≤1.25 × N	1.26–2.5 × N	2.6–5 × N	5–10 × N	>10 × N
Proteinuria	None	1+; < 0.3 gm/dl	2 to 3+; 0.3–1.0 gm/dl	4+; > 1.0 gm/dl	Nephrotic syndrome
Hematuria	None	Microscopic	Gross	Gross with clots	Obstructive uropathy
Pulmonary	None	Mild symptoms	Exertional dyspnea	Dyspnea at rest	Complete bed rest required
Fever-drug	None	Fever <38°C	Fever 38°–40°C	Fever >40°C	Fever with hypotension
Allergic	None	Edema	Bronchospasm, no parenteral therapy needed	Bronchospasm, parenteral therapy required	Anaphylaxis

Cutaneous	None	Erythema	Dry desquamation, vesiculation, pruritus	Moist desquamation, ulceration	Exfoliative dermatitis, necrosis requiring surgical intervention
Hair	None	Minimal hair loss	Moderate, patchy alopecia	Complete alopecia but reversible	Nonreversible alopecia
Infection (specify site)	None	Minor infection	Moderate infection	Major infection	Major infection with hypotension
Cardiac					
Rhythm	None	Sinus tachycardia	Unifocal PVC, atrial arrhythmia	Multifocal PVC	Ventricular tachycardia
Function	None	Asymptomatic, but abnormal cardiac sign	Transient symptomatic dysfunction, no therapy required	Symptomatic dysfunction responsive to therapy	Symptomatic dysfunction nonresponsive to therapy
Pericarditis	None	Asymptomatic effusion	Symptomatic, no tap required	Tamponade, tap required	Tamponade, surgery required
Neurotoxicity					
State of consciousness	Alert	Transient lethargy	Somnolent <50% of waking hours	Somnolent >50% of waking hours	Coma
Peripheral	None	Paresthesias and/or decreased tendon reflexes	Severe paresthesias and/or mild weakness	Intolerable paresthesias and/or marked motor loss	Paralysis
Constipation‡	None	Mild	Moderate	Abdominal distention	Distention and vomiting
Pain§	None	Mild	Moderate	Severe	Intractable

*From Miller AB, et al: *Cancer* 1981; 47:207–214. Reproduced by permission.
†N = upper limit of normal.
‡Constipation does not include constipation resulting from narcotics.
§Pain—only treatment-related pain is considered, not disease-related pain. The use of narcotics may be helpful in grading pain, depending on the tolerance of the patient.

The World Health Organization recommends standardized recording of data related to patient therapies for malignancy. Family physicians, often engaged in follow-up care of patients with malignancy, are encouraged to use this observation system.

GENERAL CARE OF THE CANCER PATIENT

TABLE 18–21.—Steps to Successful Control of Cancer Pain

1. Evaluate *physical* (visceral), *psychological* (anxiety, grief and depression), and *social* (isolation, anger and withdrawal) aspects.
2. Identify specific sources of pain (direct tumor involvement, pain of cancer therapy, or pain unrelated to tumor or therapy).
3. Assess intensity of pain—use a simple 1 to 5 scale (1 = minimal, 5 = maximal) or define by using McGill-Melzack Pain Questionnaire.*
4. Use oral medications when possible, given q4h regularly rather than PRN.
5. Always start concomitant bowel program with bulk laxative or wetting agent to alleviate constipation.
6. Administer medications in a stepwise fashion according to degree of need:

Pt's. Rating	Intensity	Medication
1–2	Mild	Nonnarcotic: ASA, acetaminophen NSAID (especially for peripheral pain or bony metastases) ± adjunct[†]
2–3	Moderate	Weak narcotic: oxycodone, codeine ± adjunct
4–5	Severe	Narcotic: morphine, hydromorphone ± adjunct

7. Antiemetic measures may be required during first 1–2 weeks of initiating narcotic therapy.

*Melzack R: *Pain* 1975; 1:277–299.
[†]Adjunct = benzodiazapine, tricyclic, and haloperidol.

CLASS	DRUG NAME	DOSE EQUIVALENTS (MG)		DURATION OF ACTION (HR)	PEAK EFFECT (HR)	USUAL ORAL DOSE (MG)	AVAILABLE FORMULATIONS	COMMENTS
Nonnarcotic								
	Aspirin	650		4–6	½–1½	650–975 q4h	Tablet, liquid, suppository	Anti-inflammatory effect GI side-effects limit use
	Acetaminophen	650		4–6	½–1½	650–975 q4h	Tablet, liquid, suppository	Lacks antiinflammatory effect, better tolerated than aspirin
Narcotic agonists		Dose equivalent to morphine 10 mg IM						
		Oral	Intramuscular					
Mild-moderate pain	Codeine	200	130	4–6	1–1½	60 q4h	Tablet, liquid, injection	Most patients will not tolerate oral doses 90 mg q4h, antitussive
	Oxycodone	30	15	3–5	1–1½	30 q4h	Tablet, liquid, injection	Antitussive, tolerated better than codeine by some patients
Moderate-severe pain	Morphine	20	10	4–6	½–1½	20 q4h	Tablet, liquid sustained release, suppository, injection	The "standard." First-pass ration oral: IM is 6:1, all doses thereafter at 2:1. Also available in liquid concentrate.

Continued.

565

TABLE 18–22.—Continued

CLASS	DRUG NAME	DOSE EQUIVALENTS (MG)	DURATION OF ACTION (HR)	PEAK EFFECT (HR)	USUAL ORAL DOSE (MG)	AVAILABLE FORMULATIONS	COMMENTS
	Methadone (Dolophine)	20	10	4–6	1–2	20 q4h	Tablet, injection	Can accumulate rapidly, somewhat more expensive than morphine
	Meperidine (Demerol)	300	100	2–3	$\frac{1}{2}$–1	75–150 q3h	Tablet, injection	Most patients will not tolerate oral doses > 150 mg
	Hydromorphone Dilaudid)	8	4	4–6	$\frac{1}{2}$–1$\frac{1}{2}$	4–8 q4h	Tablet, liquid, suppository, injection	Good potency, large dose concentrated in small volume
	Levorphanol (Levo-Dromoran)	4	2	4–8	$\frac{1}{2}$–1	2–4 q6h	Tablet, injection	Slightly longer acting than morphine, lipophilic
	Oxymorphone (Numorphan)	—	1	4–6	$\frac{1}{2}$–1$\frac{1}{2}$	10 rectally q4h	Suppository and injection	No oral form available
Mixed Agonist/ Antagonist	Pentazocine	180	60	3–4	$\frac{1}{2}$–1	280 q4h	Tablet, injection	Only oral form available in combination with naloxone, aspirin, or acetaminophen. Hallucinations in elderly, decreases narcotic effectiveness.

*From Driscoll CE: Pain management, in Driscoll CE (ed): *Primary Care: Management of the Cancer Patient.* Philadelphia, WB Saunders Co, 1987, pp 337–352. Reproduced with permission.

TABLE 18–23.—HELP FOR SPECIFIC PAIN SYNDROMES

CAUSES	INTERVENTIONS
Nerve root compression	Surgical decompression; dexamethasone 4–8 mg PO b.i.d.; nerve block.
Headache from intracranial mass	Dexamethasone 4–8 mg PO b.i.d. (dosing up to 20 mg q.i.d. may be required); palliative radiation; doxepin or amitriptyline (tertiary amines) to raise CNS serotonin levels.
Intestinal colic	Lomotil, 1–2 tablets PO q4–6 *or* loperamide 2 mg PO q6hr; stool softener; nasogastric decompression.
Bladder/rectal spasm pain	Belladonna 15 mg with opium (30 or 60 mg) in rectal suppository q4–6 h; chlorpromazine 10–25 mg q4–6h
Postherpetic neuralgia	Amitriptyline 25–150 mg PO qd; Sinemet 2 tabs t.i.d.; clonazepam 0.5 mg PO t.i.d.; other anticonvulsants such as carbamazepine, phenytoin, and valproic acid.
Phantom limb pain	Narcotics, steroids, and TENS unit; carbamazepine.
Oropharyngeal pain	Swish and swallow 15 ml 2% viscous lidocaine q2h; artificial saliva; antimonilial agent if fungal.
Muscle spasm pain	Amitriptyline 75qhs if fibromyositis; massage, heat and narcotic; inject trigger points; baclofen 5–20 mg PO t.i.d.; dantrolene sodium 24–100 mg t.i.d., cyclobenzoprine HCl 10 mg t.i.d. or diazepam 2–10 mg q.i.d.

TABLE 18–24.—MANAGEMENT OF COMMON SYMPTOMS

CONDITION	TREATMENTS
Anorexia	Frequent small feedings, high caloric supplements; sherry or wine, ½ hr a.c.; prednisone, 10–20 mg b.i.d.–t.i.d., or fluoxymesterone, 5 mg t.i.d.; Periactin, 4 mg t.i.d.
Dry or painful mouth	Mouthwash of equal parts H_2O_2, glycerine, saline, and mouthwash; carboxymethylcellulose, 5 ml PRN; lidocaine, 2% viscous, 5–15 ml swish q4h
Dysphagia	Antacids; metoclopramide, 5–10 mg q.i.d.; antifungal for candidiasis

Continued.

TABLE 18–24.—Continued

Hiccoughs	Pharyngeal irritation with dry swallow of granulated sugar, simethacone; chlorpromazine, 25–50 mg q4–6h; dexamethasone, phenytoin, or carbamazepine
Nausea/vomiting	Metoclopramide, 5–10 mg q.i.d. for gastroparesis associated with intra-abdominal tumors; prochlorperazine, 10 mg q.i.d., or haloperidol, 0.5 mg t.i.d. are first-line agents; second-line agents added to these are pyridoxine, 50 mg q.i.d., or cyclizine, 25 mg q.i.d.
Colic of intestinal obstruction	Loperamide, 2–4 mg q.i.d. dexamethasone, 8–10 mg t.i.d.
Dyspnea/cough	O$_2$, bronchodilators, opiates, hyoscine 0.4–0.6 mg sub Q, glucocorticoids
Fungating ulcers	Povidine-iodine 4% in liquid paraffin (1:1 to 1:4)— cleanse wound and apply gauze soaked in this preparation; gauze soaked in epinephrine 1:1,000 will control capillary bleeding; judicious use of collagenase or dextranomer; 1% metronidazole solution applied
Pruritus	Biliary itch may be relieved by Questran, 4 gm q.i.d.; antihistamines; steroids; crotamiton cream; tranquilizers
Decubiti	Frequent turning; egg crate mattress, water bed or sheepskin; wet lesions dried with hair dryer; magnesium and aluminum hydroxide (Maalox) topically; Op-site, Tegaderm, or Stomahesive
Urinary retention	Bethanechol, 10–30 mg t.i.d., Foley catheter
Urinary frequency	Evaluate for hypercalcemia and infection; flavoxate, 100 mg t.i.d.

19 *Nutrition*

Charles W. Smith, Jr., M.D.

NUTRITIONAL ASSESSMENT

See page 570.

TABLE 19–1.—NUTRITIONAL ASSESSMENT FOR MALNUTRITION*

	SEVERE	MILD	NORMAL
Vitamins			
Serum folate	<3.0 ng/ml	<6.0 ng/ml	≥6.0 ng/ml
Serum vitamin C	<0.2 mg/dl	<0.3 mg/dl	≥0.3 mg/dl
Anthropometrics			
Triceps skin fold[†]	<20% std.	<60% std.	M ≥ 12.5 mm, F ≥ 16.5 mm
Weight/height	<80% std.	<90% std.	(see Table 19–6)
Arm circumference[‡]	<60% std.	<80% std.	M ≥ 25.3 cm F ≥ 23.2 cm
Routine lab			
Lymphocytes	<1,200/mm^3	<1,500/mm^3	1,500/mm^3
Serum albumin	<2.8 gm/dl	<3.5 gm/dl	≥3.5 gm/dl
Hematocrit	M < 37%; F < 31%	M < 43%; F < 37%	M≥43% F ≥ 37%
Cellular immunity by mumps or *Candida* skin tests	Usually –	+ or –	Both positive

*Adapted from Weinsier R, Hunker E, Krumdieck C, et al: Hospital malnutrition, in Cunningham J (ed): *Controversies in Clinical Nutrition.* Philadelphia, George F Stickley Co, 1980, p 46.
†Skinfold measured with Lange caliper; take average of three measures.
‡Arm circumference measured at midarm with tape calibrated in millimeters.

TABLE 19–2.—Clinical Signs Used in the Physical Examination for Nutritional Assessment*

	SIGN	NUTRIENT CONSIDERATIONS
Hair	Dry, brittle Dyspigmented Easily pluckable	Protein-calorie malnutrition
Eyes	Xerophthalmia, keratomalacia	Vitamin A
	Bitot's spots	Vitamin A
	Circumcorneal injection	Riboflavin
	Conjunctival pallor	Anemia
Lips	Bilateral lesions and scars	Niacin, riboflavin
	Cheilosis	Niacin, riboflavin
Gums	Acute periodontal gingivitis (marginal redness or swelling; swollen red papillae; bleeding gums)	Ascorbic acid
Tongue	Smooth, pale, atrophic	Anemia
	Red, painful, denuded, edema	Niacin, riboflavin
	Furrows, serrations, geographic	Probably not nutritional
Face and neck	Nasolabial seborrhea	Riboflavin, niacin
	Bilateral parotid enlargement	Protein (possible)
	Goiter	Iodine
Skin	Petechiae, purpura	Ascorbic acid
	Symmetrical dermatitis of exposed skin	Niacin
	Thickened pressure points	Niacin
	Scrotal dermatitis	Riboflavin
	Follicular hyperkeratosis	Vitamin A
	"Crazy pavement" dermatitis	Vitamin A, protein
	Bilateral dependent edema	Protein, thiamin
Skeletal	Costochondral beading	Vitamin C or D
	Epiphyseal enlargement	Vitamin D
	Cranial bossing, craniotabes	Vitamin D
	Bowed legs	Vitamin D
Neurologic	Loss of vibratory sense, deep tendon reflexes, calf tenderness	Thiamin
Nails	Spoon-shaped (koilonychia) brittle, ridged nails	Iron
Teeth	Missing or erupting abnormally; gray or black spots (fluorosis); cavities (caries)	Fluoride, simple sugars

*From *Handbook of Clinical Dietetics*. New Haven, Yale University Press, 1981, p A25. Table courtesy of Mary B McCann, MD, Maine Medical Center. Reproduced by permission.

DIETS

TABLE 19–3.—Diets

Regular:
Should contain moderate amounts daily of at least one member of each of the basic four food groups:
  Meat, poultry, fish, eggs, and legumes
  Milk and milk products
  Bread and cereal
  Vegetable and fruit

Pregnancy:
Should contain recommended daily caloric allowance (1,800–2,400), plus 300 calories (see Table 19–6) and:
  3–4 servings of milk and cheese
  2–3 servings of meat, poultry, fish, or eggs
  ≥4 servings of vegetables or fruit
  ≥4 servings of bread and grain

Lactation:
Recommended caloric requirement (1,800–2,400), plus 500 calories (same distribution as in pregnancy, plus 12 cups of fluid per day) (see Table 19–6).

Infant and Pediatric:

Age	Fluids	Calories	Protein
0–6 mo.	140–160 ml/kg	kg × 117	kg × 2.2 gm
6–12 mo.	125–135 ml/kg	kg × 108	kg × 2.0 gm

Geriatric:
  Calories: 65–75-year-olds: reduce by 10%.
       >75-year-olds: reduce by 25%.
  Protein: Should be ≥12% of calories. Protein requirements don't decline with age.
  Fat: Should be ≥30% of calories.
  Vitamins/minerals: Supplementation usually indicated. Consider calcium (800–1,200 mg/day) in thin caucasian women.

Soft (mechanical soft or pureed):
For patients unable to chew, or as progression from liquid to regular diet. Is generally nutritionally adequate.

Liquid:
For postoperative or acute gastrointestinal conditions. Clear = little or no residue; "full" includes milk, strained soups, ice cream, and custard. Not nutritionally adequate.

Low Fiber (low residue):
Used for postoperative bowel surgery or acute exacerbations of inflammatory bowel disease. Contains minimal undigestible carbohydrate (e.g., cellulose and lignin), usually found in fruits, vegetables, and cereals.

Chronic Renal Failure:
Restricted protein, sodium, potassium, and fluids, depending on type and severity of CRF. Protein restriction used when creatinine clearance is 25 ml/min or less; potassium restriction if patient is oliguric or hyperkalemic. If clearance is ≤20 ml/min, use phosphate binder (e.g., Basalgel) to control hyperphosphatemia. A patient with end-stage renal disease not on dialysis should have approximately 0.6 mg/kg body wt/day of protein.

Hyperlipidemias:
Hypertriglyceridemia (type IV, ↑ VLDL):
Decrease body weight and triglyceride levels by:
Limiting CHO to 40% of caloric intake.
Using polyunsaturated fats when possible.
Restricting cholesterol and saturated fat intake.
Limiting alcohol intake.
Hypercholesterolemia (type IIa, ↑ LDL) (see TABLE 18–15):
Reduce saturated fatty acids and cholesterol by:
Decreasing ingested cholesterol to 300 mg/day.
Decreasing dairy and animal fats and substituting polyunsaturated fats.
Mixed (↑ LDL and VLDL, type IIb):
Same as for type IIa + CHO and ETOH restriction.

Sodium-Restricted Diets
4–6 gm: "No added salt"
4 gm: Cook all foods without salt.
2 gm: Eliminate foods cooked or preserved in salt or with visible salt (e.g., saltine crackers).
1 gm: Above, plus restriction of foods high in natural sodium.

TABLE 19–4.—HOW TO ESTIMATE CALORIC REQUIREMENTS*

This arithmetic equation is quickly performed and easy for patients to understand:

Weight (lb)	×	10 (light activity)
		15 (moderate activity)
		20 (heavy activity)
Age 25–34		Subtract 0
35–44		Subtract 100
45–54		Subtract 200
55–64		Subtract 300
65 +		Subtract 400

For an obese, moderately active 35-year-old woman who should weigh 110 lb, multiply 110 lb × 15 (activity factor) = 1,650. Subtract 100 (age factor) to get her daily calorie requirement (1,550).

*From Atkinson RL Jr: Nutrition vs. obesity, in Mason D, Guthrie H (eds): *The Medicine Called Nutrition.* New Jersey, Best Foods, Mazola Nutrition/Health Information Services, 1979, p 44. Reproduced by permission.

TABLE 19–5.—Common Sources of Caffeine*

PRODUCT	CAFFEINE (MG)
Coffee†	
Drip (5 oz)	146
Percolated (5 oz)	110
Instant, regular (5 oz)	53
Decaffeinated (5 oz)	2
Tea†	
One-minute brew (5 oz)	9–33
Three-minute brew (5 oz)	20–46
Five-minute brew (5 oz)	20–50
Canned ice tea (12 oz)	22–36
Cocoa and chocolate†	
Cocoa beverage (water mix, 6 oz)	10
Milk chocolate (1 oz)	6
Baking chocolate (1 oz)	35
Carbonated beverages (12-oz can)‡	
Diet Mr. Pibb	58.8
Mountain Dew	54.0
Mello Yellow	52.8
Tab	46.8
Coca-Cola	45.6
Diet Coke	45.6
Mr. Pibb	40.8
Dr. Pepper	39.6
Diet Dr. Pepper	39.6
Pepsi-Cola	38.4
Royal Crown Cola	36.0
Diet Rite Cola	36.0
Diet Pepsi	36.0

*From Department of Dietetics, Miami Valley Hospital: *Miami Valley Hospital Handbook of Nutrition.* Dayton, Ohio, 1983, p 151. Reproduced by permission.
†*Consumer Reports,* October 1981, p 598.
‡National Soft Drink Association, 1983.

VITAMINS

TABLE 19-6.—RECOMMENDED DAILY DIETARY ALLOWANCES OF VITAMINS AND MINERALS*a

	AGE (yr)	Weight (kg)	Weight (lb)	Height (cm)	Height (in.)	ENERGY (Cal)[b]	PROTEIN (gm)	Vitamin A activity (RE)[c]	Vitamin A activity (IU)	Vitamin D (IU)	Vitamin E activity (IU)[e]	Ascorbic acid (mg)	Folacin (µg)[f]	Niacin (mg)[g]	Riboflavin (mg)	Thiamin (mg)	Vitamin B6 (mg)	Vitamin B12 (µg)	Calcium (mg)	Phosphorus (mg)	Iodine (µg)	Iron (mg)	Magnesium (mg)	Zinc (mg)
Infants	0.0–0.5	6	14	60	24	kg × 117	kg × 2.2	420[d]	1400	400	4	35	50	5	0.4	0.3	0.3	0.3	360	240	35	10	60	3
	0.5–1.0	9	20	71	28	kg × 108	kg × 2.0	400	2000	400	5	35	50	8	0.6	0.5	0.4	0.3	540	400	45	15	70	5
Children	1–3	13	28	86	34	1300	23	400	2000	400	7	40	100	9	0.8	0.7	0.6	1.0	800	800	60	15	150	10
	4–6	20	44	110	44	1800	30	500	2500	400	9	40	200	12	1.1	0.9	0.9	1.5	800	800	80	10	200	10
	7–10	30	66	135	54	2400	36	700	3300	400	10	40	300	16	1.2	1.2	1.2	2.0	800	800	110	10	250	10
Males	11–14	44	97	158	63	2800	44	1000	5000	400	12	45	400	18	1.5	1.4	1.6	3.0	1200	1200	130	18	350	15
	15–18	61	134	172	69	3000	54	1000	5000	400	15	45	400	20	1.8	1.5	2.0	3.0	1200	1200	150	18	400	15
	19–22	67	147	172	69	3000	54	1000	5000	400	15	45	400	20	1.8	1.5	2.0	3.0	800	800	140	10	350	15
	23–50	70	154	172	69	2700	56	1000	5000		15	45	400	18	1.6	1.4	2.0	3.0	800	800	130	10	350	15
	51+	70	154	172	69	2400	56	1000	5000		15	45	400	16	1.5	1.2	2.0	3.0	800	800	110	10	350	15
Females	11–14	44	97	155	62	2400	44	800	4000	400	12	45	400	16	1.3	1.2	1.6	3.0	1200	1200	115	18	300	15
	15–18	54	119	162	65	2100	48	800	4000	400	12	45	400	14	1.4	1.1	2.0	3.0	1200	1200	115	18	300	15
	19–22	58	128	162	65	2100	46	800	4000	400	12	45	400	14	1.4	1.1	2.0	3.0	800	800	100	18	300	15
	23–50	58	128	162	65	2000	46	800	4000		12	45	400	13	1.2	1.0	2.0	3.0	800	800	100	18	300	15
	51+	58	128	162	65	1800	46	800	4000		12	45	400	12	1.1	1.0	2.0	3.0	800	800	80	10	300	15
Pregnant						+300	+30	1000	5000	400	15	60	800	+2	+0.3	+0.3	2.5	4.0	1200	1200	125	18+[h]	450	20
Lactating						+500	+20	1200	6000	400	15	80	600	+4	+0.5	+0.3	2.5	4.0	1200	1200	150	18	450	25

*Adapted from Schneider H, Anderson C, Coursin D: *Nutritional Support of Medical Practice*. New York, Harper & Row, Publishers, 1977, p 128. Reproduced by permission.

*a*The allowances are intended to provide for individual variations among most normal persons as they live in the United States under usual environmental stresses. Diets should be based on a variety of common foods in order to provide other nutrients for which human requirements have been less well defined.

*b*Kilojoules (kJ) = 4.2 × Cal.

*c*Retinol equivalents.

*d*Assumed to be all as retinol in milk during the first 6 months of life. All subsequent intakes are assumed to be half as retinol and half as β-carotene when calculated from international units. As retinol equivalents, three-fourths are as retinol and one-fourth as β-carotene.

*e*Total vitamin E activity, estimated to be 80% as α-tocopherol and 20% other tocopherols.

*f*The folacin allowances refer to dietary sources as determined by *Lactobacillus casei* assay. Pure forms of folacin may be effective in doses less than one-fourth of the recommended dietary allowance.

*g*Although allowances are expressed as niacin, it is recognized that on the average 1 mg of niacin is derived from each 60 mg of dietary tryptophan.

*h*This increased requirement cannot be met by ordinary diets; therefore, the use of supplemental iron is recommended.

TABLE 19–7.—MAJOR DRUG EFFECTS ON VITAMINS AND MINERALS*

THERAPEUTIC CLASS	MAJOR DRUGS	NUTRITIONAL EFFECT	CLINICAL EFFECT
Anticonvulsants and sedatives	Phenytoin, phenobarbital, glutethimide	Accelerated vitamin D and vitamin K metabolism, folic acid deficiency	Rickets Neonatal hemorrhaging Megaloblastic anemia Gingival hyperplasia Neurologic deterioration (?) Congenital malformations (?)
		Vitamin B6 deficiency	None established
Corticosteroids	Cortisone Prednisone	Accelerated vitamin D metabolism Increased vitamin C excretion Increased vitamin B6 requirement	Accelerated bone loss None established Abnormal glucose tolerance (?) Mental depression (?)
		Increased zinc excretion Increased potassium excretion Vitamin B1 deficiency	Slow wound healing Muscle weakness Wernicke's encephalopathy Korsakoff's psychosis
Alcohol		Impaired vitamin B6 activation	Peripheral neuropathy (?) Sideroblastic anemia (?) "Rum fits" (?)
		Folic acid deficiency Increased magnesium excretion	Anemia (?) ECG changes Delirium tremens

Continued.

TABLE 19–7.—Continued

THERAPEUTIC CLASS	MAJOR DRUGS	NUTRITIONAL EFFECT	CLINICAL EFFECT
Nonabsorbed antibiotics	Neomycin Kanamycin	Reduced lactase levels	Lactose intolerance
Antitubercular drugs	Isoniazid	Vitamin B_6 deficiency Niacin deficiency	Polyneuritis Pellagra symptoms
Diuretics	Hydrochlorothiazide	Increased potassium excretion Increased magnesium excretion	Muscle weakness Magnesium depletion
	Spironolactone	Reduced potassium excretion	Hyperkalemia
Hypotensives	Hydralazine	Vitamin B6 depletion	Polyneuritis
Anti-inflammatory drugs	Aspirin Indomethacin	GI bleeding	Iron deficiency anemia
	Phenylbutazone	Folic acid deficiency	Megaloblastic anemia
Oral contraceptives and estrogens	Mestranol	Vitamin B6 depletion	Mental depression Abnormal glucose tolerance
	Ethinyl estradiol		Megaloblastic anemia
	Conjugated estrogens	Folic acid deficiency	Megaloblastic cervical cytology Increased megaloblastic anemia in subsequent pregnancy
		Reduced calcium excretion	Reduced bone loss

*From Theuer R, Vitale J: Drug and nutrient interactions, in Schneider H, Anderson C, Coursin D (eds): *Nutritional Support of Medical Practice.* New York, Harper & Row, Publishers, 1977, p 298. Reproduced by permission.

General rules for the administration of an enteral feeding via the *nasogastric and gastrostomy routes,* unless otherwise indicated are

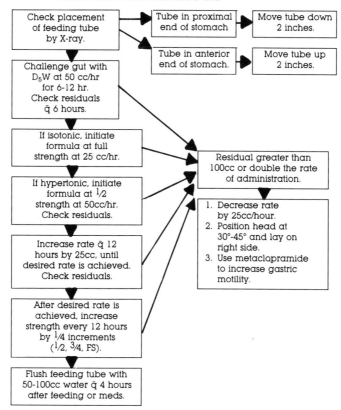

Note: Infusion rates must be reduced and individualized for pediatric patients.

FIG 19–1.

Protocol for enteral feeding. (Adapted from Ahrens L, et al: *Enteric Nutrition Handbook.* Iowa City, Iowa, University of Iowa Press, 1987, p 17.)

TABLE 19–8.—NUTRIENT ANALYSIS OF ENTERAL FORMULAS AND SUPPLEMENTS*

	MILK BASED	LACTOSE FREE				
	INSTANT BREAKFAST	ENSURE	ISOCAL	OSMOLITE HN	PROFIBER	PRECISION ISOTONIC
Calories/cc	1.0	1.06	1.06	1.06	1.0	1.0
Carbohydrate Source	Sucrose, corn syrup, lactose	Hydrolyzed corn starch, sucrose	Glucose oligosaccharides	Hydrolyzed corn starch	Hydrolyzed corn starch, soy fiber	Glucose oligosaccharides sucrose
Protein Source	Milk, sodium casinate, soybean protein isolate	Soy protein isolate, sodium and calcium caseinates	Soy protein isolate, sodium and calcium caseinates	Soy protein isolate, sodium and calcium caseinates	Sodium and calcium caseinates	Egg albumin
Fat Source	Whole Milk	Corn oil	MCT, soy oil	MCT, Corn oil, soy oil	Corn oil	Partially hydrogenated soy oil
Protein gm/liter (%)	60 (22%)	37 (14%)	34 (13%)	44 (17%)	40 (16%)	30
Fat gm/liter (%)	32 (26%)	37 (31%)	44 (37%)	37 (30%)	40 (36%)	31
Carbohydrate gm/liter (%)	144 (50%)	145 (54%)	132 (50%)	141 (53%)	132 (48%)	144
Nonprotein calories: gN	88:1	153:1	167:1	125:1	131:1	183:1
mOsm/kg water	710	450	300	310	300	300
Na/K mEq/liter	41/70	37/40	23/34	40/40	32/32	20/25
Ca/Phos mg/liter	1600/1120	549/549	634/528	761/761	667/667	680/680
Vitamins, cc to meet 100% U.S. RDA	1400	1887	1890	1321	1500	1560
Flavors	Chocolate Vanilla Strawberry	Chocolate Vanilla	Unflavored	Unflavored	Unflavored	Vanilla Orange
Form	Powder	Liquid	Liquid	Liquid	Liquid	Powder
Uses/Features	Oral Supplement, High protein	Oral Supplement	Tube feeding	Tube feeding	High fiber tube feeding (14 gm fiber/L)	Tube feeding isotonic lactose free
Manufacturer	Delmark Carnation	Ross	Mead-Johnson	Ross	Sherwood Medical	Sandoz

	LACTOSE FREE			PARTIALLY PRE-DIGESTED		
SUSTACAL	SUSTACAL WITH FIBER	VITANEED	CITROTEIN	ISOTEIN HN	PEPTAMEN	VITAL HN
1.0	1.06	1.0	0.66	1.2	1.0	1.0
Sucrose, corn syrup solids	Maltodextrin, sugar, soy fiber	Maltodextrin, fruit and vegetables, soy fiber	Sucrose, maltodextrin	Maltodextrin, fructose	Maltodextrin, starch	Hydrolyzed corn starch, sucrose
Soy protein isolate, sodium and calcium caseinates	Calcium and sodium caseinates, soy protein isolate	Beef puree, calcium and sodium caseinates	Egg albumin	Delactosed lactalbumin	Hydrolyzed whey protein	Partially hydrolyzed whey & meat & soy, free amino acids
Partially hydrogenated soy oil	Corn oil	Corn oil	Partially hydrogenated soy oil	Partially hydrogenated soy oil, MCT	Sunflower oil, MCT, lecithin	Safflower oil, MCT, mono and diglycerides
61 (24%)	46 (17%)	40 (16%)	41 (25%)	68 (23%)	40 (16%)	42 (17%)
23 (21%)	35 (30%)	40 (36%)	1.6 (21%)	34 (25%)	39 (33%)	11 (9%)
140 (55%)	141 (53%)	128 (48%)	122 (55%)	156 (52%)	127 (51%)	185 (74%)
79:1	120:1	131:1	76:1	86:1	130:1	125:1
620	450	300	495	300	260	500
41/54	31/36	30/32	31/18	27/27	22/32	20/34
1014/930	845/704	667/667	1048/1048	571/571	600/500	667/667
1080	1500	1500	1350	1770	2000	1500
Strawberry Vanilla	Vanilla	Unflavored	Fruit Punch	Vanilla	Unflavored	Vanilla
Liquid	Liquid	Liquid	Powder	Powder	Liquid	Powder
Oral Supplement, High Protein	High fiber tube feeding or supplement (6 gm fiber/L	Blenderized tube feeding	Oral Supplement, low fat, low residue	Tube feeding, high protein isotonic	Isotonic pre-digested formula with MCT oil	Tube feeding, elemental, low fat
Mead-Johnson	Mead-Johnson	Sherwood Medical	Sandoz	Sandoz	Clintec	Ross

Continued.

Table 19–8.—continued

	ELEMENTAL		HIGH CALORIC DENSITY		COMPONENTS	
	TOLEREX	VIVONEX T.E.N.	SUSTACAL HC	TWO CAL HN	MICROLIPID	POLYCOSE LIQUID
Calories/cc	1.0	1.0	1.5	2.0	4.5	2.0
Carbohydrate Source	Glucose oligosaccharides	maltodextrin and modified starch	Corn syrup solids, sugar	Hydrolyzed corn starch, sucrose	—	Hydrolyzed corn starch
Protein Source	Free amino acids	Crystalline amino acids	Sodium and calcium caseinates	Soy protein isolate, sodium and calcium caseinates	—	—
Fat Source	Safflower oil	Safflower oil	Corn oil	Corn oil, MCT	Safflower oil	—
Protein gm/liter (%)	21 (8%)	38 (15%)	61 (16%)	84 (17%)	—	—
Fat gm/liter (%)	1.5 (1%)	3 (2%)	58 (34%)	91 (40%)	500	—
Carbohydrate gm/liter (%)	231 (92%)	206 (82%)	190 (50%)	217 (43%)	—	500
Nonprotein calories: gN	281:1	139:1	134:1	125:1	—	—
mOsm/kg water	550	630	650	690	80	850
Na/K mEq/liter	20/30	20/20	37/38	46/59	—	30/2
Ca/Phos mg/liter	556/556	500/500	845/845	1053/1053	—	200/30
Vitamins, cc to meet 100% U.S. RDA	1800	2000	1180	950	—	—
Flavors	Unflavored	Unflavored	Vanilla	Vanilla	Unflavored	Unflavored
Form	Powder	Powder	Liquid	Liquid	Liquid	Liquid
Uses/Features	Tube feeding, lactose free, low fat	Jejunostomy tube feeding, high in glutamine	Oral Supplement	Tube feeding	Fat emulsion supplement	Carbohydrate supplement
Manufacturer	Norwich Eaton	Norwich Eaton	Mead-Johnson	Ross	Biosearch	Ross

*Adapted from *Recent Advances in Therapeutic Diets,* ed 4, Ames, Iowa, Iowa State University Press, 1989. Compiled by the

COMPONENTS		SPECIAL FORMULATIONS			
PRO-MIX PROTEIN	SUMACAL	GLUCERNA	HEPATIC-AID II	PULMOCARE	TRAVASORB RENAL
14.4 kcal/gm	19 cal T	1.0	1.1	1.5	1.35
—	Maltodextrin	Hydrolyzed cornstarch, fructose	Maltodextrin sucrose	Hydrolyzed corn starch, sucrose	Glucose oligosaccharides sucrose
Whey protein	—	Sodium and calcium caseinates	Amino acids	Sodium and calcium caseinates	Essential and nonessential crystaline amino acids
—	—	Hi-oleic Safflower oil, soy oil	Soybean oil, mono and diglycerides	Corn oil	MCT, sunflower oil
4 gm/T	—	42 (17%)	44 (15%)	63 (17%)	23 (7%)
0.2 gm/T	—	56 (33%)	36 (28%)	92 (55%)	18 (12%)
0.2 gm/T	5 gm/T	94 (50%)	169 (57%)	106 (28%)	271 (81%)
—	—	120:1	340:1	125:1	362:1
30	680	375	560	490	590
0.4/0.8/T 0.5/1.05	0.2/T/-	40/40	<16/<6	57/48	negligible
15/T 13/T	—	704/704	—	1040/1040	negligible
—	—	1422	—	947	2100
Unflavored	Unflavored	Unflavored	Chocolate Eggnog	Vanilla	Apricot Strawberry
Powder	Powder	Liquid	Powder	Liquid	Powder
Protein supplement	Carbohydrate supplement	Tube feeding for diabetics, Contains 14 g fiber L	Liver formula Oral supplement tube feeding 46% BCAA	Used for C.O.P.D. patients Tube feeding, high fat	Renal formular oral supplement tube feeding
Navaco	Mead-Johnson	Ross	McGaw	Ross	Travenol

Clinical Staff, Dietary Department, University of Iowa Hospitals and Clinics, Iowa City. Reproduced by permission.

ENTERAL AND PARENTERAL NUTRITION

TABLE 19–9.—Tube Feedings

Tube feedings should be used if possible prior to instituting parenteral hyperalimentation. Orders should include:
   Strength: Should approximate isotonic, if possible (300 mOsm).
   cc hr: Bolus = 300–400 cc q4–6h, or give via pump as constant infusion.
   Total Volume and Calories/24-hr. Period:
      Calories should be 1,800–3,000/day (most formulas = 1 cal/cc).
      Most commercial products are vitamin enriched.
      Water should be added for a total volume of at least 1 cc/kcal. A minimum of 2,000–2,500 cc/day should be provided.
Recommended parameters to monitor
   Weight: Weigh daily for 1 week, then once a week.
   Intake/output daily.
   Labs (initially, then every week):
      CBC
      Total protein
      Albumin
      BUN
      Sodium
      Potassium
      Glucose
      Urine for glucose and ketones (3 ×/week)

TABLE 19–10.—Complications and Suggested Treatments for Feeding

---

COMPLICATION	POSSIBLE REASON	SUGGESTED TREATMENT
Electrolyte imbalance	Composition of formula. *Other causes such as diarrhea, renal failure, or fluid status.*	Increase or decrease affected electrolytes.
Dehydration	Administration of concentrated formulas. *Other causes such as diarrhea.*	Correct any abnormal losses, provide increased free water, or adjust the formula to decrease renal solute load.
Glucosuria	Increased carbohydrate load. *Other causes such as diabetes.*	Decrease carbohydrate content of formula.
Azotemia	High-protein formula. Insufficient water to excrete waste products. *Other causes such as renal impairment, or GI bleed.*	Reduce amount of protein in formula. Increase free water for excretion.

Diarrhea and/or cramping	Medications.	Medications that can cause diarrhea are antibiotics, Maalox, KCL, and quinidine. Change to another agent if possible.
	Tube placement too low in stomach causing gastric distention with increased gastric emptying.	Check tube placement by x-ray film and adjust as needed.
	Liquid stools around impaction.	Check for impaction. An enema may be indicated. Adequate water intake or a bulking agent should be used to prevent impaction.
	Volume overload.	Reduce flow rate. Add high-fiber formula (Enrich).
	Osmotic overload (especially with transpyloric feeding).	Dilute formula with water or reduce rate of administration or change to isotonic formula.
	Decreased bulk.	Switch to formula that provides more fiber. Add high-fiber formula (Enrich).
	Inadequate intestinal flora due to antibiotic therapy.	Administer 50:50 ratio of plain yogurt and sweet acidophilus milk at 50 cc/hr for 24 hr or lactobacillus crystals t.i.d.
	Lactose intolerance.	Use lactose-free formula.
	Fat malabsorption.	Decrease fat content of feeding and/or use MCT oil.
	Insufficient osmotic pressure for absorption as indicated by low serum albumin.	Reduce enteral feeding and supplement with peripheral albumin or administer TPN until albumin is at least 2.5.
	Bacterial contamination.	Change feeding container and administration tubing every 24 hr. Use clean technique when transferring formula. Hang time not > 4 hr.

Continued.

TABLE 19–10.—Continued

Constipation	Impaction.	Check with rectal examination. Give patient a laxative or an enema.
	Decreased bulk.	Switch to formula that provides more fiber.
	Insufficient free fluid.	Increase free fluid adminstered with formula.
	Medications that decrease intestinal motility.	Change medications if possible or give stool softener, additional fluid, or laxative.
	Decreased intestinal motility due to inactivity.	Increase patient's activity or treat symptomatically.
	Complete absorption of elemental formula, resulting in minimal waste products.	Patient education and reassurance.

*From *Handbook of Clinical Dietetics.* New Haven, Yale University Press, 1981, p A25. Table courtesy of Mary B McCann, MD, Maine Medical Center. Reproduced by permission.

TABLE 19–11.—PROTOCOL FOR INITIATING CENTRAL PARENTERAL NUTRITION*

I. Run basic parenteral nutrition solution without electrolytes as listed below:
   500 ml of 50% Dextrose with 500 ml of crystalline, amino acids 8.5%
II. Suggested additions to fluids (should be modified in accordance with lab data):

Na	40–50 mEq/L (as acetate or chloride)
K	30–40 mEq/L (as acetate or chloride)
$MgSO_4$	4–8 mEq/L
Ca	4–5 mEq/L (as gluconate)
PO	10–15 mEq/L (as sodium or potassium)
MVI_{12}	1 ampule/day
Zn	4 mg/day
Cu	2 mg/day (liver function should be monitored)

NOTE: Exclusive use of chloride may result in hyperchloremic metabolic acidosis

III. IV rate
   40 ml/hr for first 24 hours.
   80 mg/hr for next 24 hours.
   120 ml/hr thereafter.
   May be increased as tolerated up to 250 ml/hr, on physician's order only.
   Do not increase IV rate if you get behind.
IV. IM medications
   10 mg vitamin K weekly or as indicated by prothrombin time.

V. Parameters to watch
   Accurate input/output.
   Finger-stick glucose 3–4 × /d.
   Urine for sugar and acetone q6h; call if greater than 2 + .
   Orders for sliding scale insulin.
   Urine for specific gravity.
   Weigh daily.
VI. Lab studies

	During first 7 days or when patient is ill or unstable	After first 7 days and when patient is stable
Electrolytes	Daily	3× weekly
Plasma osmolarity	Daily	3× weekly
Glucose	Daily	3× weekly
Prothrombin time	Initially	Weekly
Chemistry profile (BUN, proteins, calcium phosphorus, uric acid, SGOT)	3× weekly	weekly
Mg^{++}	3× weekly	weekly
Ammonia	2× weekly	weekly
Blood pH	2× weekly	weekly
CBC	Weekly	weekly
Transferrin	Weekly	Weekly
Ferritin	Weekly	Weekly
Zinc	Weekly	Weekly

VII. Insulin
   Human regular insulin given either subcutaneously or in the intravenous
      solution is indicated in the following cases:
   Known diabetes mellitus.
   Elderly patients (5–25 units).
   Pancreatic disorders.
   Posttraumatic period when insulin response is depressed.
   Critically ill, nutritionally depleted patients in whom positive caloric
      balance is deemed urgent for survival.
VIII. Catheter care (central line)
   Change IV tubing daily.
   Change dressing Monday, Wednesday, and Friday:
      Use antiseptic ointment.
      Dressing must be occlusive.
   Do not give medications, draw blood, or measure CVP through central
      catheter unless double lumen catheter is utilized.

Continued.

TABLE 19–10.—Continued

IX. Intravenous fat emulsion 10% or 20%

Occasional infusions may be necessary to prevent essential fatty acid deficiency.

When used as a caloric supplement, 500 ml may be infused daily.

Cautious administration is recommended if hepatic dysfunction, blood dyscrasia, or a respiratory disorder exists.

X. Discontinuing hyperalimentation

It is recommended that hyperalimentation be tapered over 24–48 hours prior to cessation.

If central hyperalimentation is suddenly discontinued, a peripheral IV of D5W should be started and the patient observed for signs of hypoglycemia.

*Adapted from the Department of Dietetics, Miami Valley Hospital: *Miami Valley Hospital Handbook of Nutrition.* Dayton, Ohio, 1983, pp 38–40.

TABLE 19–12.—FOUR STANDARD FORMULAS FOR PARENTERAL NUTRITION*

	CENTRAL FORMULA† (Protein Source, L-amino acid 5.5%)	CENTRAL FORMULA (Protein Source, L-amino acid 8.5%)	PERIPHERAL FORMULA (Protein Source, L-amino acid 3.5%)	RENAL FAILURE FORMULA (Central Line Only) (Protein Source, L-amino acid 8.5%)
Amino acids, 500 ml	27.5 gm	42.5 gm	35.14 gm	Amino acids, 125 ml, 10.6 gm
Dextrose, 500 ml D50	250 gm	Dextrose, 500 ml D50, 250 gm	Dextrose, 500 ml D20, 100 gm	Dextrose, 500 ml D50, 250 gm
Sodium	35 mEq	35 mEq	25 mEq	3 mEq
Potassium	30 mEq	30 mEq	14 mEq	0 mEq
Magnesium	5 mEq	5 mEq	5 mEq	0 mEq
Chloride	35 mEq	35 mEq	25 mEq	34.3 mEq
Acetate	50 mEq	68 mEq	54 mEq	6.6 mEq
Phosphorus	15 mm	15 mm	15 mm	0 mm
Calcium gluconate	—	—	—	0
MVI concentrate	—	—	—	1

Continued.

589

TABLE 19–12.—Continued

	CENTRAL FORMULA[†] (Protein Source, L-amino acid 5.5%)	CENTRAL FORMULA (Protein Source, L-amino acid 8.5%)	PERIPHERAL FORMULA (Protein Source, L-amino acid 3.5%)	RENAL FAILURE FORMULA (Central Line Only) (Protein Source, L-amino acid 8.5%)
Total kcal	960	960	380	938
Ratio (CHO:N)	184:1	118:1	—	527:1
Grams of N	4.63 gm	7.15 gm	28 gm	1.8 gm
Grams protein eq.[‡]	28.94 gm	42.5 gm	18.44 gm	11.3 gm
Osmolarity	1,920	1,920	450	1,010
Approx. volume	1,000 ml	1,000 ml	1,000 ml	625 ml

*Adapted from Cannon J, Welsh J, Whang R: Gastrointestinal system and nutrition, in Papper S (ed): *Manual of Medical Care of the Surgical Patient*. Boston, Little, Brown & Co, 1981, p 73.
†Can also be used peripherally by adding 50 ml D10. This solution would contain 50 gm dextrose and have an osmolarity of approximately 680.
‡Grams of protein equivalent are computed by multiplying 6.25 times the grams of nitrogen.
D10 = 10% glucose; D50 = 50% glucose; CHO = carbohydrate; N = nitrogen.

TABLE 19–13.—METABOLIC PROBLEMS ASSOCIATED WITH TOTAL PARENTERAL NUTRITION*

	PROBLEM	DIAGNOSIS	POSSIBLE CAUSES	TREATMENT
Glucose metabolism	Hyperglycemia	Increased blood sugar Glycosuria	Excessive rate of infusion Inadequate insulin	Adjust rate of infusion Administer regular insulin
	Hyperosmolar nonketotic coma	Increased blood sugar Increased serum and urine osmolality Glycosuria Coma	Excessive total glucose load or rate of infusion: inadequate insulin, glucocorticoids, latent diabetes, sepsis, pancreatic disease, acute or chronic renal failure	Appropriate fluids and insulin therapy
	Ketoacidosis in the diabetic	Increased blood sugar Acidosis Ketones	Inadequate endogenous insulin response; inadequate exogenous insulin therapy	Appropriate fluids and insulin
	Postinfusion hypoglycemia	Confusion Coma Decreased blood sugar	Unusual in nondiabetic patient; seen in patients with liver depleted of glycogen who have been in severe negative nitrogen balance Persistence of endogenous insulin production by stimulated islet cells	Gradually taper glucose infusion prior to termination

Continued.

591

TABLE 19–13.—Continued

PROBLEM	DIAGNOSIS	POSSIBLE CAUSES	TREATMENT
Amino acid metabolism			
Hyperchloremic metabolic acidosis	Increased serum chloride Acidosis	Excessive chloride and monohydrochloride content of certain crystalline amino acid solutions	Provide a portion of sodium and potassium as acetate salts rather than chlorides
Hyperammonemia	Increased blood ammonia Lethargy	Pediatric age group and patients with cirrhosis are at high risk May be due to relative arginine deficiency which decreases effectiveness of urea cycle: ornithine, aspartic, and/or glutamic acid deficiencies have been implicated	Add 2 mM/kg/day of arginine glutamate or 3 mM/kg/day of arginine hydrochloride
Prerenal azotemia	Increased BUN	Excessive protein hydrolysate or amino acid infusion	Adjust rate of administration
Essential fatty acid deficiency	Dermatitis, hair loss, thrombocytopenia, poor wound healing	Abnormal plasma lipid patterns, serum deficiency of phospholipid linoleic and/or arachidonic acids	Inadequate essential fatty acid administration; inadequate vitamin E administration	Infusion of IV fat emulsion Vitamin E administration

Calcium phosphorus metabolism	Hypophosphatemia 1. Decreased erythrocyte 2,3-DPG 2. Increased affinity of hemoglobin for oxygen 3. Aberrations of erythrocyte metabolism	Decreased serum phosphorus	Inadequate phosphorus administration, redistribution of serum phosphorus into cells and bone	Add phosphorus to TPN regimen
	Hypocalcemia	Decreased serum calcium Tetany, muscle spasm	Inadequate calcium administration Profound in patients who have phosphorus replacement without calcium replacement Hypoalbuminemia	Add adequate calcium to TPN regimen
	Hypercalcemia	Increased serum calcium	Excessive calcium administration with or without high doses of albumin; excessive vitamin D administration	Adjust calcium in TPN regimen Adjust vitamin D dosage
Potassium imbalance	Hypokalemia	Decreased serum potassium	Inadequate potassium intake relative to increased requirements or protein anabolism; diuresis	Potassium replacement
	Hyperkalemia	Increased serum potassium	Excessive potassium administration particularly in metabolic acidosis and renal decompensation	Decreased potassium in the total parenteral nutrition regimen

Continued.

TABLE 19–13.—Continued

PROBLEM		DIAGNOSIS	POSSIBLE CAUSES	TREATMENT
Trace metal deficiencies	Hypomagnesemia	Neuromuscular irritability; disorientation, tremor, and seizure Low urinary excretion of magnesium	Inadequate magnesium administration relative to increased requirements for protein anabolism and glucose metabolism	10–20 mEq magnesium per day added to the TPN regimen
	Zinc	Skin lesions, loss of hair, poor wound healing, diarrhea	Inadequate zinc administration	Zinc acetate
	Copper	Anemia, leukopenia, hypoproteinemia	Inadequate copper replacement	Add copper to total parenteral nutrition
Vitamin deficiencies	Folic acid deficiency	Anemia	Inadequate replacement	5 mg/week IV
	Vitamin B_{12} deficiency			1,000 μg/month IM
	Vitamin K	Bleeding	Inadequate administration	10 mg/week IM or SQ

*Adapted from Cannon J, Welsh J, Whang R: Gastrointestinal system and nutrition, in Papper S (ed): *Manual of Medical Care of the Surgical Patient.* Boston, Little, Brown & Co, 1981, pp 74–76.

TREATMENT OF HYPECHOLESTEROLEMIA

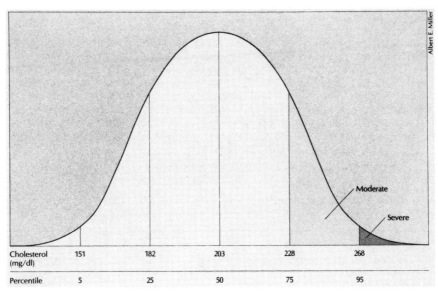

FIG 19–2.
Epidemiologic studies show an increased risk of CAD for persons with serum cholesterol levels >180 mg/dl. Thus, the distribution curve of cholesterol levels in white men 40 to 44 years of age reveals the 75th percentile to be a more realistic predictor of risk than the statistical upper limit of normal, the 95th percentile. (From Levy RI: *Hosp Pract* 1988; 23[suppl 1]:15. Reproduced by permission.)

TABLE 19–14.—COMPONENTS OF DIETS RECOMMENDED
FOR CHOLESTEROL REDUCTION*

	STEP 1 DIET[†]	STEP 2 DIET[†]
Total fat	<30% total calories	<30% total calories
Saturated fat	<10% total calories*	<7% total calories*
Polyunsaturated fat	<10% total calories	<10% total calories
Monounsaturated fat	10%–15% total calories	10%–15% total calories
Carbohydrates	50%–60% total calories	50%–60% total calories
Protein	10%–20% total calories	10%–20% total calories
Cholesterol	<300 mg/day	<200 mg/day
Total calories	As necessary to achieve and maintain desirable weight	

*From Griffin GC, Castelli WP: *Postgrad Med* 1988; 84(3):56, as adapted from National Cholesterol Education Program: *Arch Intern Med* 1988; 148:36–69. Reproduced by permission.
†Step 1 diet recommended for patients with cholesterol >240 mg% or >200 mg% if high risk for CAD. Step 2 diet recommended if step 1 ineffective or is used by high-risk patients with total cholesterol >240 mg%.

TABLE 19–15.—NATIONAL CHOLESTEROL EDUCATION PROGRAM GUIDELINES*

SERUM CHOLESTEROL LEVEL	DEGREE OF RISK	RECOMMENDATION
<200 mg/dl	Low	Recheck cholesterol every 5 yr
200–239 mg/dl without CAD or other risk factors[†]	Borderline high	Restrict dietary saturated fat, cholesterol, and calories, if overweight
		Recheck cholesterol annually
		Lipoprotein profile optional
200–239 mg/dl with CAD or at least two other risk factors[†]	High	Obtain lipoprotein profile[‡]
		Goals of therapy are based on LDL cholesterol; begin with diet
		If LDL cholesterol remains >190 mg/dl after diet, prescribe drugs
≥240 mg/dl	High	Same as above

*Adapted from Levy RI: *Hosp Pract* 1988; 23(suppl 1):17, as adapted from National Cholesterol Education Program: *Arch Intern Med* 1988; 148:36.
†Male sex, family history of early CAD, cigarette smoking, hypertension, diabetes mellitus, >30% overweight, HDL cholesterol <35 mg/dl.
‡Treatment is based on the concentration of serum LDL cholesterol: <130 mg/dl, desirable range; 130–160 mg/dl, borderline high risk; >160 mg/dl, high risk.

TABLE 19–16.—SATURATED FAT AND CHOLESTEROL IN COMMON FOODS*†

	SATURATED FAT (GM)	CHOLESTEROL (MG)
Bread (most varieties, per slice)	0.2	0
Bun or roll	0.5	0
Butter (1 T)	7	30
Margarine (1 T)	2	0
Soft diet margarine (1 T)	1	0
Angelfood cake	0	0
White cake with frosting	3	20
Cream cheese (1 oz)	5	30
Cheese (1 oz)	6	30
Weight Watchers Cheese Product (1 oz)	<1	2
Donut	5	20
Oatmeal (without milk) (1 c)	0.4	0
Egg custard (1 c)	7	275
Instant pudding (with skim milk) (1 c)	0.3	0
Egg	1.7	275
Egg yolk	1.7	275
Egg white	0	0
Egg Beaters egg substitute	0	0
Spaghetti (plain)	Trace	0
Potato (baked, plain)	0	0
French fries (1 order)	7	15
Homogenized milk (1 c)	5	30
Nonfat skim milk (1 c)	0.3	Trace
Creamy yogurt (1 c)	5	30
Nonfat yogurt (1 c)	0.3	Trace
Olive oil (1 T)	2	0
Canola oil (1 T)	1	0
Peanut oil (1 T)	2.3	0
Salad dressing (1 T)	1.5	Trace
Poultry (3 oz light meat, skinless)	1	70
Fried chicken nuggets (9 pieces)	14	125
Ice cream (1 c)	9	60
Blended fruit ice	0	0
Nonfat frozen yogurt (1 c)	0.3	Trace
Salmon (coho) (3 oz)	1	35
Ground beef (3 oz, 27% fat)	7	80
Extra-lean beef (3 oz)	4	50
Cream soups (1 c)	5	20
Vegetable soup (1 c)	0.3	0
Vegetables	0	0
Fruits	0	0
Beans, rice, legumes (1 c)	Trace	0

*From Griffin GC, Castelli WP: *Good Fat Bad Fat: How to Lower Your Cholesterol and Beat the Odds of a Heart Attack.* Tucson, Ariz, Fisher Books, 1988. Reproduced by permission.
†T = tablespoon; c = cup.

TABLE 19-17.—Currently Available Lipid-Modifying Drugs*

	NICOTINIC ACID	CLOFIBRATE	GEMFIBROZIL	BILE ACID SEQUESTRANTS	PROBUCOL
Mechanism of action	↓VLDL production ↑HDL	↑Intravascular catabolism of VLDL, IDL	↑Intravascular catabolism of VLDL, IDL ↑HDL	↑LDL removal	↑LDL removal (receptor independent)
Indications	↑VLDL, IDL (in types III–V) ↑LDL (in type II)	↑VLDL, IDL (in types III–V)	↑VLDL, IDL (in types III–V)	↑LDL (in type II)	↑LDL (in type II)
Dosage Initial	100 mg t.i.d.	1 gm b.i.d.	300 mg b.i.d.	4 gm b.i.d. (cholestyramine) 5 gm t.i.d. (colestipol)	250 mg b.i.d.
Maintenance	1–3 gm t.i.d.	1 gm b.i.d	600 mg b.i.d.	8–16 gm b.i.d. (cholestyramine) 5–10 gm t.i.d. (colestipol)	500 mg b.i.d.

Major side effects				
Flushing, pruritus, nausea	Nausea, diarrhea	GI distress, rash	Constipation, nausea	Diarrhea, nausea
Other side effects				
GI distress, glucose intolerance, hyperuricemia, hepatotoxicity, skin changes	Cholelithiasis, myositis, ventricular ectopy, abnormal liver function tests, (?) sometimes ↑LDL	Glucose intolerance, leukopenia, (?)cholelithiasis, (?)sometimes ↑LDL	Liver function abnormalities, hyperchloremic acidosis (rare), steatorrhea (rare), ↑VLDL	(?)↓HDL (long residence in body) QT interval prolongation
Drug interactions	Vasodilation by ganglioplegic antihypertensive agents	Displacement of acidic drugs from albumin-binding sites; enhances effect, toxicity of some drugs (e.g., warfarin, phenytoin)	Potentiation of oral anticoagulants	↓ Absorption of phenylbutazone, thiazides, tetracycline, phenobarbital, digitalis, warfarin, propranolol	(?)

*Adapted from Levy RI: *Hosp Pract* 1988; 23(suppl 1):18.

20 Endocrinology

Charles W. Smith, Jr., M.D.

DIABETES MELLITUS

TABLE 20–1.—DIAGNOSIS OF DIABETES MELLITUS*

	FASTING PLASMA GLUCOSE	2-HR POSTPRANDIAL PLASMA GLUCOSE
Normal	< 115 mg/dl	< 140 mg/dl
Impaired glucose tolerance	< 140 mg/dl	140–200 mg/dl
Diabetes mellitus	≥ 140 mg/dl (on more than one occasion)	≥ 200†

*Adapted from Cahill GF, et al: Diabetes mellitus, in Rubenstin E, Federman DD (eds): *Metabolism in Scientific American Medicine.* New York, Scientific American Inc, 1987, p VI-7.
†Not required if fasting level is ≥ 140

TABLE 20–2.—INSULIN PREPARATIONS*

SPEED OF ACTION	TYPE	ONSET (HR)	PEAK (HR)	DURATION (HR)
Rapid	Regular	0.5–1	3–6	6–10
	Semilente	0.5–1	4–6	12–16
	Humulin R	0.5–1	2.5–5	6–8
Intermediate	NPH	1.5–3	6–12	18–24
	Lente	1–3	6–12	24–48
	Humulin N	1–1.5	4–12	24
	Humulin L	1–2.5	7–15	24
Long-acting	PZI	4–6	14–24	>36
	Ultralente	4–6	18–24	>36

*Adapted from Clutter WE: Diabetes mellitus and hyperlipidemia, in Campbell JW, Frisse M (eds): *Manual of Medical Therapeutics.* Boston, Little, Brown & Co, 1983.

TABLE 20–3.—HYPOGLYCEMIC AGENTS*

DRUG	DURATION (HR)	FREQUENCY	DAILY DOSE RANGE
Tolbutamide (Orinase)	6–12	b.i.d.–t.i.d.	1–2 gm
Chlorpropamide (Diabinese)	48–60	q.d.	125–500 mg
Acetohexamide (Dymelor)	12–24	q.d.–b.i.d.	250–500 mg
Tolazamide (Tolinase)	10–16	q.d.–b.i.d.	100–500 mg
Glyburide (Diabeta, Micronase)	≥16	q.d.–b.i.d.	2.5–20 mg
Glipizide (Glucotrol)	6–24	q.d.–b.i.d.	5.0–40 mg

*Adapted from Levin SE: Diabetes mellitus and hypoglycemia, in Hershman JM (ed): *Management of Endocrine Disorders*. Philadelphia, Lea & Febiger, 1980.

TABLE 20–4.—INITIATION OF INSULIN TREATMENT

Education: Must include injection techniques, characteristics of insulin, monitoring urine and/or blood sugar, diet, and importance of weight control and exercise.

Hospitalization: Indicated for ketoacidosis, severe hyperglycemia (>300–350), infection, or pregnancy.

Insulin dose and frequency (see Table 20–5):
1. NIDDM (type II): Give insulin only to control symptoms. Patients usually do well with a single A.M. dose of NPH.
2. IDDM (type I): Usually requires split dose; ⅔ of total dose is given in A.M.; ⅓ in P.M.; tight control may require additional regular insulin.
3. Adjustments should be made every 3–7 days. Look for patterns of urine or blood sugar responses, not single daily fluctuations. Limit dose increments to 5 units initially, decreasing to 2- to 3-unit increments as better control is attained.

TABLE 20–5.—APPROACH TO CONTROL PROBLEMS IN DIABETES MELLITUS

PROBLEM	TREATMENT
Fasting hyperglycemia	Give evening dose of NPH (5–10 units) and reduce A.M. dose
Late morning hyperglycemia	Add regular (~5 units) to A.M. dose
Late evening hyperglycemia	Add regular (~5 units) before dinner (give bedtime snack)
Hypoglycemia (if unexplained by exercise or meal delay)	Reduce insulin in 2- to 5-unit decrements

TABLE 20–6.—INSULIN RESISTANCE

Definition:
Requirement of >200 units/day for 2 days without ketoacidosis.
Possible causes:
Obesity, infection, steroid treatment (or Cushing's syndrome), or insulin-binding antibodies (most common).
Treatment approaches:
1. Change to purified pork or Humulin®.
2. Use multiple doses of regular, not intermediate or long-acting insulin.
3. Prednisone, 60 mg/day PO, taper as insulin requirements decrease.
4. Use sulfated insulin (modified for less antigenicity).

TABLE 20–7.—HOME GLUCOSE MONITORING

Indications
Pregnancy, "brittle" patients, and in cases where urine testing is unreliable or impractical. Also useful if tight control is desired.
Patient options
1. Chemstrip bG: Read as color comparison. Most convenient, least expensive, but less accurate.
2. Reflectance meter (Stat Tek, Accucheck, etc.) requires periodic calibration. Portable battery-powered units available.
Technique
Obtain a drop of blood (with Autolet), place it on reagent area of strip, leave for 60 seconds, wash, then read.

TABLE 20–8.—TREATMENT OF DIABETIC KETOACIDOSIS

Fluids
1 L/hr of normal saline. Decrease rate according to patient response (begin 5% Dextrose when glucose is 250–300 mg/dl).
IV insulin
0.33 units/kg as IV bolus, then 10 units/hr, prepared as follows:
100 units regular insulin, diluted with 500 cc of 0.45% NaCl.
Run 100 cc through IV line to allow insulin adsorption to tubing.
This makes a solution of .2 unit/cc. A rate of 50 cc/hr = 10 units/hr.
IM insulin
Can be used as an acceptable alternative to constant infusion, as follows:
Give 20 units of regular insulin as IV bolus, plus 10–15 units IM.
Give 5–10 units IM every hour.
Blood sugar level (with either method) should fall by 60–120 mg/100 cc/hr.
Electrolytes
Na^+: As 0.9% NaCl (1 L/hr).
K^+: Hold if urine output <30 cc/hr; give 40 mEq/L KCl to a total of 100–300 mEq in the 1st 24 hours.

PO_4^-: Follow phosphate levels as glucose falls; if necessary, give 40–60 mEq/L as potassium phosphate instead of KCl if phosphorus is less than 3 mg/dl.

HCO_3^-: Give 80–100 mEq in 100 cc of 0.45% NaCl over 1 hour if arterial ph is 7.1 or less.

Measurements (use flow sheet)

Vital signs, mental status, fluid intake and output every 30 minutes initially, then every 1–2 hours as indicated.

Glucose, sodium, potassium, bicarbonate, and anion gap hourly initially then every 2–4 hours as indicated.

Serum ketones (with Acetest Tabs) every 2–3 hours.

Creatinine, BUN, Ca^{++}, arterial blood gas, phosphorus, osmolality, ECG, chest x-ray, urinalysis and culture, and blood cultures should be obtained initially and repeated only if indicated.

Tubes

Endotracheal if patient is comatose.

Foley only if unable to void or otherwise unable to determine output.

Nasogastric tube if distention, nausea, or vomiting occurs.

CVP should be placed if patient is elderly or debilitated.

TABLE 20–9.—DIABETIC MANAGEMENT OF SURGICAL PATIENTS

Sliding scales based on urines should *not* be used.

If NIDDM (type II) and diet is controlled, follow preop. and postop. blood sugar and treat only if values are above 300 mg/dl.

If NIDDM (type II) and patient is taking an oral agent, D/C on day of surgery and:
Minor surgery: treat only if BS > 300 mg/dl.
Major surgery: Give 15–20 units of NPH on day of surgery plus 5% Dextrose at 100–125 ml/hour. Give additional insulin as required.

If on insulin, begin 5% Dextrose preop. and give one-half usual daily dose as subcutaneous NPH. Run IV at 125–150 cc/hr and give additional regular insulin as indicated by frequent (~q2–3h) evaluation of blood sugar levels.

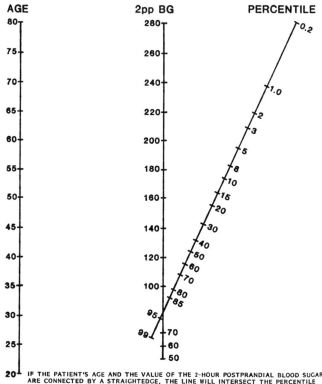

IF THE PATIENT'S AGE AND THE VALUE OF THE 2-HOUR POSTPRANDIAL BLOOD SUGAR ARE CONNECTED BY A STRAIGHTEDGE, THE LINE WILL INTERSECT THE PERCENTILE LINE AT A POINT WHICH INDICATES THE PERCENTAGE OF PATIENTS OF THAT AGE WHO HAVE NORMAL BLOOD VALUES AT THAT LEVEL AND DO NOT HAVE CLINICAL DIABETES.

FIG 20–1.
Nomogram for interpreting 2-hour postprandial blood sugar in relation to patient age. (Adapted from *Patient Care,* June 15, 1974. Darien, Conn, Patient Care Communications.)

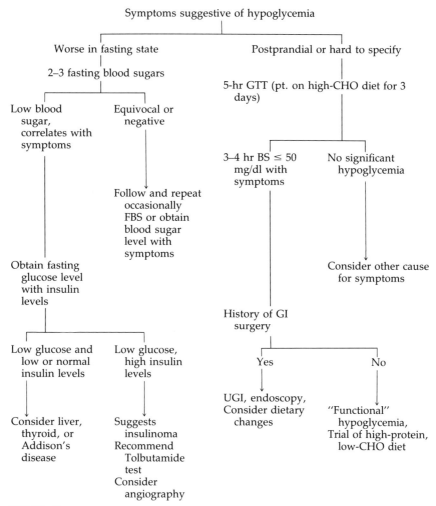

FIG 20–2.
Evaluation of hypoglycemia.

THYROID

TABLE 20–10.—COMMON TESTS OF THYROID FUNCTION

TEST	SUBSTANCE MEASURED	NORMAL VALUES	INDICATION	COMMENT
Serum T$_4$	Total thyroid hormone (99.97% bound)	5–12 ng/dl	Screening for thyroid disease	False pos. usually due to increased TBG (see Table 20–11)
Free T$_4$	Unbound thyroid hormone	2 ng/dl	Confirmation of questionable case	Cumbersome assay, not very precise
T$_3$ uptake	Relative saturation of thyroid-binding proteins	25%–35%	Combined with T$_4$ to give thyroid index	Useful as indirect measure of TBG
Free T$_4$ index (FT$_4$I)	Calculated product of T$_4$ and T$_3$ uptake	1–4 ng/dl	Screening for thyroid disease	Most useful single indicator of thyroid status
Serum T$_3$	Triiodothyronine concentration (bound and unbound)	115–190 ng/dl	Evaluation for "hyperthyroid" state, if thyroid index is normal	Often confused with T3 uptake test; if + Dx. is "T3 toxicosis"
Serum TSH	Total thyroid-stimulating hormone	2–11 μU/ml	Most useful screen for primary hypothyroidism	Use new high-sensitivity test
TRH test	Capacity of pituitary to respond to thyrotropin-releasing hormone	Raises TSH severalfold	Good test to resolve borderline cases	If no rise in TSH Hyperthyroid state exists

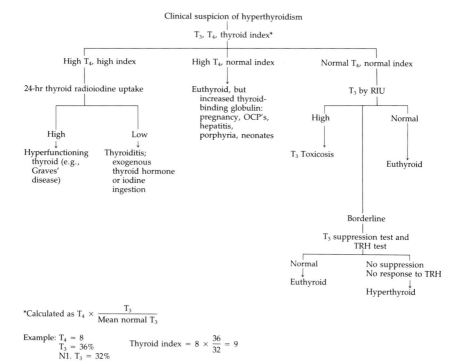

$$\text{*Calculated as } T_4 \times \frac{T_3}{\text{Mean normal } T_3}$$

Example: $T_4 = 8$
$T_3 = 36\%$ Thyroid index $= 8 \times \dfrac{36}{32} = 9$
N1. $T_3 = 32\%$

FIG 20–3.
Evaluation of hyperthyroidism.

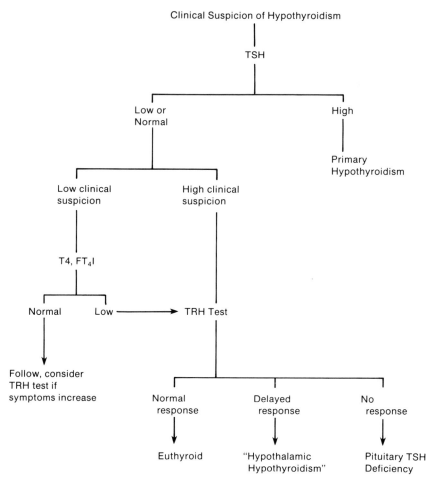

FIG 20–4.
Evaluation of hypothyroidism.

TABLE 20–11.—THYROID-BINDING GLOBULINS

	INCREASED TBG	DECREASED TBG
Causes	Estrogens	Androgens
	Acute hepatitis	Chronic liver disease
	Genetic	Protein loss
	Porphyria	Genetic
	Neonates	
Effect on T_4	Increased	Decreased
Effect on T_3 uptake	Decreased	Increased
Effect on TSH	None	None

TABLE 20–12.—TRH TEST*

The TRH test evaluates the pituitary-thyroid axis. It is a helpful test to resolve previously difficult clinical problems such as:
Borderline hypothyroidism with minimal elevation of TSH
Clinical hypothyroidism with normal TSH
Suspected "hypothalamic hypothyroidism"
Borderline hyperthyroidism

Procedure:
Draw baseline TSH
Give 500 μg of TRH as IV bolus.
Draw TSH at 15-, 30-, 45-, and 60-minute intervals.
Interpretation: Baseline should double, peaking at 30 minutes;
Primary hypothyroid = high baseline and exaggerated response
"Hypothalamic hypothyroid" = delayed peak
Pituitary failure = no response
Hyperthyroid = no rise in TSH

*Adapted from Watts NB, Keffer JH: The thyroid gland, in *Practical Endocrine Diagnosis*. Philadelphia, Lea & Febiger, 1978.

ADRENAL GLAND

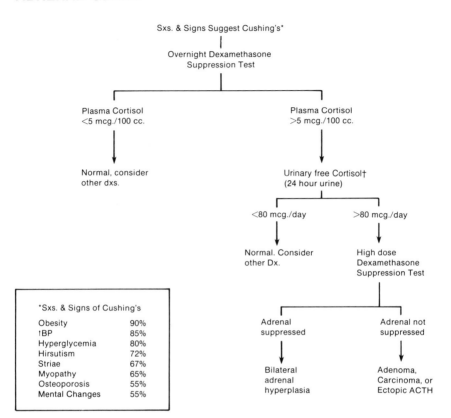

FIG 20–5.
Evaluation of Cushing's syndrome.

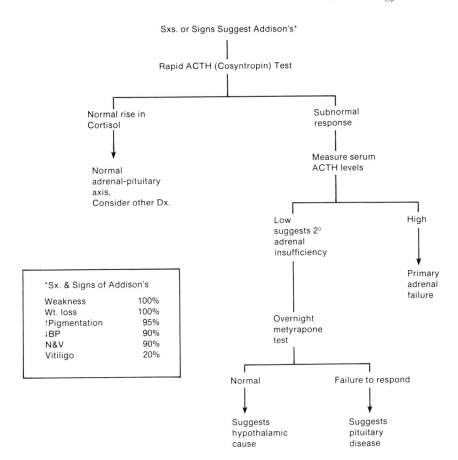

FIG 20–6.
Evaluation of Addison's disease.

TABLE 20–13.—EVALUATION OF ADRENAL FUNCTION

Dexamethasone suppression test:
  Give dexamethasone 1 mg and a sedative at bedtime.
  Draw fasting cortisol next A.M.
  Make sure sleep hasn't been disturbed.
  Failure to suppress cortisol to <5 µg/100 cc suggests Cushing's syndrome.
High-dose dexamethasone suppression test:
  Collect daily 24-hr urines for 4 days for free cortisol and creatinine (first 2 days
    are baseline measurements).
  Measure plasma cortisol at 8 A.M. and 8 P.M. for diurnal variation (optional).
  At 8 A.M. on day 3, start dexamethasone, 2 mg PO q6h for 48 hr.
  Measure plasma cortisol at 8 A.M. on day 5 (concludes test).
  Plasma and urinary cortisol levels are suppressed in presence of bilateral hy-
    perplasia, but not in other conditions.
Rapid ACTH (Cosyntropin) test:
  Measure baseline plasma cortisol.
  Give 250 µg of Cosyntropin (synthetic ACTH) after getting baseline cortisol
    value.
  Obtain cortisol levels at 30 and 60 minutes after injection.
  Normal = rise in cortisol >70 µg/100 cc with a peak response of >18 µg/100
    cc.
Overnight metyrapone test:
  Give 3 gm of metyrapone as a single oral dose at bedtime with food (to delay
    absorption).
  Measure plasma 11-deoxycortisol at 7 A.M. the next day.
  Normal = >7 µg/100 cc rise in 11-deoxycortisol.
Furosemide stimulation test:
  Give Lasix, 60 mg PO in A.M.
  Maintain patient in upright posture for 5 hours.
  Draw blood into iced tube for plasma renin.
  Renovascular hypertensives = 5× normal values. Normal value on "normal"
    sodium diet in supine position = 1.6 ng/ml/hr. (Suppressed values = ½
    normal.)

TABLE 20–14.—PERIOPERATIVE STEROID REPLACEMENT*

	INTRAVENOUS HYDROCORTISONE	INTRAMUSCULAR HYDROCORTISONE	ORAL HYDROCORTISONE
Operation day	300 mg plus	50 mg preop 50 mg postop	—
Postoperative day			
1	200 mg plus	50 mg q12h	—
2	150 mg plus	50 mg q12h	—
3	100 mg plus	50 mg q12h	—
4	—	50 mg q12h plus	25 mg q6h
5	—	25 mg q12h plus	25 mg q6h[†]
6	—	25 mg daily	
7	—	—	25 mg q6h
8–10	—	—	25 mg q8h
11–20	—	—	25 mg q12h
21–	—	—	20 mg 8 A.M. 10 mg 4 P.M.

*Adapted from Tuck M: Adrenal disease, in Hershman JM (ed): *Management of Endocrine Disorders.* Philadelphia, Lea & Febiger, 1980.

[†]Add fludrocortisone, 0.05–0.2 mg orally daily. Adjust dose depending on blood pressure, body weight, and serum electrolytes.

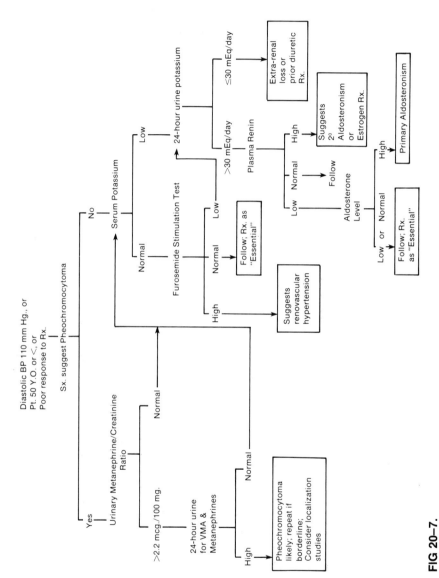

FIG 20–7.
Evaluation of secondary and "endocrine" hypertension.

Appendices

Barry L. Carter, Pharm. D.

TABLE A–1.—Temperature
Conversion, Fahrenheit/
Centigrade*

°F	°C	°F	°C
97.0	36.1	102.0	38.9
97.5	36.4	102.2	39.0
98.0	36.7	102.4	39.1
98.2	36.8	102.6	39.2
98.4	36.9	102.8	39.3
98.6	37.0	103.0	39.4
98.8	37.1	103.2	39.6
99.0	37.2	103.4	39.7
99.2	37.3	103.6	39.8
99.4	37.4	103.8	39.9
99.6	37.6	104.0	40.0
99.8	37.7	104.2	40.1
100.0	37.8	104.4	40.2
100.2	37.9	104.6	40.3
100.4	38.0	104.8	40.4
100.6	38.1	105.0	40.6
100.8	38.2		
101.0	38.3		
101.2	38.4		
101.4	38.6		
101.6	38.7		
101.8	38.8		

*Fahrenheit to Centigrade: $5(°F - 32)/9 = °C$. Centigrade to Fahrenheit: $(°C × 9)/5 + 32 = °F$.

TABLE A–2.—Conversion Factors for Length and Weight

Length: Inches to centimeters: inches × 2.54.
Weight: Calculation of lean body weight (LBW) in lb:
      Females: LBW = 100 lb + 5 lb for each inch over 5 feet.
      Males: LBW = 110 lb + 6 lb for each inch over 5 feet.

TABLE A–3.—Equivalent Fat Content as a Percentage of Body Weight for the Sum of Four Skin Folds (Biceps, Triceps, Subscapular, Suprailiac)*

SUM OF SKIN FOLDS (mm)	MALES (AGE, YR)				FEMALES (AGE, YR)			
	17–29	30–39	40–49	50+	16–29	30–39	40–49	50+
15	4.8	. . .	. . .	. . .	10.5	. . .	. . .	. . .
20	8.1	12.2	12.2	12.6	14.1	17.0	19.8	21.4
25	10.5	14.2	15.0	15.6	16.8	19.4	22.2	24.0
30	12.9	16.2	17.7	18.6	19.5	21.8	24.5	26.6
35	14.7	17.7	19.6	20.8	21.5	23.7	26.4	28.5
40	16.4	19.2	21.4	22.9	23.4	25.5	28.2	30.3
45	17.7	20.4	23.0	24.7	25.0	26.9	29.6	31.9
50	19.0	21.5	24.6	26.5	26.5	28.2	31.0	33.4
55	20.1	22.5	25.9	27.9	27.8	29.4	32.1	34.6
60	21.2	23.5	27.1	29.2	29.1	30.6	33.2	35.7
65	22.2	24.3	28.2	30.4	30.2	31.6	34.1	36.7
70	23.1	25.1	29.3	31.6	31.2	32.5	35.0	37.7
75	24.0	25.9	30.3	32.7	32.2	33.4	35.9	38.7
80	24.8	26.6	31.2	33.8	33.1	34.3	36.7	39.6
85	25.5	27.2	32.1	34.8	34.0	35.1	37.5	40.4
90	26.2	27.8	33.0	35.8	34.8	35.8	38.3	41.2
95	26.9	28.4	33.7	36.6	35.6	36.5	39.0	41.9
100	27.6	29.0	34.4	37.4	36.4	37.2	39.7	42.6
105	28.2	29.6	35.1	38.2	37.1	37.9	40.4	43.3
110	28.8	30.1	35.8	39.0	37.8	38.6	41.0	43.9
115	29.4	30.6	36.4	39.7	38.4	39.1	41.5	44.5
120	30.0	31.1	37.0	40.4	39.0	39.6	42.0	45.1
125	30.5	31.5	37.6	41.1	39.6	40.1	42.5	45.7
130	31.0	31.9	38.2	41.8	40.2	40.6	43.0	46.2
135	31.5	32.3	38.7	42.4	40.8	41.1	43.5	46.7
140	32.0	32.7	39.2	43.0	41.3	41.6	44.0	47.2
145	32.5	33.1	39.7	43.6	41.8	42.1	44.5	47.7
150	32.9	33.5	40.2	44.1	42.3	42.6	45.0	48.2
155	33.3	33.9	40.7	44.6	42.8	43.1	45.4	48.7
160	33.7	34.3	41.2	45.1	43.3	43.6	45.8	49.2
165	34.1	34.6	41.6	45.6	43.7	44.0	46.2	49.6
170	34.5	34.8	42.0	46.1	44.1	44.4	46.6	50.0
175	34.9	. . .	. . .	. . .	. . .	44.8	47.0	50.4
180	35.3	. . .	. . .	. . .	. . .	45.2	47.4	50.8
185	35.6	. . .	. . .	. . .	. . .	45.6	47.8	51.2
190	35.9	. . .	. . .	. . .	. . .	45.9	48.2	51.6
195	. . .	. . .	. . .	. . .	. . .	46.2	48.5	52.0
200	. . .	. . .	. . .	. . .	. . .	46.5	48.8	52.4
205	. . .	. . .	. . .	. . .	. . .	. . .	49.1	52.7
210	. . .	. . .	. . .	. . .	. . .	. . .	49.4	53.0

*Adapted from Durnin JVGA, Womersley J: *Br J Nutr* 1974; 32:77–97.

Men 25-59 Years

Height (feet/ inches)	Small Frame (pounds)*	Medium Frame (pounds)*	Large Frame (pounds)*
5' 2''	128-134	131-141	138-150
5' 3''	130-136	133-143	140-153
5' 4''	132-138	135-145	142-156
5' 5''	134-140	137-148	144-160
5' 6''	136-142	139-151	146-164
5' 7''	138-145	142-154	149-168
5' 8''	140-148	145-157	152-172
5' 9''	142-151	148-160	155-176
5'10''	144-154	151-163	158-180
5'11''	146-157	154-166	161-184
6' 0''	149-160	157-170	164-188
6' 1''	152-164	160-174	168-192
6' 2''	155-168	164-178	172-197
6' 3''	158-172	167-182	176-202
6' 4''	162-176	171-187	181-207

*in indoor clothing weighing 5 lbs, shoes with 1'' heels

Women 25-59 Years

Height (feet/ inches)	Small Frame (pounds)*	Medium Frame (pounds)*	Large Frame (pounds)*
4'10''	102-111	109-121	118-131
4'11''	103-113	111-123	120-134
5' 0''	104-115	113-126	122-137
5' 1''	106-118	115-129	125-140
5' 2''	108-121	118-132	128-143
5' 3''	111-124	121-135	131-147
5' 4''	114-127	124-138	134-151
5' 5''	117-130	127-141	137-155
5' 6''	120-133	130-144	140-159
5' 7''	123-136	133-147	143-163
5' 8''	126-139	136-150	146-167
5' 9''	129-142	139-153	149-170
5'10''	132-145	142-156	152-173
5'11''	135-148	145-159	155-176
6' 0''	138-151	148-162	158-179

*in indoor clothing weighing 3 lbs, shoes with 1'' heels

FIG A–1.

Height-weight correlations for adults.

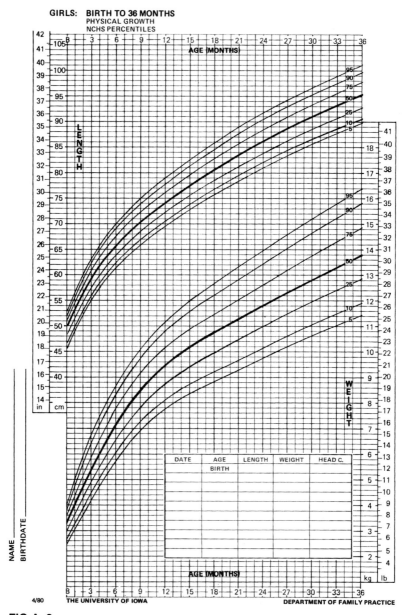

FIG A–2.
Length, weight, and age correlations for girls aged 0–36 months.

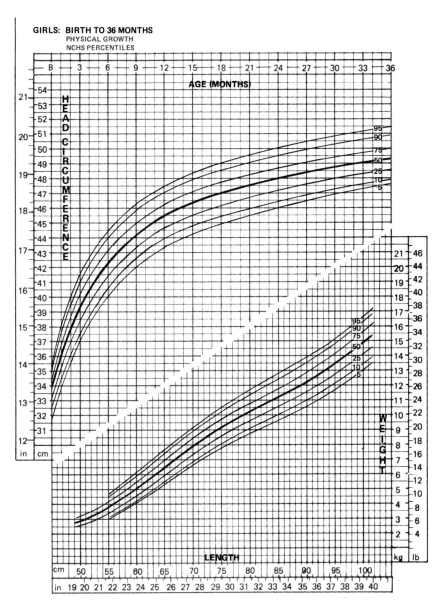

FIG A–3.
Length, weight, age, and head circumference correlations for girls aged 0–36 months.

GIRLS: 2 TO 18 YEARS
PHYSICAL GROWTH
NCHS PERCENTILES

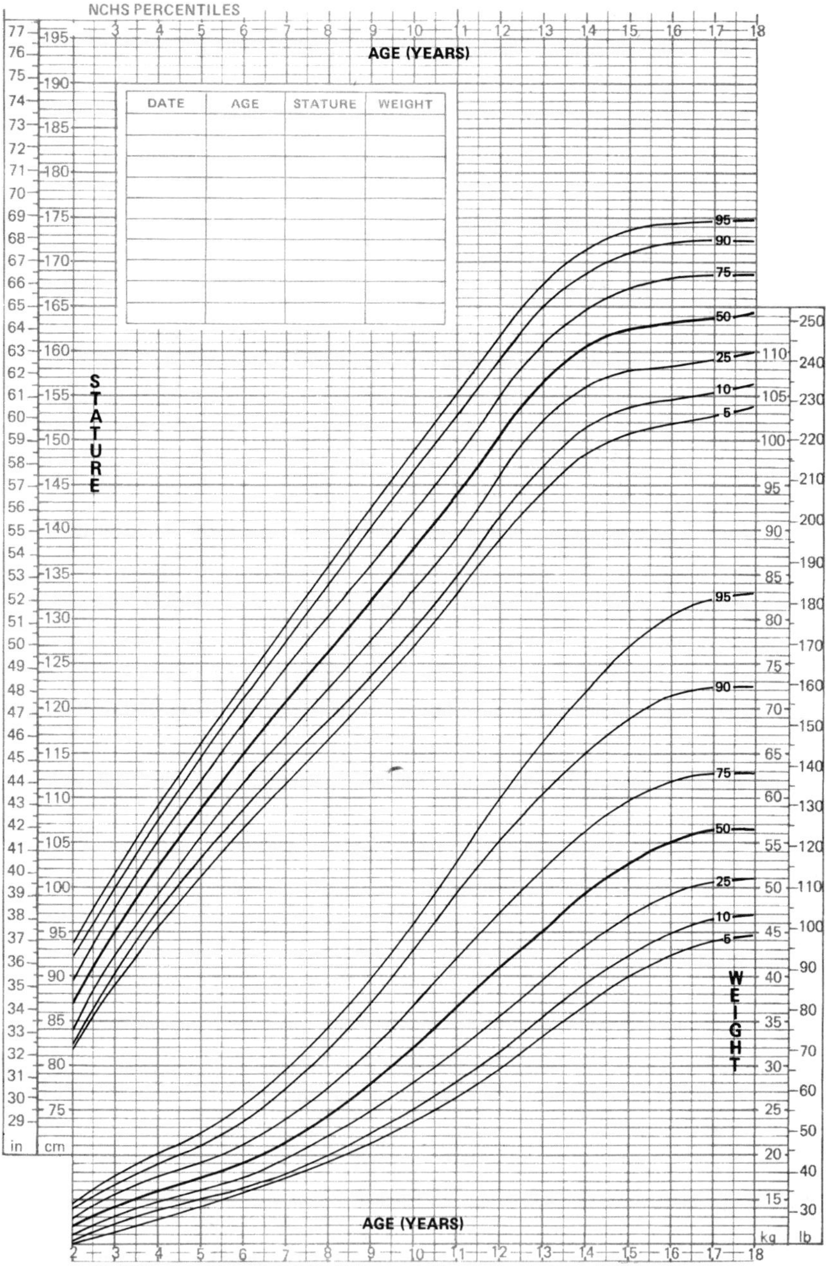

FIG A–4.
Growth profile for girls aged 2–18 years.

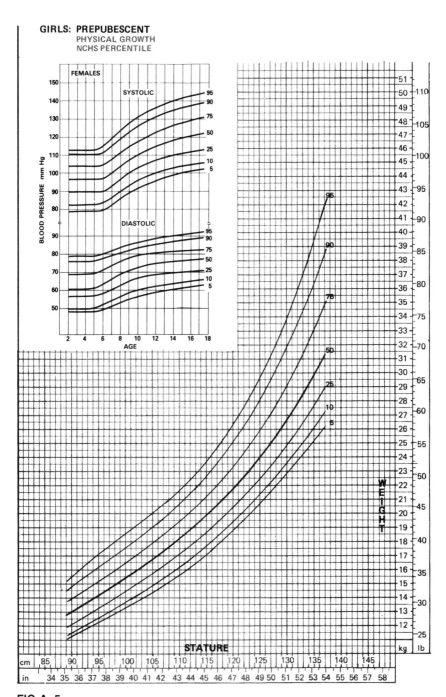

FIG A-5.
Prepubescent growth profiles for girls.

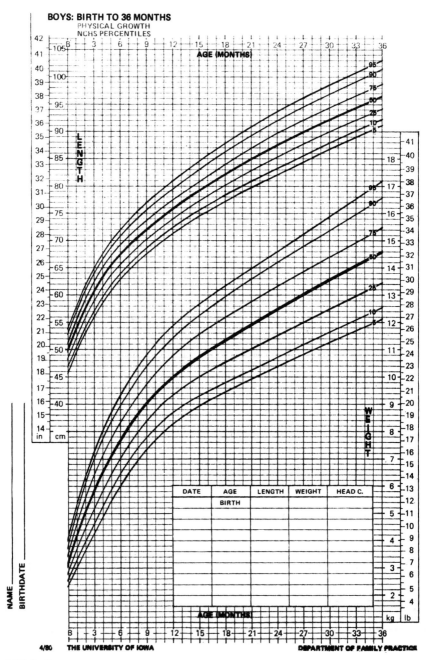

FIG A–6.
Length, weight, and age correlations for boys aged 0–36 months.

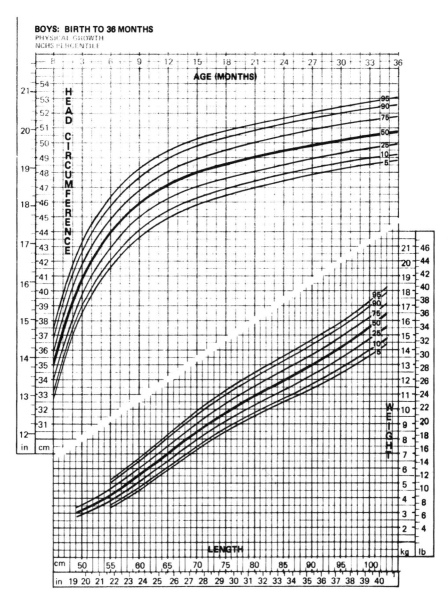

FIG A–7.
Length, weight, age, and head circumference correlations for boys aged 0–36 months.

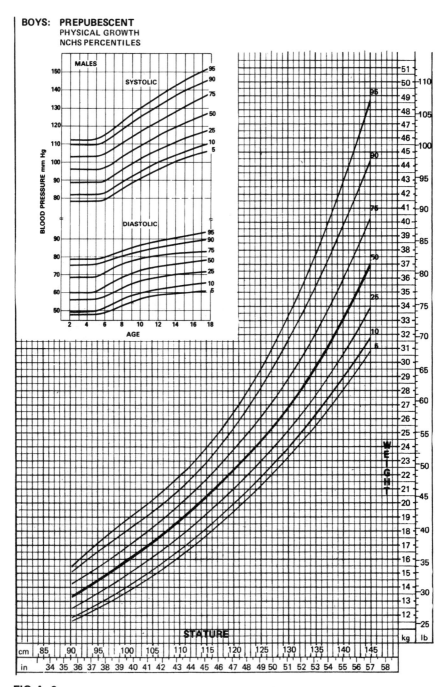

FIG A–8.
Prepubescent growth profiles for boys.

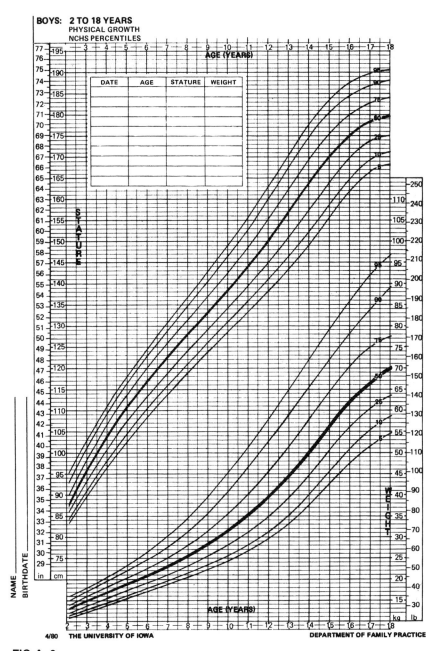

FIG A–9.
Growth profiles for boys aged 2–18 years.

TABLE A–4.—FLUID AND ELECTROLYTE MAINTENANCE THERAPY*

| | LOSSES | | | | REQUIREMENTS | |
	Urine (ml)	Stool (ml)	Insensible (ml)	Total (ml)	ml/person	ml/kg
Infant (2–10 kg)	200–500	25–40	75–300 (1.3 ml/kg/hr)	300–840	330–1,000	100–165
Child (10–40 kg)	500–800	40–100	300–600	840–1,500	1,000–1,800	45–100
Adolescent or adult (60 kg)	800–1,000	100	600–1,000 (0.5 ml/kg/hr)	1,500–2,100	1,800–2,500	30–45

*Adapted from Trunkey D: Fluid and electrolyte therapy, in Schrock TR (ed): *Handbook of Surgery*, ed 15. Greenbrae, Calif, Jones Medical Publication, 1982, p 92.
Values are for a patient in a normal state of hydration. Daily water losses and water requirements are those for healthy persons not working or sweating.

TABLE A–5.—VOLUME AND COMPOSITION OF GASTROINTESTINAL
SECRETIONS AND SWEAT*

FLUID	AVG. VOLUME (ml/24 hr)	ELECTROLYTE CONCENTRATIONS (mEq/L)			
		Na$^+$	K$^+$	Cl$^-$	HCO$_3^-$
Blood plasma		135–150	3.6–5.5	100–105	24.6–28.8
Gastric juice	2,500	31–90	4.3–12	52–124	0
Bile	700–1,000	134–156	3.9–6.3	83–110	38
Pancreatic juice	>1,000	113–153	2.6–7.4	54–95	110
Small bowel (Miller-Abbott suction)	3,000	72–120	3.5–6.8	69–127	30
Ileostomy: Recent	100–4,000	112–142	4.5–14	93–122	30
Adapted	100–500	50	3	20	15–30
Cecostomy	100–3,000	48–116	11.1–28.3	35–70	15
Feces	100	<10	<10	<15	<15
Sweat	500–4,000	30–70	0–5	30–70	0

*Adapted from Trunkey D: Fluid and electrolyte therapy, in Schrock TR (ed): *Handbook of Surgery,* ed 15. Greenbrae, Calif, Jones Medical Publisher, 1982, p 94.

TABLE A–6.—ACID-BASE BALANCE

Normal values: CO$_2$ 24–30 mM/L
      Arterial pH   7.38–7.42
      Arterial P$_{CO_2}$ 35–45 mm Hg
      Serum chloride   96–106 mEq/L
      Arterial P$_{O_2}$ 80–90 mm Hg
Anion gap = (serum Na$^+$ + serum K$^+$) − (serum Cl$^-$ + serum HCO$_3^-$)
    Normal anion gap = 12–14 mEq/L
Bicarbonate deficit − Bicarbonate dose (mEq) = 0.5 × Weight (kg) × Desired
   increase in serum HCO$_3^-$ (mEq/L)
   or
   (25 − observed bicarbonate) × 0.5 (weight in kg) = total deficit

TABLE A–7.—Common Causes of Hyperchloremic
Metabolic Acidosis*

Excess acid load
  Hyperalimentation
  Acidifying agents (ammonium chloride, arginine HCl, lysine HCl)
  Chloride exchange resin-cholestyramine
Losses of alkaline fluids
  Diarrhea
  Ileostomy
  Colostomy
  Pancreatic fistula
Decreased renal acid excretion
  Renal tubular acidosis
  Acetazolamide (Diamox®)
  Uremia
  Hypoaldosteronism

  *Associated with a normal anion gap.

TABLE A–8.—Common Causes of Acid-Base Disorders

ACIDOSIS	ALKALOSIS
Metabolic	
Renal failure	Nasogastric suction
Diabetic ketoacidosis	Vomiting
Alcoholic ketoacidosis	Diuretics
Starvation ketosis	Glucocorticosteroids
Lactic acidosis	Cushing's disease
Uremic acidosis	Chloride restriction
Drugs (salicylates, ethylene glycol,	Alkali therapy
methanol, paraldehyde)	Antacid use
Respiratory	
CNS depression	Hyperventilation
Obstructive lung disease	Sepsis
Mechanical hypoventilation	Salicylate intoxication
Status asthmaticus	Mechanical overventilation
Pneumothorax	Pneumonia
Abdominal distention	High altitude

TABLE A–9.—CREATININE CLEARANCE ESTIMATES*†

Cockroft-Gault equation:

$$CrCl = \frac{(140 - Age) \times Weight\ (kg)}{72 \times S_{cr}}$$

Multiply by 0.85 for females.

Weight: Lean weight in kg
CrCl: Creatinine clearance
S_{cr}: Serum creatinine

NOTE: A 75-year-old woman (60 kg/lean) who has a "normal" serum creatinine value of 1.0 may not have "normal" renal function:

$$\frac{(140 - 75) \times 60\ kg}{72(1.0)} \times 0.85 = 46\ cc/min$$

*Adapted from Cockroft DW, Gault MH: 16:31–41. 1976; *Nephron.*
†In young healthy persons with stable renal function. May be less accurate in the elderly.

TABLE A–10.—SODIUM AND CALORIE CONTENT OF FOODS*

FOOD	QUANTITY	mg	mEq	kcal
Snacks				
Salted peanuts	1 tbsp	69	3	95
Unsalted peanuts	1 tbsp	trace	. . .	95
Green olives	2 olives	312	13.6	15
Black olives	2 olives	150	6.5	35
Potato chips	5 chips	34	1.5	60
Pretzels (ring)	1	87	3.8	25
Dairy Products				
Butter, salted	1 pat	99	4.3	45
Butter, unsalted	1 pat	1	. . .	45
American cheese	1 oz	318	13.8	110
Cottage cheese	3 oz	229	10.0	90
Egg	1 large	66	2.9	80
Milk (whole)	8 oz	122	5.3	160
Margarine (salted)	1 pat	99	4.3	45
Vegetables				
Green beans	1 cup			
Fresh		5	0.2	40
Canned		295	12.8	40
Beets	½ cup			
Fresh		36	1.6	55
Canned		197	8.6	55
Broccoli, fresh	⅔ cup	10	0.4	25
Cabbage, raw	1 cup	20	0.9	17
Carrots				
Raw	1 large	47	2.0	40
Canned	⅔ cup	236	10.3	30

Continued.

TABLE A–10.—Continued

FOOD	QUANTITY	mg	mEq	kcal
Celery	1 outer stalk	63	2.7	7
Corn				
Fresh	1 ear	trace	. . .	70
Canned	½ cup	196	8.5	70
Peas				
Fresh	⅔ cup	1	. . .	75
Canned	¾ cup	236	10.3	90
Frozen	3½ oz	115	5.0	. . .
Potatoes, boiled	1 medium	3	. . .	65
Sauerkraut	⅔ cup	747	32.5	20
Tomatoes				
Raw	1 medium	4	. . .	27
Canned	½ cup	130	5.7	25
Meats				
Bacon	1 strip	71	3.1	45
Hamburger	¼ lb	41	1.8	325
Chicken (broiler)	3½ oz	78	3.4	180
Frankfurter (beef)	⅛ lb	550	23.9	130
Ham, cured	¼ lb	518	22.5	325
Pork chop	6 oz	52	2.3	600
Sausage	3½ oz	740	32.2	325
Salmon canned (water)	3½ oz	387	16.8	130
Sardines canned (oil)	3½ oz	510	22.2	200
Tuna canned (oil)	3½ oz	800	34.8	180
Tuna canned (water)	3½ oz	41	1.8	90
Other				
Bread, white	1 slice	117	5.1	60
Corn flakes	1 cup	165	7.2	110
Noodles, Rice		3	. . .	. . .
Fruit juices	6–8 oz	2–4	. . .	. . .
Fresh fruits	3½ oz	1–5	. . .	. . .

*Sodium restrictions: 2 gm of salt (NaCl) = 800 mg of sodium = 34 mEq Na^+.

TABLE A–11.—Potassium Content of Foods

FOOD	QUANTITY	mg	mEq	kcal
Meats				
Hamburger	3 oz	290	7.4	245
Beef round	3 oz	340	8.7	245
Chicken (fryer)	4 oz	710	18.2	180
Turkey	4 oz	350	9.0	180
Fruits, vegetables				
Banana	1 medium	628	16.1	100
Brussel sprouts	1 cup	300	7.7	56
Cauliflower raw	1¼ cup	500	12.8	30
Dates	1 cup	1,390	35.6	
Fruit cocktail, canned (syrup)	8 oz	410	10.5	170
Grapefruit	1 cup	380	9.7	40
Peach	1 medium	180	4.6	40
Raisins	2 tbsp	144	3.7	60
Spinach	1 cup	600	15.4	40
Sweet corn	1 cup	230	5.9	150
Tomato	1 medium	340	8.7	27
Watermelon	½ slice of ¾ in. × 10 in.	380	9.7	100
Wheat germ	100 gm	737	18.9	
Beverages (8 oz)				
Apricot juice		250	9.5	
Coffee, instant	2 gm	238	6.1	. . .
Grapefruit juice, canned		405	10.4	78
Milk, whole (high sodium)		356	9.1	160
Milk, nonfat (high sodium)		278	7.1	90
Orange juice, fresh		496	12.1	120
Prune juice, canned		563	14.4	184
Tea		66	1.7	. . .
Tomato juice, canned (high sodium)		544	14.0	48

TABLE A–12.—Salt Substitutes*

VARIETY	mg	mEq
Adolph's salt substitute, 1 packet	430	11.0
Co-salt, 1 gm	450	11.5
Diasal, 1 gm	442	11.3
Nu-salt, 1 gm	404	10.4
Saltfree, 1 gm	548	14.1
Morton salt substitute, 1 gm	493	12.6
Morton Lite salt, 1 gm†	260	6.6

*Adapted from Knoben JE, et al: Miscellaneous data, in *Handbook of Clinical Drug Data,* ed 5. Hamilton, Ill, Drug Intelligence Publication, 1983, p 49.
†Morton light salt is high in sodium (50% sodium chloride). One tablespoon = approximately 5 gm.

TABLE A–13.—NORMAL HEMATOLOGY VALUES*

Hematology (adults)		
Carboxyhemoglobin		0.05 of total
Erythrocytes		
Males		$4.6-6.2 \times 10^{12}/L$
Females		$4.2-5.4 \times 10^{12}/L$
Children (depends on age)		$4.5-5.1 \times 10^{12}/L$
Leukocytes, total		$4.5-11.0 \times 10^{9}/L$
Band neutrophils	3%–5%	150–400/cu mm
Segmented neutrophils	54%–62%	3,000–5,800/cu mm
Lymphocytes	25%–33%	1,500–3,000/cu mm
Monocytes	3%–7%	300–500/cu mm
Eosinophils	1%–3%	50–250/cu mm
Basophils	0–0.75%	15–50/cu mm
Platelets		150,000–350,000/cu mm
Reticulocytes		25,000–75,000/cu mm
		(0.5%–1.5% of erythrocytes)
MCH		27–31 pg
MCV		$80-96 \ \mu^3$
MCHC		32%–36%
Hematocrit		
Males		40–54 ml/dl
Females		37–47 ml/dl
Hemoglobin		
Males		14–18 gm/dl
Females		12–16 gm/dl
Hemoglobin, fetal		<1% of total
Hemoglobin, A1C		3%–5% of total
Methemoglobin		0–130 mg/dl
Sedimentation rate (Wintrobe)		
Males		0–5 mm/hr
Females		0–15 mm/hr
Sedimentation rate (Westergren)		
Males		0–15 mm/hr
Females		0–20 mm/hr

Bone marrow differential
Myeloblasts	0.3%–5.0%
Promyelocytes	1.0%–8.0%
Myelocytes	
Neutrophilic	5.0%–19.0%
Eosinophilic	0.5%–3.0%
Basophilic	0–0.5%
Metamyelocytes	13.0%–32.0%
Polymorphonuclear neutrophils	7.0%–30.0%
Polymorphonuclear eosinophils	0.5%–4.0%
Polymorphonuclear basophils	0–0.7%
Lymphocytes	3.0%–17.0%
Plasma Cells	0.0–2.0%
Monocytes	0.5%–5.0%
Reticulum cells	0.1%–2.0%
Megakaryocytes	0.3%–3.0%
Pronormoblasts	1.0%–8.0%
Normoblasts	7.0%–32.0%

*Adapted from Conn RB: Laboratory reference values of clinical importance, in Rakel RE (ed): *Current Therapy.* Philadelphia, WB Saunders Co, 1988, pp 1043–1044.

TABLE A–14.—Normal Hematology Values for Children*

AGE	HEMOGLOBIN (gm/dl)			RBC COUNT (millions/mm²)	HEMATOCRIT (PACKED RBC VOLUME/dl) (%)	MEAN CORPUSCULAR VOLUME (MCV) (μm^3)	MEAN CORPUSCULAR HEMOGLOBIN (MCH) (pg)	MEAN CORPUSCULAR HEMOGLOBIN CONCENTRATION (MCHC) (%)
	TERM BABIES	PREMATURE BABIES (1,200–2,400 gm)	SMALL PREMATURE BABIES (<1,200 gm)					
Birth (cord values)	13.6–19.6	17.0	15.6	5.4	56.6	106	38	38
1 day	21.2			5.6	56.1	106	38	38
1 wk	19.6	15.3	14.8	5.3	52.7	101	37	37
2 wk	18.0			5.1	49.6	96	35	36
3 wk	16.6	13.2	12.0	4.9	46.6	93	34	36
4 wk	15.6	9.6	8.2	4.7	44.6	91	33	35
2 mo.	13.3			4.5	38.9	85	30	34
3 mo.	12.5	9.8	8.1	4.5	38.0	84	29	34
4 mo.	12.4	9.8	9.0	4.5	36.5	79	27	34
6 mo.	12.3			4.6	36.2	78	27	34
8 mo.	12.1			4.6	35.8	77	26	34
10 mo.	11.9			4.6	35.5	77	26	34
1 yr	11.6	11.0	11.0	4.6	35.2	77	25	33
2 yr	11.7			4.7	35.5	78	25	33
4 yr	12.6			4.7	37.1	80	27	34
6 yr	12.7			4.7	37.9	80	27	33
8 yr	12.9			4.7	38.9	80	27	33
10–12 yr	13.0			4.8	39.0	80	27	33
Adult men	16.0			5.4	47.0	87	29	33
Adult women	14.0			4.8	42.0	87	29	34

*From Lanzkowsky P, Hoekelman RA, Blatman S, et al (eds): *Primary Pediatric Care.* St Louis, CV Mosby Co, 1987, p 860. Reproduced by permission.

TABLE A–15.—Normal Laboratory Values: Vitamins

VITAMIN	AGE	VALUE
Folates (serum)	Newborn	7–32 ng/ml
	Thereafter	1.8–9.0 ng/ml
Thiamin (whole blood)		1.6–4.0 µg/dl
Vitamin A (serum)	Newborn	35–75 µg/dl
	Child	30–80 µg/dl
	Thereafter	30–65 µg/dl
Vitamin B2 (riboflavin) (urine, per gm creatinine)	Adult	80–269 µg/gm
	Pregnancy	90–120 µg/gm
Vitamin B12 (serum)	Newborn	175–800 pg/ml
	Thereafter	100–700 pg/ml
Vitamin C (plasma)		0.6–2.0 mg/dl
Vitamin D3 (25-hydroxy)	Summer	15–80 ng/ml
	Winter	14–42 ng/ml
Vitamin D3 (1,25-dihydroxy)		25–45 pg/ml
Vitamin E (tocopherols)		5–20 µg/ml

TABLE A–16.—Normal Blood and Serum Chemistries[*][†]

	Age	Normal Value	
Ammonia nitrogen (whole blood)	Jaundiced infant	100–200 µg/dl	
	Newborn	90–150 µg/dl	
	Child	40–80 µg/dl	
	Adult	15–45 µg/dl	
Amylase (serum)	All	25–125 units/L	
(urine, 24 hr)		1–17 units/hr	
α_1-Antitrypsin (serum)	Newborn	145–270 mg/dl	
	Adult	78–200 mg/dl	
Aspartate aminotransferase (AST, SGOT) (serum)	Infant	15–60 units/L	
	Adult	8–20 units/L	
Base excess (whole blood)	Newborn	−10 to −2 mmol/L	
	Infant	−7 to −1 mmol/L	
	Child	−4 to +2 mmol/L	
	Adult	−2 to +3 mmol/L	
Bicarbonate (serum)			
Arterial		21–28 mmol/L	
Venous		22–29 mmol/L	
Bilirubin, total (serum)		Premature (mg/dl)	Full-term (mg/dl)
	Cord	<2	<2
	0–1 day	<8	<6
	1–2 days	<12	<8
	2–5 days	<16	<12
	Thereafter	<2	0.2–1.0

Continued.

TABLE A–16.—Continued

	Age	Normal Value
Bilirubin, direct (conjugated)		0–0.2 mg/dl
Bilirubin, indirect (unconjugated)		0.2–0.7
Calcium, ionized (serum)	Cord	5.2–5.8 mg/dl
	Newborn	4.3–5.1 mg/dl
	Adults	4.48–4.92 mg/dl
Calcium, total (serum) (varies with protein concentration)	Child	8.8–10.8 mg/dl
	Adult	8.4–10.2 mg/dl
Carbon dioxide, partial pressure, PCO_2 (whole blood)	Infant	27–41 mm Hg
	Adult M	35–48 mm Hg
	Adult F	32–45 mm Hg
Carbon dioxide (serum) (total CO_2)	Cord	14–22 mmol/L
	Premature	14–27 mmol/L
	Newborn	13–22 mmol/L
	Child	20–28 mmol/L
	Adult	23–29 mmol/L
Carbon monoxide (whole blood)		
	Nonsmokers	<2%
	Smokers	<10%
	Symptoms	>20%
	Lethal	>50%
Catecholamines (24 hr, urine)		
Norepinephrine	1–4 yr	0–29 μg/day
	4–10 yr	8–65 μg/day
	Adult	0–100 μg/day
Epinephrine	1–4 yr	0–6 μg/day
	4–10 yr	0–10 μg/day
	Adult	0–15 μg/day
Catecholamines, free (plasma)		
Norepinephrine		104–548 pg/ml
Epinephrine		88 pg/ml
Ceruloplasmin (serum)	Newborn	1–30 mg/dl
	6–12 mo.	15–50 mg/dl
	1–12 yr	30–65 mg/dl
	Adult	15–60 mg/dl

Chloride (serum)		98–106 mmol/L
(urine)	Infant	2–10 mmol/day
	Child	15–40 mmol/day
	Adult	110–250 mmol/day
(sweat)	Normal	0–35 mmol/L
	Marginal	30–60 mmol/L
	Cystic fibrosis	60–200 mmol/L
Cholesterol, total (serum)	Cord	45–100 mg/dl
	Newborn	53–135 mg/dl
	Infant	70–175 mg/dl
	Child	120–200 mg/dl
	Adolescent	120–200 mg/dl
	Adult (desirable)	140–200 mg/dl
Cholinesterase (serum)		0.5–1.3 pH units
(erythrocytes)		0.5–1.0 pH units
Copper (serum)	Newborn	20–70 μg/dl
	6 yr	90–190 μg/dl
	12 yr	80–160 μg/dl
	Adult M	70–140 μg/dl
	Adult F	80–155 μg/dl
(urine)		15–30 μg/dl
Cortisol (plasma)	8 A.M.	5–23 μg/dl
	4 P.M.	3–15 μg/dl
Creatine kinase (CPK)	Newborn	10–200 μ/L
(serum)	Adult M	12–80 μ/L
	Adult F	10–55 μ/L
	>70 yr M	22–90 μ/L
	>70 F	16–80 μ/L
Isoenzymes serum	(MB fraction)	<4%–6% of total
Creatinine (serum)	Cord	0.6–1.2 mg/dl
	Child	0.3–0.7 mg/dl
	Adult M	0.6–1.2 mg/dl
	Adult F	0.5–1.1 mg/dl
Creatinine clearance	Newborn	40–65 ml/min/1.73 m^2
(urine)	Child M	90–150
	Child F	95–125
	Adult M	90–130
	Adult F	80–120
	Normal pregnancy	Up to 200
Estradiol (serum)	Adult M	8–36 pg/ml
	F: follicular	10–90 pg/ml
	midcycle	100–500 pg/ml
	luteal	50–240 pg/ml
	postmenopausal	10–30 pg/ml

Continued.

TABLE A–16.—Continued

	Age	Normal Value	
Estriol (E3) (serum)	Gestation (wk)	Free (µg/L)	Total (ng/ml)
	25	3.5–10.0	30–170
	28	4.0–12.5	40–220
	30	4.5–14.0	40–220
	32	5.0–16.0	40–220
	34	5.5–18.5	60–280
	36	7.0–25.0	60–280
	37	8.0–28.0	80–350
	38	9.0–32.0	80–350
	39	10.0–34.0	80–350
	40–41	10.5–25.0	80–350
(urine, 24 hr)	30		6–18 mg/day
	35		9–28
	40		13–42

Decrease of >40% of previous value suggests fetus at risk

Estrogens, total (serum)	Adult M	40–115 pg/ml
	F: cycle	
	Day 1–10	61–394 pg/ml
	Day 11–20	122–437 pg/ml
	Day 21–30	156–350 pg/ml
	Prepubertal or postmenopausal	<40 pg/ml
Estrogen receptor assay (0.5–1 gm tissue)	Negative	<3.0 fmol/mg
	Borderline	3–10 fmol/mg
	Positive	>10.0 fmol/mg
Fatty acids, total (serum)		190–420 mg/dl
Ferritin (serum)	Newborn	25–200 ng/ml
	1 mo.	200–600 ng/ml
	2–5 mo.	50–200 ng/ml
	6 mo.–15 yr	7–140 ng/ml
	Adult M	15–200 ng/ml
	Adult F	12–150 ng/ml
Follicle stimulating hormone (FSH) (serum)	M, adult:	4–25 IU/L
	F, premenopause	4–30 IU/L
	Midcycle peak	10–90 IU/L
	Pregnancy	Low
	Postmenopause	40–250 IU/L

(urine)	<1 yr, F	<1.4 IU/day
	1–8 yr, M	<4.5 IU/day
	1–8 yr, F	<4.0 IU/day
	9–10 yr, M	1–5 IU/day
	9–10 yr, F	1–4 IU/day
	11–12 yr, M	1.5–5 IU/day
	11–12 yr, F	1–8 IU/day
	13–14 yr, M	2–12 IU/day
	13–14 yr, F	1–10 IU/day
	Adult M	4–18 IU/day
	Adult F	3–12 IU/day
	Higher in males, >60 yr	
Free thyroxine index	1–3 days	9.3–26.6
(FT$_4$I) (serum)	1–4 wk	7.6–20.8
	1–4 mo.	7.4–17.9
	4–12 mo.	6.1–14.5
	1–6 yr	5.7–13.3
	>6 yr	5.5–10.0
γ-Glutamyl-transferase	M	8–37 μ/L
(GGT) (serum)	F	6–24 μ/L
Gastrin (serum)		0–100 pg/ml
Glucose (serum)	Cord	45–96 ng/dl
	Neonate	30–60 ng/dl
	>1 day	50–80 ng/dl
	Child	60–100 ng/dl
	Adult	70–105 ng/dl
	>60 yr	80–115 ng/dl
Glucose tolerance test, oral (serum)	Adults	Normal (mg/dl)
	Fasting	70–105
	60 min	<200
	90 min	<200
	120 min	<140
Growth hormone (serum or plasma)	Cord	10–50 ng/ml
	Newborn	15–40 ng/ml
	Child	<1–20 ng/ml
	Adult M	<2 ng/ml
	Adult F	<10 ng/ml
	>60 yr M	0.4–10 ng/ml
	>60 yr F	1–14 ng/ml

Continued.

TABLE A–16.—Continued

	Age		Normal Value
Immunoglobulin levels (serum)	IgG (mg/dl)	IgM (mg/dl)	IgA (mg/dl)
Cord	760–1,700	5–24	0–5
Newborn	700–1,480	5–30	0–2.2
< 6 mo.	300–1,000	15–109	3–82
6 mo.–2 yr	500–1,200	43–239	14–108
2–6 yr	500–1,300	50–199	23–190
6–12 yr	700–1,550	50–260	29–270
Adult	600–1,600	40–345	76–390
Insulin, fasting (RIA) (serum)	Newborn	3–20 μIU/ml	
	Adult	6–24 μIU/ml	
Iron-binding capacity (serum)	Newborn	60–175 μg/dl	
	Infant	100–400 μg/dl	
	Thereafter	250–400 μg/dl	
	Elderly	200–300 μg/dl	
Iron, total (serum)	Newborn	100–250 μg/dl	
	Infant	40–100 μg/dl	
	Child	50–120 μg/dl	
	Adult M	50–160 μg/dl	
	Adult F	40–150 μg/dl	
	Elderly	40–80 μg/dl	
Lactate			
Venous whole blood		4.5–19.8 mg/dl	
Arterial whole blood		4.5–14.4 mg/dl	
Lactase dehydrogenase (LDH) (serum)	Newborn	160–450 U/L	
	Neonate	300–1,500 U/L	
	Infant	100–250 U/L	
	Child	60–170 U/L	
	Adult	45–90 U/L	
LDH isoenzymes			
LDH_1 (heart)		14%–26% of total	
LDH_2		29%–39%	
LDH_3		20%–26%	
LDH_4		8%–16%	
LDH_5 (liver, skeletal muscle)		6%–16%	

Luteinizing hormone (serum)	M, 10–13 yr	4–12 IU/L
	12–14 yr	6–12 IU/L
	12–17 yr	6–16 IU/L
	15–18 yr	7–19 IU/L
	Adult	6–23 IU/L
	F, 8–12 yr	2.0–11.5 IU/L
	9–14 yr	2.0–14.0 IU/L
	12–18 yr	3.0–29.0 IU/L
	F, Follicular	5–30 IU/L
	Midcycle	75–150 IU/L
	Luteal	3–30 IU/L
	Postmenopausal	30–130 IU/L
(urine)	11–13 yr	0.48–11.28 IU/day
	13–15 yr	2.6–27.6 IU/day
	15–17 yr	4.6–24.0 IU/day
	M, adult	13–60 IU/day
	F, follicular:	7.2–23.5 IU/day
Magnesium (serum)		1.3–2.2 mEq/L
Osmolality (serum)		275–295 mOsm/kg
(urine, random)		50–1,400 mOsm/kg, depending on fluid intake
		>850 mOsm/kg after 12 hr fluid restriction
(urine, 24 hr)		300–900 mOsm/kg
Oxygen pressure (whole blood arterial) (Po_2)	Newborn	65–80 mm Hg
	Thereafter	83–100 mm Hg (decreases with age)
Oxygen saturation		
Whole blood arterial	Newborn	40%–90%
	Thereafter	95%–98%
Whole blood venous	Newborn	30%–80%
	Thereafter	25%–29%
pH (37° C) (whole blood arterial)	Premature	7.35–7.5
	Newborn	7.27–7.47
	Thereafter	7.35–7.45
Phenylalanine (serum)	Premature	2.0–7.5 mg/dl
	Newborn	1.2–3.4 mg/dl
	Adult	0.8–1.8 mg/dl
Phosphatase, acid (serum) (RIA)		<3.0 ng/ml
Phosphatase, alkaline ρ-nitrophenylphosphate, carbonate buffer)	Newborn	50–165 U/L
	Child	20–150 U/L
	Thereafter	20–70 U/L
Phospholipids (serum)	Newborn	75–170 mg/dl
	Infant	100–275 mg/dl
	Child	180–295 mg/dl
	Thereafter	125–275 mg/dl

Continued.

TABLE A-16.—Continued

	Age	Normal Value
Phosphorus, inorganic (serum)	Cord	3.7–8.1 mg/dl
	Premature (1 wk)	5.4–10.9 mg/dl
	Newborn	4.3–9.3 mg/dl
	Child	4.5–6.5 mg/dl
	Thereafter	3.0–4.5 mg/dl
Placental lactogen (hPL) (serum)	At term	5.5–6.5 µg/dl
Porphobilinogen (urine, 24 hr)		0–2.0 mg/day
Potassium (serum/plasma)	Premature (cord)	5.0–10.2 mmol/L
	Premature (48 hr)	3.0–6.0 mmol/L
	Newborn (cord)	5.6–12.0 mmol/L
	Newborn	3.7–5.9 mmol/L
	Child	3.4–4.7 mmol/L
	Thereafter	3.5–5.1 mmol/L
(urine, 24 hr)		25–125 mEq/day
Pregnanediol (urine, 24 hr)	Child	0.5 mg/day
	Adult M	0.6–1.5 mg/day
	F, Follicular phase	<1 mg/day
	Luteal phase	2–7 mg/day
	Pregnant	5–63 mg/day
	Postmenopause	0.2–1.0 mg/day
Pregnanetriol (urine, 24 hr)	Newborn/child	<0.5 mg/day
	Thereafter	<2.0 mg/day
Progesterone (serum)	M: Stage 1	0.11–0.26 ng/ml
	Adult	0.12–0.3 ng/ml
	F: Stage 1	0–0.3 ng/ml
	Stage II	0–0.46 ng/ml
	Stage III	0–0.6 ng/ml
	Stage IV	0.05–13.0 ng/ml
	Follicular	0.02–0.9 ng/ml
	Luteal	6.0–30.0 ng/ml
Prolactin (serum)	M, Adult:	Up to 20 ng/ml
	F, Follicular	Up to 23 ng/ml
	Luteal	5–40 ng/ml
	Pregnancy:	
	1st Tri.	<80 ng/ml
	2d Tri.	<160 ng/ml
	3d Tri.	<400 ng/ml
	Newborn:	>10-fold adult levels
Protein, total (serum)	Premature	3.6–6.0 gm/dl
	Newborn	4.6–7.0 gm/dl
	Child	6.2–8.0 gm/dl
	Thereafter	6.0–8.0 gm/dl
(urine, 24 hr)		1–14 mg/dl
(urine, at rest)		50–80 mg/day
(urine, exercise)		<250 mg/day

Semen analysis (ejaculate)	Volume	2–6 ml
	Count	>20 million/ml
	Motility	>50% 2 hr after collection
	Morphology	>60% normal forms
	Liquefaction	30 min after ejaculation
Sodium (serum)	Newborn	134–146 mmol/L
	Infant	139–146 mmol/L
	Child	138–145 mmol/L
	Thereafter	136–146 mmol/L (diet-dependent)
Specific gravity (urine, random)		1.002–1.030
(urine, 24)		1.015–1.025
T_3 resin uptake (serum)	Newborn	25%–37%
	Adult	24%–34%
Testosterone (serum)	Child	0.03–0.05 ng/dl
	Adult M	5.6–10.2 ng/dl
	Adult F	0.24–0.38 ng/dl
Thyroid-stimulating hormone (hTSH) (serum)	Cord	3–12 μIU/ml
	Newborn	3–18 μIU/ml
	Thereafter	2–10 μIU/ml
Thyroxine-binding, globulin (serum)		15–34 μg/ml
Thyroxine, total (serum)	Cord	8–13 μg/dl
	Newborn	11.5–24 μg/dl
	Neonate	9–18 μg/dl
	Infant	7–15 μg/dl
	1–5 yr	7.3–15 μg/dl
	5–10 yr	6.3–13.3 μg/dl
	Thereafter	5–12 μg/dl
	>60 yr M	5.0–10.0 μg/dl
	>60 yr F	5.5–10.5 μg/dl
	Pregnancy (last 5 mo.)	6.1–17.6 μg/dl
Transferrin (serum)	Adults	220–400 mg/dl
	>60 yr	180–380 mg/dl
Triiodothyronine (T_3 RIA, total) (serum)	Cord	30–70 ng/dl
	Newborn	75–260 ng/dl
	1–5 yr	100–260 ng/dl
	5–10 yr	90–240 ng/dl
	10–15 yr	80–210 ng/dl
	Thereafter	115–190 ng/dl
	>60 yr M	105–175 ng/dl
	>60 yr F	108–205 ng/dl
Triiodothyronine, reverse (rT_3) (serum)	Cord	98–174 ng/dl
	Thereafter	21–61 ng/dl

Continued.

TABLE A–16.—Continued

	Age	Normal Value
Tyrosine (serum)	Premature	7.0–24.0 mg/dl
	Newborn	1.6–3.7 mg/dl
	Thereafter	0.8–1.3 mg/dl
(urine)		8.0–20.0 mg/dl
Urea nitrogen (serum/ plasma)	Cord	21–40 mg/dl
	Premature (1 wk)	3–25 mg/dl
	Newborn	4–12 mg/dl
	Infant/Child	5–18 mg/dl
	Thereafter	7–18 mg/dl (higher with high-protein diet)
Uric acid (serum/plasma)	Child	2.0–5.5 mg/dl
(uricase method)	Thereafter: M	3.5–7.2 mg/dl
	F	2.6–6.0 mg/dl
(urine)		<420 mg/day (lower with low-purine diet)
Urobilinogen (urine)	Urine, 2 hr	0.1–0.8 EU/2 hr
	Urine, 24 hr	0.5–4.0 EU/day
Uroporphyrin (urine, 24 hr)		<50 µg/day
Vanillylmandelic acid	Newborn	<1 mg/day
(VMA) (urine)	Neonate	<1 mg/day
	Infant	<2 mg/day
	Child	1–5 mg/day
	Adolescent	1–5 mg/day
	Thereafter	2–7 or 1–7 µg/mg creatinine

*Adapted from Mabry CC, Tietz NW: Tables of normal laboratory values, in Behrman RE, et al: (eds): *Textbook of Pediatrics,* ed 13. Philadelphia, WB Saunders Co, 1987, pp 1835–1858, and Elin RJ: Reference ranges and laboratory values of clinical importance, in Wyngaarden JB, Smith LH (eds): *Textbook of Medicine,* ed 18. Philadelphia, WB Saunders Co, 1987, pp 2395–2402.
†Reference values may vary according to analytic method used.

TABLE A–17.—Amniotic Fluid

Amniotic fluid		
Amniotic fluid analysis absorbance at 450 nm bilirubin	28 wk	0.0–0.048 A
	40 wk	0.0–0.020 A
	28 wk	0.0–0.075 mg/dl
	40 wk	0.0–0.025 mg/dl
Creatinine		>2.0 mg/dl generally indicates fetal maturity when maternal serum creatinine is normal

Lecithin/spingomyelin (L/S) ratio		2.0–5.0 indicates probable fetal lung maturity
Lecithin phosphorus		>0.10 mg/dl indicates probable adequate fetal lung maturity
Osmolality	28 wk	255–275 mOsm/kg
	40 wk	241–264 mOsm/kg
pH		6.96–7.20
Sodium	28 wk	124–148 mmol/L
	40 wk	115–139 mmol/L
Volume	10 wk	Approx. 25 ml
	40 wk	300–1,700

TABLE A–18.—SPINAL FLUID

Lumbar CSF		Polymorphonuclear	WBCs/mm³ Mononuclear	RBCs/mm³
Albumin/globulin ratio			16.2–2.2	
Albumin, quantitative			10–30 mg/dl	
Calcium			4.2–5.4 mg/dl	
Cell count			WBCs/mm³	
	Premature	0–100*	0–25*	0–1,000
	Newborn	0–70*	0–20*	0–800*
	Neonate, early	0–25	0–5	0–50
	Neonate, late	0–5	0–5	0–10
	Thereafter	0	0–5	0–5
Chloride	Newborn		108–122 mmol/L	
	Thereafter		118–132 mmol/L	
Cholinesterase			13–21 mU/ml	
Glucose (40%–60% of blood or serum glucose level)	Newborn		30–80 mg/dl	
	Infant/child		60–80 mg/dl	
	Thereafter		40–70 mg/dl	
Immunoglobulins			IgG: 0.8–6.4 mg/dl	
			IgA: 0.4–0.6 mg/dl	
			IgM: Negative	
Lactate			0.1–1.0 mmol/L	
Lactate dehydrogenase (LDH) (1 → p; 30°C)	Newborn		2.3–8.4 U/L	
	Child		0.0–20.0 U/L	
	Adult		6.3–30.0 U/L	
Magnesium			2.2–3.0 mmol/L	
Pandy test			Negative	
pH (37°C)			7.33–7.42	
Potassium			2.8–4.1 mmol/L	

Continued.

TABLE A–18.—Continued

Protein, total	Premature	40–300[†] mg/dl
	Newborn	45–100
	Child	10–20
	Adolescent	15–30
	Thereafter	15–45 (turbidometric method)
		8–32 (column method)
Protein electrophoresis		Prealbumin, 2.9%–5.3%
		Albumin, 56.8%–68.0%
		α_1-globulin, 4.1%–6.4%
		α_2-globulin, 6.2%–10.2%
		β-globulin, 10.8%–14.8%
		γ-globulin, 6.1%–8.3%
Sodium		138–150 mmol/L
Specific gravity		1.007–1.009
Transaminases:		
Aspartate aminotransferase (SGOT, AST; 30°C)		2–10 U/L
Alanine aminotransferase (SGPT, ALT; 30°C)		None detected
Xanthochromia*		Absent

*Number of cells greater than observed in older infants' CSF occurs in many newly born infants who grow and develop normally.
†Values greater than 100 mg/dl are seen in many prematurely born infants who grow and develop normally.

TABLE A–19.—Urine[*†]

Urinalysis and Urine Chemistry

Specific gravity	1.015–1.025
pH	4.6–8.0
RBCs	2–5 per HPF
WBCs	0–5 per HPF
Ammonia	30–50 mEq/24 hr
Amylase (Somogyi)	35–260 units/hr
Calcium (200 mg calcium diet)	<7.5 mEq or <150 mg/24 hr
Catecholamines	<100 μg/24 hr
Creatinine	1.0–1.6 gm/24 hr
Glucose	50–300 mg/24 hr
Ketones (mean ± 1 SD)	50.5 ± 30.7 mg/24 hr
Lactic dehydrogenase	560–2,050 units/8 hours
Protein	<50 mg/24 hr
Porphobilinogen	0
Potassium	25–100 mEq/24 hr (varies with diet)
Sodium	100–260 mEq/24 hr (varies with diet)
Urobilinogen	1–3.5 mg/24 hr
Vanillylmandelic acid (VMA)	0.7–6.8 mg/24 hr

*Adapted from Mabry CC, Tietz NW: Tables of normal laboratory values, in Behrman RE, et al (eds): *Textbook of Pediatrics,* ed 13. Philadelphia, WB Saunders, 1987, pp 1835–1858; and Elin RJ: Reference ranges and laboratory: Values of clinical importance, in Wyngaarden JB, Smith LH (eds): *Textbook of Medicine,* ed 18. Philadelphia, WB Saunders Co, 1987, pp 2395–2402.
†Reference values may vary according to analytic method used.

Index